TRAVELS THROUGH A TOXIC SHOCK NIGHTMARE

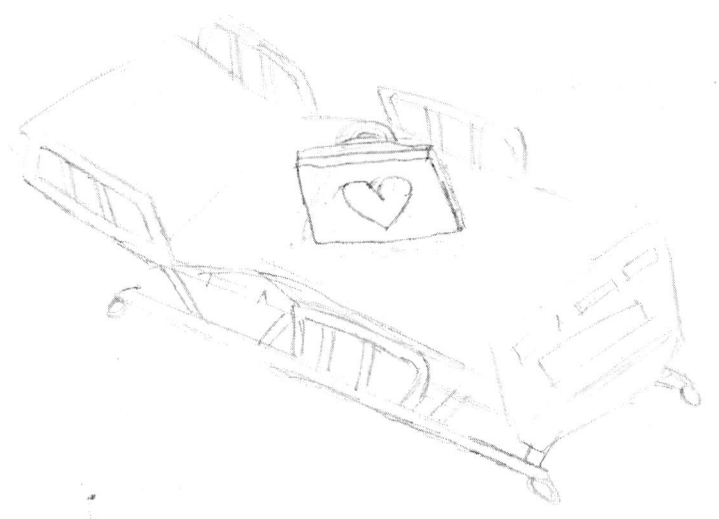

HOWARD HOOVER

Travels through a Toxic Shock Nightmare

All Rights Reserved © 2013 by Howard Hoover
Artwork Copyright © 2013 by Kate Hoover, Phoebe Hoover, and Henry Hoover

No part of this book may be reproduced or transmitted in any form or by any means, graphic, electronic, or mechanical, including photocopying, recording, taping, or by any information storage retrieval system, without the permission in writing from the publisher.

Copyright © Howard W. Hoover, 2013

ISBN: 1492966940
ISBN 13: 9781492966944
Library of Congress Control Number: 2013919303
CreateSpace Independent Publishing Platform
North Charleston, South Carolina

FOR MY FAMILY

Contents

Author's Notes ix
Foreword xi
Preface xvii
The Progression xix

Part I: A Beginning

January 15, 2009
Chapter 1   911 1

January 13, 2009
Chapter 2   My Life 7

January 14, 2009
Chapter 3   Start Line 15

January 14, 2009
Chapter 4   Descent 19

January 15, 2009
Chapter 5   Checking Out 22

Part II: I'm Miles Away[15]

January 15 – 26, 2009
Chapter 6   Bearings 29
Chapter 7   Frequent Flyer 42
Chapter 8   Body of Work 53

Chapter 9	Uncertainty of the Past	75
Chapter 10	Lessons	91
Chapter 11	South Dakota	100

Part III – A Delicate Brand of Reality

<u>January 27 - 31, 2009</u>

Chapter 12	Historic Site	131
Chapter 13	Slow Return	140
Chapter 14	London	156
Chapter 15	Hazy Care	159

<u>February 1 - 3, 2009</u>

Chapter 16	Theories	169
Chapter 17	Questionable Companion	181
Chapter 18	Trust	196
Chapter 19	Interactions	211
Chapter 20	Tough Love	224

<u>February 4 - 9, 2009</u>

Chapter 21	Speech	241
Chapter 22	New Normal	248
Chapter 23	Field Trip	268
Chapter 24	Questionable Freedom	287
Chapter 25	Relief and Fear	301
Chapter 26	My Room	313

Part IV: I Thought I Heard "Pomp and Circumstance"

<u>February 9 - 18, 2009</u>

Chapter 27	Moving On	333
Chapter 28	Reunion	348
Chapter 29	Temper	362

CONTENTS vii

Chapter 30	Awakening	374
Chapter 31	Community	387
Chapter 32	Failure/Success	398
Chapter 33	Back	421
Chapter 34	Sharper	439

Part V: Closer to My Home[151]

<u>February 18 – 25, 2009</u>

Chapter 35	Final Steps	467
Chapter 36	Closer	482
Chapter 37	Vanity	505

<u>February 26, 2009</u>

| Chapter 38 | Farewell | 519 |

Epilogue: A Suitable Ending, I Think 523
January 15, 2010, 5:00 a.m. HST
February 3, 2010

*Top Eleven Things I Learned During My
Time with Toxic Shock Syndrome* 529
Afterword 535
Acknowledgements 537
About the Author 541
Bibliography 543
Discography 545
Notes 555

Author's Notes

This is the story of just one sepsis survivor.

Similarities of persons living or dead with characters in this book are real, unimagined, and intended. Only the names have been changed to protect the slightly embarrassed.

With a few exceptions the names of places and locations have been altered with little imagination.

Apologies for some strong language, it captures the feeling of the time.

Foreword

In an era of increasing antibiotic-resistant bacteria, decreasing pharmaceutical research for effective antibiotics, and increasing patient complexity, the diagnosis of sepsis takes on the specter of a health care epidemic. Sepsis is responsible for the highest healthcare dollar spent in the US today. It kills 1 in 4 presenting with the diagnosis and is the most frequent diagnosis resulting in hospital readmission.

The critical care community has focused on sepsis for greater than a decade with outstanding research regarding early identification and treatment. Despite these efforts, even the hospitals that have been identified as the best for implementing codified protocols for treatment are successful in complying with all the elements of treatment only 40% of the time. Why do hospitals fail? Early recognition is often difficult (presentation in the first few hours can be deceptive as the patient does not appear ill despite objective measures suggesting the development of a serious physiologic problem) and adequate treatment requires a choreographed team to perform multiple tasks simultaneously. Once identified, the hospital team needs 24/7 access to a critical care team that includes critical care physicians, nurses, and respiratory therapists. Unfortunately, surveys of hospital staffing across the US find that the availability of these 24/7 teams is the exception rather than the rule as our country faces a shortage of critical care providers.

So, where is the good news? Large healthcare systems understand the current predicament and have instituted system-wide initiatives directed at early identification through education and easy-to-use protocols, have developed unique staffing models utilizing remote monitoring of all ICUs by critical care physicians and nurses, and have developed triage protocols making certain patients are in the right location to receive the care required.

Which brings us to the more recently recognized problem of sepsis – what happens to the patient during and after effective treatment of sepsis? The sepsis community has started to focus on the impact of all the technology and treatments on the recovering septic patient. Prolonged time (often days or weeks) on a ventilator (breathing life support), with medications attempting to allow for sedation and pain control, often result in delirium and muscle weakness. It is estimated that 80% of the survivors suffer from "Post Intensive Care Syndrome" – cognitive dysfunction and weakness often lasting greater than one year.

The author provides a detailed, and often disturbing, account of the mental and physical impact of surviving sepsis – vivid hallucinations, out-of-body experiences, and severe physical weakness – that would be trying for any individual to tolerate without longstanding emotional and mental impact. His story is one that should be read by every critical care provider to better understand the implications of every action taken during the care of the critically ill patient. Not only is it important that the critical care team perform the necessary actions that result in the most likely ability to survive, it must also continue to better understand the impact of every medication used and every intervention performed. Empathy, hope, clarity, and humor must be a part of every encounter by every healthcare provider. The healthcare system needs to rapidly develop an initiative to address the post intensive care syndrome utilizing education, research, and therapy teams.

Scott Lindblom, MD
Medical Director, CHS Critical Care Network
Section Chief, Pulmonary & Critical Care Medicine

The Last Time Around[1]

The Del-Vetts

Well - I'm sittin' here sinking on deeper down
My head is a-spinning around and 'round I can't seem to shake this feelin'
Oh - my body is a-rockin' and reelin'
Oh - it's such a funny feelin'
Well - I know this is the last time around for me - oh yeah

Oh I'm sinking - oh - I'm sinking on deeper down
My eyes are blurred and I can't hear a sound
Fight it - help me fight it
'cause I know this is the last time around for me - oh yeah

Oh - it's taken me over and swallowed me up
I'm caught in a landslide - I can't bend or duck
I've run out of time and I've run out of luck
I know this is the last time around

Oh - yeah
Last time around

Well - I know this is the last time around for me

Preface

TAMPA STADIUM
JANUARY 1, 1991

I was standing in the old Tampa Bay Center mall parking lot (don't look for it; it's not there) after Clemson shellacked Illinois 30-0 in the Hall of Fame Bowl in Tampa Stadium (don't look for it; it's not there). I was with my parents and sister, and we were talking to some old family friends. Suddenly, as if on cue, I felt something hit my shoulder. Upon further examination it appeared to be bird shit. I timidly gazed upward, half seriously thinking that the offender was still hanging around to hit me in the eye. Once I looked up, I saw nothing but sky. I looked to my right, and saw what must have been the offending culprit, a seagull with a cocky flap in its wings, leaving the scene of the crime with no other seagull, bird, or unidentified flying object of any kind in sight.

I thought, *million to one shot, Jonathan Livingston, million to one shot.*

The Progression

SEPSIS
PRONUNCIATION (SEP'SIS, -SĒZ)
The presence of various pathogenic organisms, or their toxins, in the blood or tissues, septicemia is a common type of sepsis.[2]
[G. *sēpsis*, putrefaction]

Septic shock is a medical emergency caused by decreased tissue perfusion and oxygen delivery as a result of severe infection and sepsis, though the microbe may be systemic or localized to a particular site. It can cause multiple organ dysfunction syndrome (formerly known as multiple organ failure) and death. Its most common victims are children, immunocompromised individuals, and the elderly, as their immune systems cannot deal with the infection as effectively as those of healthy adults.[3]

Toxic shock syndrome (TSS) is a potentially fatal illness caused by a bacterial toxin. Different bacterial toxins may cause toxic shock syndrome, depending on the situation. The causative bacteria include *Staphylococcus aureus* and *Streptococcus pyogenes*. Streptococcal TSS is sometimes referred to as **toxic shock-like syndrome (TSLS)** or **streptococcal toxic shock syndrome (STSS)**.[4]

"There is a thin line that separates laughter and pain, comedy and tragedy, humor and hurt."
—Erma Bombeck

Part I: A Beginning

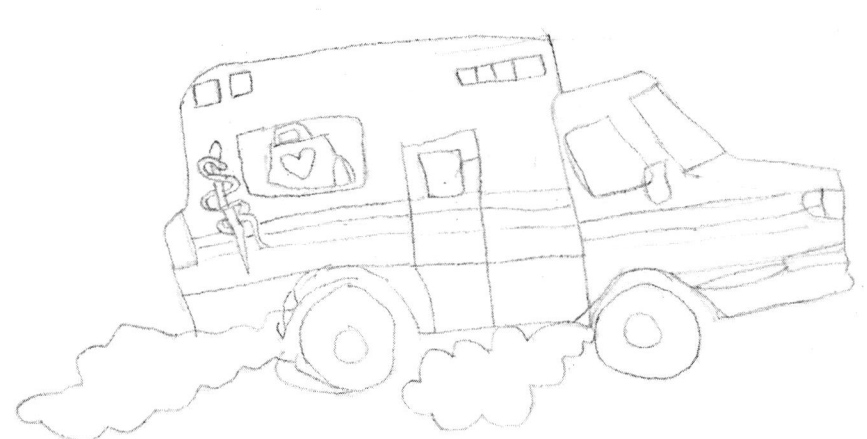

CHAPTER 1

911

Sepsis is a clinical condition characterized by systemic inflammation and widespread tissue injury due to infection. There is a continuum of illness severity ranging from sepsis to severe sepsis to septic shock to toxic shock syndrome.[5]

JANUARY 15, 2009
11:30 A.M.

SO HOLD ON, HERE WE GO [6]

Lying face down on the floor I only had one thought, *where am I?* The sound of heavy footsteps and male voices coming up the stairs clued me in that all was not right. I theorized that I had fallen from the attic as I tried to turn my head to look up. However, my head would only turn a couple of degrees, as if someone had tapped me on the shoulder, and I was none too eager to know who it was. I had no memory of what had transpired before this as I lay on the floor of the upstairs hallway of my house. I was just outside my bedroom, and I could not move. As the footsteps and voices got closer I felt I was in a dream, or the victim of a cruel practical joke. The voices and steps continued to approach through a haze. I had no fear of them. Perhaps they could get to the bottom of this.

I could feel someone kneel close to where I lay.

"Can you move?" a man asked.

I could feel his hot breath next to my ear. I thought this was a rather familiar distance, but I was in no condition to question issues of personal space. It made me feel like an injured football player when the training staff comes sprinting onto the field. The conversation that is taking place in their small world was always something that I could only imagine until now.

The power of voice had escaped me. I could only moan hoarsely, and perhaps shake my head.

"What's your name?" he asked.

Even if I could speak I would have still said nothing, because I couldn't be sure. I had no answers.

I heard a garbled world of voices and felt activity around me until a clear voice said, "We're going to turn you over."

They somehow turned my limp body over, and an oxygen mask was soon attached to my face. The blast of air was so soothing and refreshing, but only to a certain point. It felt like it was just a stop-gap measure in helping me. No way could I continue with this on my face. I just took the relief it gave without another question because I was having definite troubles without it.

"Do you know where you are?"

I thought it was my house; however it really didn't feel like my house. It felt like I was in another decade. I still had no answer.

I saw the hallway wall in a blurred, spotted way but could not make out any faces. I heard only voices during this exchange. I felt like I was in another world, hoping my responses or lack of them would make all of this go away.

"We're going to need the gurney that can get him down these stairs," the interviewer said to someone.

There was a lull in the proceedings. I had no idea where my wife Becky was, she had to be around here somewhere. I just couldn't tell where. Every time I opened my eyes I was met with this horrible tunnel vision coupled with a feeling of being underwater. Every act, every motion was in a start, pause mode.

I heard the gurney brought up the stairs, and a lot of help was needed to get my prone body onto it. I am six feet four, weigh around 210 pounds, and may be even full of muscle during good times, but I hadn't eaten in a day and a half. This as dead weight is a challenge to move, even for the burliest of fellows. A sedated rhino on the Serengeti gets less attention than I was getting now. Perhaps I would just be tagged and left to roam around the house.

"This is a big guy; we need all you guys to help out," said the interviewer.

Many hands were brought under me as I was lifted. The straps were tightened, and I was brought to a reclined position. They began to roll me toward the top of the stairs. The stairs have two ninety degree turns and surprisingly I was barely jostled while I was brought down to the foyer. The scary part was I could not move, nor could I feel a thing. I just knew something was wrong, then again I felt like I was in some other guy's body. That feeling might have been a pretty good indicator that something was wrong. This couldn't be me; but it was. Adding to my woes was my thought that the stairs were being scratched up with this gurney. I could hear the grunting of the firefighters straining to get me down, and I was a little embarrassed by all of the attention.

I was whisked outside into the January air. The blast of cold air woke me up for a bit. I was surprised over this fuss like I was a thousand pound shut-in that had to be rescued from himself. Yet would I eventually be able to wash myself with a towel wrapped around a stick? The ambulance and fire engine were outside on the street. I could sense a crowd had started to gather as I was rolled down the driveway.

"We're neighbors. What's wrong with Howard?" someone asked. I could not hear the response.

"We're going to take him to St. Hubbins," said the ambulance driver.

"OK," I heard Becky say somewhere behind me.

My house is equidistant between two of the largest hospitals in Charlotte and possibly the state of North Carolina. We are a couple of miles from both hospitals: St. Hubbins and General Hospital.

In hindsight, had I weighed the two hospitals on aesthetic grounds, I would have preferred St. Hubbins's emergency room. I went there a few years ago to tend to a wound I had received on my forehead by clumsily opening a window in the upstairs bathroom. It was the window's fault, not mine. The waiting room there had a big screen TV and cushy chairs that would provide a comfortable environment for me while I waited my turn. In comparison, the visit I had to the ER of General Hospital with my youngest daughter, who was three months old at the time, was comparable to a scene from *Independence Day*. However that was six years ago, and the one significant point in comparing the two was that General Hospital has a higher-rated trauma center. Plus, with Dr. Noah Drake, Luke, and Laura, how could I go wrong?

Usually when I hear Emergency Room I think there will be a large investment of time, an IV, a replacement of fluids, some paperwork, an annoying ER bill, and I would be good to go. Quite frankly, I had shit to do. There was some project I had been working on for work for some place that was due at some unspecified time for someone that I didn't know. It was that important. Amazingly, I thought of none of that as I was rolled to the ambulance. As I was slid into the unfamiliar space I could continue to make out the neighbors asking about me, but I could not hear the answers they were being given.

Once I was in the ambulance I felt myself going. There was a force weighing me down that I could not fight. I heard voices around me, and the central point in my decreasing field of vision was the interior of the doors, with blurry faces outside looking on.

As I lay in the ambulance, I consoled myself by repeating in my head, *they'll make this go away; all of this will go away.* The doors then closed on me; my eyes closed; and there was darkness.

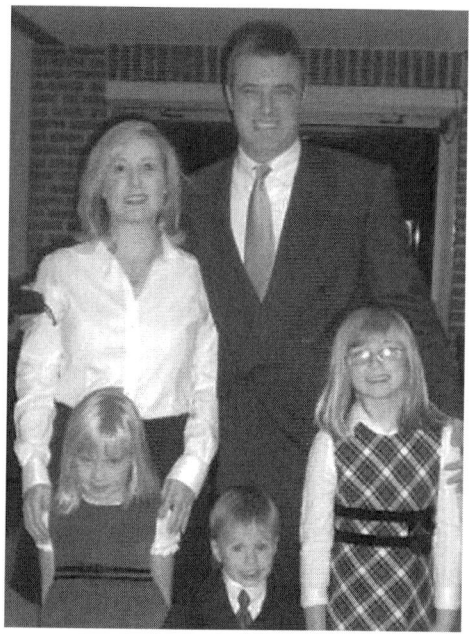

December 2008

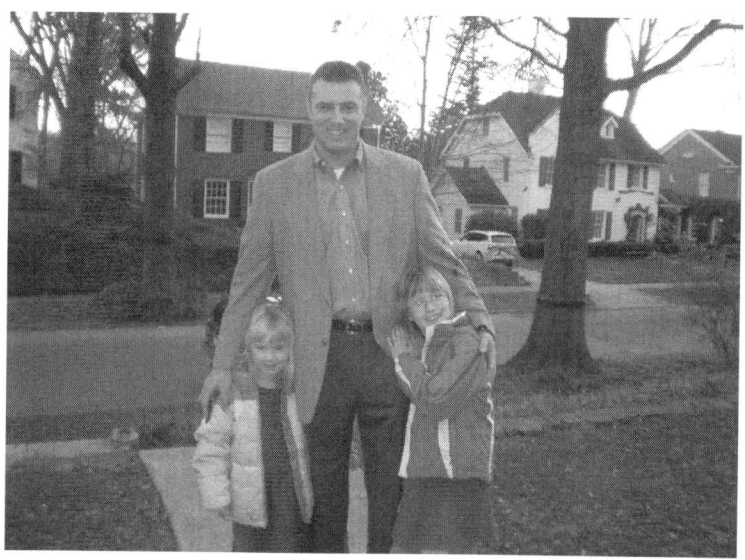

January 9, 2009

CHAPTER 2

My Life

Group A streptococcus (GAS, eg, Streptoccocus pyogenes) less commonly causes invasive diseases, which is complicated by toxic shock syndrome (TSS) in approximately one-third cases.[7]

TUESDAY JANUARY 13, 2009
11:00 A.M.

EVERY TIME YOU HEAR THAT WHISTLE BLOW[8]

The call came around 11:00 AM on Tuesday, January 13. I recognized the number on the phone: LES. Local Elementary School was where my two daughters, Kate and Phoebe, were in second grade and kindergarten, respectively. As any parent knows, it isn't usually good to get a call during the day from your child's school.

"Hello," I answered.

"This is Mrs. Dustin at Local Elementary School. Phoebe is sick and needs to be picked up," she said.

"What's the matter?"

"She's thrown up and is now in the Nurse's office. She has a fever as well."

"OK, I'll be there to get her." I hung up.

These were the times that I was happy I worked from home. I became a contract employee in September 2006 working from home with a reduced workload, and so I was the self-proclaimed World's Greatest King of Flexibility. There is an award I gave to myself on the wall stating such. I requested this position when my oldest daughter was beginning kindergarten. The days of Kate being at daycare for a full workday were finally at an end. She had been there for five years and now real school would be starting. Becky and I just didn't feel right about having her in after-school programs as we have always been paranoid, as I am sure all parents are with their first child. All of these "firsts" tended to make us a little crazy, and this was once again a "first." I could see Kate being in a rough and tumble group of older kids, and either being beaten up regularly or worse, and learning bad habits, as if this wouldn't happen during the regular school day.

Local Elementary School is less than a mile from our house in Charlotte, so the pick-up is pretty painless. It was a beautiful almost spring-like day to be the middle of January. I felt a little irritated since I had some work to do, and I was supposed to tutor later that morning. I had begun tutoring the year before when Kate's first-grade teacher said during Parents' Night at the beginning of the year what a wonderful experience being a tutor was. She regaled us parents with touching tales of how fulfilling it was for other parents from past classes who had volunteered. Her talk moved me, and I have never really been one to raise my hand or to get up while others sat; but I went to the sign-up sheet after the meeting and signed up to be a tutor. I was nervous as hell during the first few sessions, yet as it turned out, I did enjoy it;

PART I: A BEGINNING - MY LIFE

and I stuck with it through the entire year. Fortunately, my horrible performance as a first-grade student had not come back to haunt me.

As good fortune had it, I ended up tutoring for Kate's teacher, and it was wonderful to talk with her before the students got back into the classroom from recess. She mentioned during our conversations how she had overcome cancer a few years before that caused her to lose her hair, and her recovery had been very difficult. I remembered thinking how horrible it all sounded, and how fortunate I was to not have had any experiences like that. I couldn't really relate with what she had gone through, only that I was thankful that I had my health. Still, I took it all for granted. So this academic year I volunteered once again and coincidentally I was tutoring the same students I had the year before. While they didn't seem to always appreciate my help, I was nonetheless undeterred in being an annoying presence to them.

As I walked into the office to pick up Phoebe, I saw one of the students that I was supposed to tutor later that morning. Her mother was there with her, and the little girl was not feeling well. I walked behind the counter and saw Phoebe in the nurse's room lying down. Sometimes Phoebe will act sick and not really be sick, as I am sure all little kids do when the pressures of the day become overwhelming. I know I faked the stomach ache in the car as my dad would drop me off when I was in first grade in order to avoid another awful day with Miss Devil. She was a real old curmudgeon of a teacher that made learning the worst experience imaginable. However, this time Phoebe had really thrown up, and I would be taking her home.

As we walked out of the office, I said to the little girl's mother, "Needless to say, I won't be tutoring your daughter today."

This was understood, and I walked Phoebe out the door.

I got Phoebe home, planted her in front of the TV, made her comfortable, and phoned Becky's mom who is always on standby in these cases, or at least I assume so. I assume a lot in these cases. She moved up from Tallahassee, Florida in April 2006 once she retired and our youngest, Henry, was born. All of the family she knew in Tallahassee had either passed or moved away so this was a wonderful time in her life to be near her grandchildren. I was actually busy at this time and had two projects going on so she was definitely going to be needed today.

Working from home is nice; I have always tried to squeeze work in between the hours of 9:00 a.m. and 3:00 p.m. so that I can get the kids from school. I have found that there is an inverse relationship between productivity and the number of times the washer and dryer chime. On occasion, when there is a second wind that comes cascading through my internal sails, I will work after dinner once the kids are put to bed. Not to stress too much the importance of this and how it cuts into my "On My Ass" time, but such levels of work remind me of Paul McCartney. He mentioned during an interview in 2001 that after the Beatles had broken up and kids had come into their lives, he and Linda would head to the studio to get to work after the kids were fed, bathed, and put to bed. Well, this was kind of like that except instead of recording music for the album *Ram*, I was looking over a financial model for Winston-Salem, North Carolina. In other words, my work was not being awaited by millions of adoring fans, just a handful of people with the ability to utilize the "Track Changes" feature in Word.

Grandma came over and watched Phoebe as I continued to work. I went back to school, and got Kate at 3:30 p.m. The afternoon was pretty uneventful. Becky was out of town in New York for a meeting for the day, so I also had to get Henry from daycare as well. Since Becky would not be home for dinner, the fan-favorite meal that I always brought out on nights like this was spaghetti and meatballs. A real gut buster if you aren't careful, especially when garlic bread is added to the mix.

Actually, I can make more than just spaghetti and meatballs. For instance, there was the night I made the huge pot of split pea soup. Becky was there to partake on the first night, but she was going out of town for the rest of the week. As George Costanza's mother from *Seinfeld* might have said, "What am I going to do with all of this split pea soup?" I knew. I would serve it again the next night. There were some long faces at the table when it was put in front of them. Not having learned my lesson from that night, and with so much leftover, I decided to have it again. I thought, *I am the dada; they will do as I say.*

It didn't turn out that way though. When the split pea soup was brought out again they acted like Regan from *The Exorcist* had just thrown it up all over the walls. I had never seen a six-year-old and a four-year-old so passionate about such an injustice. If they were big enough, and had the know-how, they would have strung me to the car and dragged me through the neighborhood as a warning to others not to make the same mistake. For some reason I was defensive about this. How can you say that having split pea soup the third night in a row is so terrible? Well, it was. Even I had to agree. I learned my lesson that night. I have made the big pot of split pea soup since that time, but I only forced it on myself for lunch after the first night. Bleh. So why do I keep making split pea soup? Because when it is cold outside it always seems like a wise decision. Afterward it turns out to be an unwise decision.

As evening fell, Becky's mom helped with getting the kids ready for bed, and thankfully cleaned the kitchen. On spaghetti night I have a fear of going back into the breakfast room since it can at times be the messiest of the messes to clean with a seven, five, and two-year-old. However, by this time, I was beginning to not feel right, so much so that I would have let the mess the fat lady left behind in the spaghetti dinner dream sequence from the Beatles' film flop *Magical Mystery Tour* just sit. I simply didn't care.

There is just a general fatigue one gets at the onset of a sickness, or at least I do. It is like a road sign flashing "Sickness Ahead." At times you are making good time, and don't wish to slow down. Other times you just know that Sheriff Lobo from TV's *BJ and the Bear*, and the smash spin-off TV's *Sheriff Lobo*, might be behind that billboard ready to give pursuit. So you heed the sign. At this moment I had no choice, this felt different, more pronounced, like a governor had been installed on my body. There was a dizziness and general malaise that I had not felt before; I was slowing down. I struggled through reading stories that evening and quickly put everyone to bed. Kiss, Kiss, Good Night, maybe the *Die Hard* trilogy is on TNT again.

Becky's mom said her farewell that evening after the lights were turned off. I was planning to do some more work but at this point my internal sails were listless, and the thought of it was too much. I had taken on the Winston-Salem project just the day before. There were quite a few things that I had to do before I went into the office the next day, Wednesday; yet there was no desire, no urge, and I had no sense of what I would say. I had made notes but nothing in electronic format, plus I had not done the larger of the two tasks which could be time consuming even when I am at my peppiest. There was nothing about that task that made me feel peppy.

So as expected, I parked it in front of the TV, awaiting John McClane to take my pain away. My fatigue was very pronounced at this point, like there was twice the earth's gravity on that couch. I just prayed that if one of the kids had a dilemma they could figure it out because I had one more trip up those stairs left in me. I couldn't really focus on what was on TV. It was as if someone had just sat me in front of it and turned it on for me. I felt that this was disrespectful, especially when TV's brightest stars had come out to shine.

As I battled to sit there trying to figure out this internal puzzle, the headlights came up the driveway. It was going on 9:00 p.m., and Becky was home from NYC. As I sat there, I had a general disinterest in the proceedings, not only on TV but on her safe arrival home, forgetting that she had even been out of town. I heard the car door shut, her footsteps on the sidewalk, and her approach to the front door. The key went into the lock, jangling as usual since the original seventy-year-old lock is still on the door and is nothing less than finicky. I just sat there motionless as the door opened. She came inside, and I didn't even look over at her. It was as if I was being angry at her over something, but I wasn't. The truth was that I felt as if her arrival was like something on TV, and I could not interact with it either. I could have been floating somewhere in the room for all I knew. I could feel that Becky saw my supposed lack of interest, said a short hello, and proceeded to get settled. I was playing the part of the aloof husband; all I was missing was a bottle of Scotch (single malt, not blended, what am I a caveman?) in hand, turning ignoring your spouse into an art form.

After a while Becky joined me on the couch, and I didn't even turn to look at her as I said a meek almost formal, "Hello." By this point I was too tired to care, and after a few minutes I said, "I'm tired, I'm going to bed." I think Becky took this as dismissive of her presence, and I can't blame her for being sore about it or taking it the wrong way. It was also unusual for me to head upstairs before 9:15. It was a tradition for me to make one last round of the channels and continue to watch nothingness.

I headed upstairs like a zombie, and not one of those fleet of foot *Return of the Living Dead* zombies but a true dyed-in-the-wool *Night of the Living Dead* zombie, only without the moans. I found myself standing beside the bed, and then I just fell into it in my favorite Chippewas Football sweatshirt and sweat pants. No pre-bed ritual for me on this night; something was happening.

CHAPTER 3

Start Line

Severe invasive GAS infections are defined as bacteremia, pneumonia, or any other infection associated with the isolation of GAS from a normally sterile body site.[9]

WEDNESDAY, JANUARY 14, 2009
3:20 A.M.

TELL ME, TELL ME WHAT'S WRONG WITH ME[10]

I awoke at 3:00 a.m., actually, 3:18 a.m. As I recalled this was around the same time that all of the demons, ghosts, mummies, C.H.U.D.s, and pigs would get frisky in the *Amityville Horror*. I was in such discomfort that I could not just lie there and go back to sleep. I hadn't felt this bad since July 5, 2000, when I downed about ten Krystal hamburgers after a hard July 4th of drinking bad beer at a downtown music festival. That night's entertainment offered Rick Springfield, so this evening was still looking up for me. Becky had called into work that day for me to say I had gotten into some bad hamburger and would be unable to come in. All I ended up getting for my trouble was a viewing of the dramatic re-telling of the Monkees story on VH-1 that day. I would rather have had the split pea soup a fourth time.

I didn't recall having any bad hamburger at this ungodly hour, and I hadn't been digging in the garbage for any either so I slowly got up. I knew that I was going to upchuck, and I had to get to a bathroom. There are a few things I hate, and kissing the porcelain god is one of them. I know others hate it too, but I hate it with a passion. It is my least favorite thing to do. When I see my kids do it I think, "Oh. It's OK. Tough it out." When I'm going through it I think, *Oh, woe is me!* I sound like a spoiled princess/sleestack hybrid when the event finally occurs, after much preening and hand to the forehead. The noise that comes out of me is not of this earth.

Realizing this, I left the bedroom, and walked out to the landing. I was a bit dizzy and weak so I held onto the railing as I made a drunken eighty-five-year-old man look like former Los Angeles Laker great James Worthy on a fast break. Below was a drop of about ten feet to the foyer so I had to be careful but care was not in my mind at the time. I stood at the top of the stairs knowing I had to get to my study bathroom, and somehow isolate the sounds I would soon be making. For some reason as I looked down those dark stairs I thought that I would be unable to make the trip, I would tumble head over heels, and that would be the end. So I sat down on my bottom, and I rode down those stairs that I had tap danced up and down so many times before. It was a bumpy ride but it was all I knew to do.

As I got to the bottom of the stairs, there was the foyer on my right and the study on the left. I slowly rode down the two steps to the study, shut the door, and crawled into my bathroom for some unpleasant me time. I tried to crouch by the toilet to wait out the final countdown. My weakness didn't even allow me to do that. It is a half-bath so there was no room to lie down. I got good and familiar with the toilet as I melted to the floor which would be my home for the remainder of the night. I knew it would be a long night but somehow I could not sit there anymore. My discomfort was increasing. The dizziness, the nausea, just an overwhelming feeling of helplessness was overtaking me. Reaching for some comfort based on historic precedent, I kept telling myself that like all of the times in the past that I had felt sick it would soon be over. I lay down with my head at the foot of the toilet, and my feet hanging out the bathroom door. I cannot recall if I actually got sick that night or not. I must have made a noise because I heard Becky's voice, so my Sleestack impression must have carried up the stairs on notes so lovely and sweet.

"Howard, are you OK?" she asked. When she was serious about something she always called me by me Christian name.

"Yes," I said. "I just feel weak."

She then got me a pillow, and I lay back down. By this time this was more of a passing out and not a sleep. I don't recall getting back up to get sick or not. At 7:00 a.m. Becky woke me up, and I knew I would be unable to go into the office as was requested of me the previous day. I pulled myself up in the desk chair just relieved that the night was over and that daylight had come. The daylight would chase this away, I told myself. I just needed to get back to bed. I slowly typed out an e-mail to my office contact:

Office Contact,

Phoebe was sick yesterday and unfortunately I got it. I believe they are flu likw symptoms and I would rather not come into the office today. I am almost through the fin proj model for both QA/

QC and assumptions. I will try to come in tomorrow or e-mail you my notes (must transcribe first). I don't think at this point I can do the feas model compsrison.

Let me know what you think and I apologize for springing this on you.

Howard

I have always been proud to say that there are only two misspellings in this entire message, excluding the abbreviations and shorthand. Also, there was no way I was transcribing my notes. Even healthy I would find this task unpleasant. Notwithstanding the unpleasantness of the task, the one thing that I have always been struck by in this message is "flu-like symptoms." When I hear that anymore I think sepsis, and since this time I have heard the same condition described in the deaths of Brittany Murphy and Corey Haim. I had not gotten my flu shot since I always thought such a thing was a waste of time. I am healthy. Only kids and the elderly need to worry about such things. I was very unprepared.

I turned off the computer and went upstairs, knowing full well I would not be able to do the little I had promised. I was actually able to walk at this point. I was a bit shaky but I got to the bed, and collapsed again.

CHAPTER 4

Descent

Twenty percent of patients have an influenza-like syndrome characterized by fever, chills, myalgia, nausea, vomiting, and diarrhea.[11]

WEDNESDAY, JANUARY 14, 2009
7:00 A.M. – 10:00 P.M.

YOU MUST NOT BE DRINKING ENOUGH[12]

"Howard, you're not drinking; you need to drink something."

It was Becky, and it was later that day. I looked over at the cup full of Gatorade, lemon/lime, not my favorite, and took a sip. It was not what I wanted so I went back to sleep. I think I heard the kids getting up and running around downstairs. Then, the door sensor chimed a few times and silence. Becky was taking them to school. It was something I usually did and enjoy, but I was missing it today. The day passed from morning into afternoon. I had no recollection except for the light turning fainter and fainter outside.

I don't remember when the kids came home or if the usual activity of homework and TV watching was taking place downstairs with one exception: I was awakened by the sound of the door creaking slowly open. Tiny footsteps came in, and then stopped. There was a little presence in there, and it had to be the very stealthy two-year-old Henry. Everyone says Henry is me at that age but I think that he resembles Becky more in the eyes and eyebrows. I could feel Henry examining the situation with the unmoving lump in the bed that was me; he said nothing. I simply could not raise my head to offer comfort, and I did not want him catching what I had. So I lay there silently. Besides, Henry is a talker and had I acknowledged him then a conversation with an almost three-year-old over the level of sickness I felt would be in the offing. I knew if a conversation of this magnitude, even my attempts to allay it, would weaken me more and more so I played possum. Rudeness for self-presevation.

Becky came to the door, and whispered, "Henry, don't bother Daddy; he's not feeling well."

"But I wanted to say hello, and check on him," Henry replied in his most caring voice.

"Come on out of there, let's go downstairs."

The door quietly closed.

That night I woke up with a start. I heard rustling in the room, I managed to raise myself up onto my arms and look over the foot of the bed. Becky was lying on the floor with a pillow and blanket. I managed to utter, "Why are you down there?"

"Because I don't want to get what you have or disturb you," she said

I agreed with this assessment but felt bad for her having to handle everything with work, the kids, and the house, and ending the day with sleeping on the floor. It seemed much like the days when we had a newborn in the house. These feelings were fleeting as I dropped back to my prone position. Usually with the flu I would feel great aches and pain, while uncomfortable it still made me feel alive, but with this there was nothingness, a complete absence of being. It was a feeling like I was losing touch with my body.

CHAPTER 5

Checking Out

Confusion is present in 55 percent of patients and coma or combativeness may be manifest in some patients.[13]

THURSDAY, JANUARY 15, 2009
9:00 A.M. – 11:30 A.M.

BUT SOON COMES MISTER NIGHT
CREEPIN' OVER[14]

I was downstairs. It was well into the morning, and I really gave that observation no further consideration. I don't know how I got out of bed, down the stairs or why I felt I had to get up. Something must have motivated me. I guess I just wanted to get away from what was making me feel bad, whatever that may be. When I was growing up my family had a dog named Deacon, and on a few occasions when he felt really sick he would wander off in the backyard where we couldn't find him. One alarming time we searched and searched, and finally found him under the deck. From what I had gathered he felt so bad that anyplace was better than where he was. This was how I felt, like a dog just finding a place to get away from his tormentor.

My tunnel vision was kicking in full time at this point as I wandered into the living room. I thought I was alone until I heard Becky tapping away on her laptop, so I sat down slowly. I don't know how I did this without collapsing. My vision was hindered like I had a piece of cheese cloth covering my face and blinders on. Alarm was seeping through the indifference brought on by my strength-sapping condition.

As I tried to act normal through this trial Becky asked, "Do you want to watch some TV?"

I nodded absently; my mouth was inoperable, perhaps it was agape. I had no sense of what countenance my body had decided to wear. The TV was already on, I noticed, and this still did nothing to improve my mood. Perhaps it's because daytime TV is something I really abhor, especially network TV. I never have it on during the day while I am working. Seeing ads for truck-driving school, Technical Institutes, and the Barbazon School of Modeling depresses me with the thought that these ads are geared toward a certain audience: the bored housewife, the unemployable, the surrendered. It also harkens back to those long summer days during those three plus interminable years my family lived in Brandon, Florida in the late 70s. Long before cable came to that part of Florida, when there was nothing to do; all we had was daytime TV and those ads. Even with all of 2009's viewing options now at my disposal, TV was still rubbing me the wrong way.

I looked at the screen, trying to get my bearings; I could see the picture but could not focus on the conversation. I think it was *Ellen* with the show's namesake, Ellen, being glib with the full support of her obviously drugged studio audience. I knew it was some awful gabfest where guests pause for a sip from some mug filled with something. They talk about their latest achievements or who is wonderful to work with, and how I can only imagine the wonders of their life and their exclusive club.... You know, I really don't give a shit. You want to help? Make me feel better; there you go, get on it. Of course they wouldn't have given a shit about me, especially while caught in mid-sentence over how they hang out with Ellen or any host for that matter. Bullshit, they haven't met until now. They could have dropped dead right at that moment and my expression would not have changed.

As alarm continued to fight indifference, I realized I couldn't take sitting there anymore. The illness, my tormentor, had found me and my stillness, and I had to go away again. I just had to move. I don't know where I went but I went somewhere.

I was in the bed when Becky found me later. She said, "I made an appointment for you to go to the doctor after lunch."

I suddenly rose to the occasion by saying sternly, "Why would you do that? No! No!" It was as if she had told me we were going to all of my school reunions simultaneously. I was quite annoyed that I was being disturbed, and I knew there was no way I could break out of this lethargy in which I found myself to get out of bed much less get in a car and wait in a waiting room. I couldn't imagine how I and my "New Improved Tunnel Vision (Now with More Spots)!" would do on a road trip. The thought of such actions was simply too overwhelming. I weakly held on to the pillow for dear life hoping the idea would take on a human form and go to the doctor on its own.

Later, Becky came back in the room and said, "I have had your appointment moved up so we are going at noon."

Well, this annoyed me to no end knowing that the road trip was nigh. What little energy I had left was doomed. I had little fight left

PART I: A BEGINNING - CHECKING OUT

in me. I just lay there still hoping I had become invisible. All the hope could not eliminate the knowledge that the jig was up, and I was going to have to somehow get in the car. It was for the best because I had to get out of this mess in which I had somehow found myself. My last outburst left me unable to respond at this point.

I lay there forgetting all that occurred before, so I had to be reminded that it was finally time to go to the dreaded doctor appointment. I occasionally went to the doctor and would every other year get a physical but rarely did I go when I was sick. Like Teddy Roosevelt might have said, a strong will and discipline would help me fight through it, and my tormentor would be dispatched after twenty-four hours... usually. Just stay at home and it would work its way out of my body. This was something that I was taking for granted. Why wasn't that concept working this time? When had the rules changed? I thought, *wait until Dr. Phillips gets a load of this.*

Becky came back in the room and announced that it was time to get ready for the appointment. She slowly sat me up in the bed as I struggled to get my sweatshirt off since I simply couldn't go into the doctor looking like this. I must have looked a fright. I had not been in the bed this long, even when I was seventeen. I needed to get on something other than sweatpants and a sweatshirt; perhaps there might be time to iron a tuxedo T-shirt?

Becky said, "Don't worry about your sweatshirt, just leave it on."

I stood up slowly like the bedridden victim that I had become.

"Are you OK?"

I nodded with as much bravado as I could muster. I looked at the alarm key pad by the bedroom door. The light from the display panel somehow offered me hope. I couldn't take my eyes off of it. I could actually see it. See what it said. It offered some steady state of normalcy as if to say, *we can do this!* Instead I felt doubt, and thought, *what is going on with me? Will this ever go away? What will the end of this feel like?* It felt so bad that I couldn't imagine my world without it.

Becky was waiting for me at the top of the stairs as I shuffled my way out of the bedroom and onto the landing like that old dude Tim Conway used to play on *The Carol Burnett Show*. I could see her figure in focus, then out of focus. I just couldn't see the detail for some reason. I stood there waiting for some force to continue my journey for me. I couldn't move.

"Howard? Are you OK?" she said with great alarm. I guess I didn't look too great; my body had decided on a facial expression that she was not accustomed to.

"Just sit down. Do I need to call 911?" she yelled.

I felt it was time to give up and call in the big guns. I needed more than a doctor office visit. When anything would happen to the kids, we never hesitated to call 911, yet I think of that day as the day when emergency help was true to its meaning.

I tried to lower myself to the floor with great style but my legs simply gave way under me, and I collapsed with my feet toward the stairs. I could see Becky unmoving at the top of the stairs as I fell. It was more of a blurred vision of things. Then there was darkness.

Part II: I'm Miles Away[15]

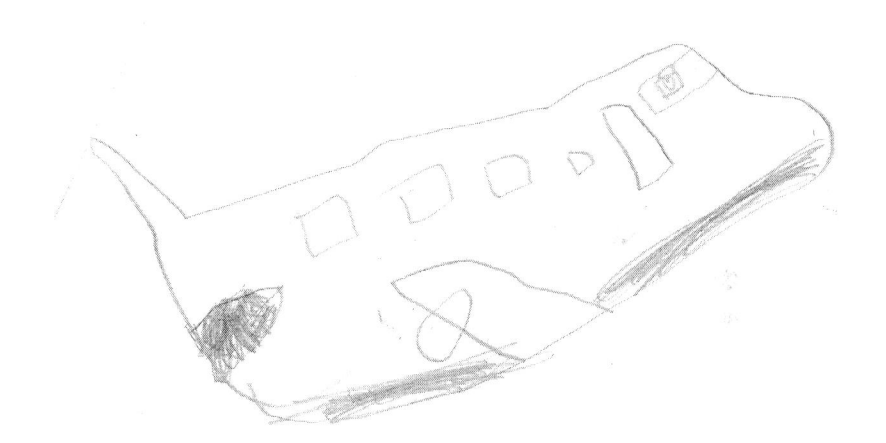

CHAPTER 6

Bearings

Nearly 50 percent of patients are normotensive on presentation or admission, but become hypotensive within the subsequent 4 hours.[16]

JANUARY 15 – 26, 2009
GENERAL HOSPITAL EMERGENCY ROOM AND
MEDICAL INTENSIVE CARE UNIT

I WONDER WHAT'S GONNA HAPPEN TO YOU/
YOU WONDER WHAT HAS HAPPENED TO ME[17]

It was a medical care facility I was rolling through: the fluorescent lighting, the clean antiseptic walls, the white, the glare. There was no mistaking it. Brown doors on either side of me in the hallway passed in a blur. Where this facility was exactly, where I was at this moment, I had no idea. Flat on my back, I could not imagine a time when I wasn't like this. The thought of this put an unholy fear in me as the "gurney/bed on wheels/contraption with wheels/who the hell knows" rolled away taking me to some destination that maybe it hadn't even yet determined.

As this journey continued, through the blur I could hear voices above me, two female voices. The voices sounded young and surprisingly cheerful. This demeanor was at odds with the fear residing deep in my thoughts, and I could not reconcile the two. Why were they so cheerful, so cavalier? I determined that they had to be nurses assigned to me, doing something with me.

The blur of the voices finally began to dissipate, and I could make out words, sentences. I could sense exertion in their voices as one of the female nurses complained about the lack of steering on the contraption they were pushing, and breathlessly recounted a story. "I remember once we had one of these contraptions that you couldn't steer, and it ran over one of the nurses I was with's toes. She screamed and screamed. She ended up losing the toe."

The nurse laughed, but it was a nervous laugh as if she was trying really hard to lighten the moment, and wished mightily that the same fate would not befall her.

I tried to take the story in stride; however I was struck with even more fear. Not only was my situation untenable in this contraption, it was unsafe outside it as well. I was in some sort of maul machine. A dismemberment story about a past co-worker was not lightening the mood.

The hallway still passed by quickly. My escort was urgently trying to get me somewhere, as if they were afraid that the contraption was eyeing their toes. There was no end to the facility. Hallways ran into lobbies, reception areas, exposed areas that made me feel vulnerable. We just kept going and going and going. There was finally a respite from the lighting when we exited the hospital briefly and entered a dimly lit parking deck. The cold air hit my face and hands while the rest of my body was bundled up. I thought, *we must be up north*

PART II: I'M MILES AWAY[15] - BEARINGS

somewhere, but where? What city is this? People were shuffling out of the way as if they could sense the urgency surrounding the contraption and my situation. One older gentleman hurried out of the way as if he knew the contraption's past, and what it was capable of. There was no stopping it, and I was unable to yell to warn them, and the possessors of the female voices seemed to have other issues on their minds.

Where in the world could I have been up north? What city could it have been? I thought, *I must be in Pierre, South Dakota.* It just appeared out of the blur. A theory came to me that somehow I did some vacationing in Pierre, South Dakota and really screwed up. Something had gone horribly wrong, and now I was here at the mercy of two voices, and their inability to steer. Of course, I have never been to Pierre, South Dakota, at least I didn't think so. Nevertheless here I was so there was no arguing with my situation, and what that was, I had no idea.

What I did know was that now I was being wheeled all the hell over this huge-ass hospital and its parking decks. The alternating pattern of fluorescent lighting and its annoying warmth with the dimly-lit parking deck and its unbearable cold had no end.

My thoughts turned to my family. *I have a family right? Do I still? Did I ever? Does anyone know I'm here? Where is Becky? What happened to her?* I was at the mercy of this contraption, the female voices that favored dismemberment stories, and ultimately the location that this set up was taking me to. I couldn't explain any of this; it was just happening and I couldn't stop it.

The breathless chuckling female voices, the contraption, and I finally slowed down as I figured that we had reached our destination. I could see we were outside a bank of elevators, the light was dim and for some reason we just stayed there and didn't move. I waited for one of the elevators to open and swallow us, but instead something was being wheeled out to me that appeared to be an MRI machine or a CatScan. As if fear had not found the tightest clutch in which to hold me, it was getting closer when I realized that I was unable to speak or move. This was fear, realizing that even if I had wanted to make a remark or move during my journey, I couldn't have. I was a helpless being, and that was all.

However, this helplessness, this fear felt more pronounced than that. Besides the speechlessness and paralysis, I was overcome with the feeling that I was being judged, and that this would be a time when I had to shine. I had to make a case for my life or it was all over. The body of evidence that I was going to have to provide was whether I really ever existed or not.

I heard a male voice and surmised that a doctor had entered the area. I supposed the judgment would now commence when he said, "We're going to run some tests on you. Is there anything you can tell us? Any memory you have that may let us know that you're who you think you are?"

I was wondering if he knew that he was speaking to a mute paralyzed guy that suddenly realized that he was a mute paralyzed guy. Of course I was who I thought I was, always had been, should always be. I tried to remember something, anything, a memory that proved my existence. Then something popped into my head that could be embarrassing during a lighter moment but at this time was a life ring, and I grabbed it. I remembered a song that I once sang to my oldest daughter, Kate, when she was two. The entire performance was caught by Becky on film unbeknownst at the time to me. There I am on film in dark slacks and an undershirt standing by the kitchen garbage can putting a new bag in. I was singing the world–wide hit *Feelings* by Morris Albert to her. Music from 1977 may be a tough pill to swallow for some; however, I should get some leeway. It is Morris Albert.

The scene begins with me singing one line, "Feelings," to her.

She repeats in her little precious voice, "Feelings," to me.

"Nothing more than feelings."

"Nothing more than feelings"

"Trying to forget my"

"Trying to forget my"

"Feelings of love"

"Feelings of love"

I played the entire scene in my head. I could hear her voice singing to me, and I was starting to get more upset. I thought *where is Kate? What has happened to her? Why isn't she here with me?* I had always known where my children were at any given moment, but I was at a total loss to explain where she was. What was she doing? Was she out of harm's way? Did she ever exist? Had I dreamt her life? Had I dreamt that memory? I needed to know. I needed to bust out of this uncertainty but it held me in, and I was its unwilling victim.

I tried to ask but could not. I was really getting frustrated. I couldn't make them know, and they went about their jobs not realizing the total distress and torture that was occurring inside of me. Somehow I was able to relay to the doctor this memory yet was unable to communicate the name of the song to him. It was as if they were keeping a tab on my brain waves, monitoring them for some glimmer. Suddenly, a stringed instrument, something resembling a zither with only five strings, was produced, and placed above my face. I could see the name *Fender* on the instrument, but I had no idea what kind of instrument it was.

Slowly, I slid inside the machine. The doctor spoke up and said, "OK, we need you to play on this instrument the tune of the song you sang to your daughter."

I had no idea why the name of the song was so important; why were they digging further? To irritate me? Was this song the key to my freedom? Of course I had not even considered the notion of how the hell I was supposed to play this thing.

The only body part I could come up with that a mute paralyzed guy might be able to use was my tongue since the strings hovered over my mouth. Oh God, if only I could get the words out. I heard the slow humming of the machine as it began scanning my brain and its faulty memory. The test was going to take too long, and meanwhile Kate was in grave danger. I had to let them know who I was, who she was so someone could help her.

The name of the song came through the haze of my mind, but it was too late. I was already in the tube, and they couldn't hear me. The humming was impregnable. My thoughts even seemed overwhelmed by it.

The doctor said, "I'm going to have to do some research on this over the weekend."

This poor guy had to sit by a piano, and come up with a tune. How could he possibly know? Was this guy a doctor or George Gershwin? Plus, why was I feeling sorry for him?

Somehow, I was able to move my arms and hands. They did not feel attached to my body. They felt like they were someone else's as if they had a mind of their own, and they started beating on the inside of the tube. My desire to let them know outweighed the potential embarrassment that I ever sang such a song. I was screaming. I could hear my voice. I could see arms that might be mine banging helplessly. I may have been embarrassing myself, overreacting but I had to let them know. I screamed, "I remember the name of the song! I remember the name of the song!" as I continued banging on the sides of the tube. My life depended on the banging.

The incessant whirring of the machine stopped. The silence was an eerie presence in my little space. I could hear movement and voices as the lights went back on. Did they hear me or was this just the end of the test? How they would be amazed when they heard me speak and relay my memory. I would get out of this. I would prove my life was there; it happened. Success. I would tell them everything now but as soon as the lights came on, the scene went dark.

***

EVERY NIGHT I HAVE THE SAME DREAM[18]

My eyes opened. I was in another hallway; it might have been the same hospital, the sounds, the smell, the look. I couldn't be sure. There was commotion going on around me, outside of my field of vision. I saw no one. The goal of knowing why I was here was still not realized. Flat on my back, I was alone against a wall. Out of the corner of my eye I could see a desk that could be a nurse's station. There were voices. I was placed here for some reason, and I could not move. Was my answer helpful? Did I prove my right to exist? Did the memory I had save me?

As I pondered my dilemma something caught my eye, a placard that was white with blue lettering and a picture in the center. I could have reached out to touch it if I could only have moved. I studied it more closely; my blurry vision taking it in slowly, and I heard it before I figured out what it was. It made a squealing sound, and as I focused

I could see it was a picture of a fetus staring right back at me, wiggling slightly. I looked away in horror but had to look back at it to make sure what I saw was true. It was still there, and I was still horrified. What kind of hospital was this? Someone had put me in front of this horrible photograph. Who did these people think they were? Perhaps it was telling me of its right to exist. I couldn't help it; I didn't want to deal with it. Even with my obvious discomfort, it kept calling out with its bone-chilling squeal. I tried to look away from it. It was too shocking, too brutal, and I just stared at it, studying it as the awful sound it made continued. All I could do was offer it an unwilling audience, someone it could talk to, someone that was thinking *please someone move me, please move me now!* I closed my eyes.

***

TRYING TO REMEMBER WHERE IT ALL BEGAN[19]

I was in a hospital room or was it a gate at an airport? Was I in a hospital waiting to get on a flight? There was a lot of movement in the room. I could see people enter a doorway to my right and leave through a doorway on my left without missing a step or even pausing. I just lay there and took in all the activity. I didn't know if I was invisible, what my purpose was in this area, or if I was even safe here. I noticed a lady standing behind a podium at the foot of my bed. She must have been the gate agent or gate keeper. She was taking something from the people as they passed by her without an exchange of a pleasantry or even a glance. As the last group passed by her, she continued to occupy herself with some papers on the podium. Then, as if sensing my gaze she paused, looked up, her eyes met mine, and said "Your parents are here."

My parents are here? You called them here to Pierre? Why did I think I was in Pierre? How did I get here? Why was I here? Nevertheless, it was great that they were here; they'll get me out of here. The lady looked to her left as if to acknowledge their approach. I couldn't make them out, they were walking too fast. All I could see were dark human forms. I couldn't tell if that was really them or someone was pulling my leg. Worry filled me about why they were really there, and the shape I must be in. Before I could even tell if that was really them, they walked right by the gate agent and through the door. I waited and waited for them to return through the door or come through the other door but they didn't. They had disappeared. Were they really here or was that gate agent full of lies?

I heard a different voice say as if I had not taken notice the first time, "Your parents are here."

Yes, I know that, you already told me. Like a replayed scene I saw two more figures walk into the room. What was this about? They had already walked in here. Well, were they here or weren't they? People kept going through the door to the jet way, pausing briefly so the gate agent could take their boarding passes.

Then a third frustrating time I heard an announcement, "Your parents are here with Dr. So and So, we hear he is the best doctor in the hospital."

Do I have a play-by-play person in the room now? Is the 80s NBC broadcast announcing team of Bob Trumpy and Charlie Jones calling this horrible late afternoon NFL west coast game? I saw Dr. So and So walk in with the figures that must be my parents. He wasn't looking at me. He was looking down at the ground, reflecting. I couldn't make out a face but I knew he must be the hospital's resident delicate genius.

Objections to this situation came to me immediately. First of all they had no idea why I was here. Second if he was so great then why was I here? And third, I doubted if this hospital's finest could cure whatever ailment had brought me here. By the way, why wouldn't anyone tell me what that ailment was?

Dr. So and So was a white haired gentleman, so I had to trust that he knew what was wrong, and that Pierre, South Dakota know how could get me out somehow. I was not optimistic; they looked rather grave. I had a sinking feeling that I was at the bottom of the heap looking to the top for help, and there was no higher power in existence that I could go to. This guy was it. I hoped beyond all hope that he was some sort of wizard or judge who could wave his wand and get me the hell out of here; but it wasn't like that. Something bad had happened.

***

BUT DON'T LET MY SHOW CONVINCE YOU[20]

Later, I woke up to find my mom standing there with someone that I should know but didn't recognize. Suddenly, a young doctor came bursting through the door as if he were the answer to all of the questions that hung in the air. He stopped, and looked at me in an overdramatic sudden fashion. He held his chest in mock pain, adoration, affection. I didn't know exactly what he was going for emotionally, he seemed to be trying to make a big entrance or receive the *Robin Williams Award for Overacting*. I politely stared, but the comedy wasn't working with me. I tried to look amused; I simply didn't have it in me.

PART II: I'M MILES AWAY[15] - BEARINGS

I still couldn't figure out why I was here, why was I in South Dakota? I swore I was from somewhere else, and I had never been in the state before now.

The young doctor made some senseless jokes with my mom and the other person and was off. Wonderful, I guess his work was done here. Was this too hard a case, not challenging enough? What was it? My expectations were being lowered and lowered by the minute.

As he turned to leave the room he hesitated as if he had forgotten something. Yes? Yes? Something you remembered that will get me out of here perhaps? Were you holding on to the answer this entire time, something to hold over me?

He turned, and said in mock reflection, "I'll return with something you'll need."

My mom said, "I know exactly what he's going to do. This is a joke; I've seen it before." with a very knowing air.

My expectations were hitting a rocky shore with this statement. What I thought might spring me was just a joke perhaps learned in The Clown Institute of Clownery. Not the kind of clown higher education a prospective student would find in the phonebook, but one with ivy on the outside of the buildings, and clowns wearing leather elbow patches on their grossly oversized polka dot outfits whilst they stuff each other in Audis. Or to put it another way if I was awaiting the reenactment of a scene from *Patch Adams* then I was simply fucking out of here.

I thought in exasperation, *fill us in on the joke, what is he doing? Why are you keeping it to yourself? Why the hell are you acting so light hearted when this is it for me? Fuck the joke! Get me the hell out of here! Because this situation isn't funny!* I continued in a more subdued tone, *OK, I get the joke. It was funny and now I'm drained. Ha Ha. Stop the joke now, let's move on and I hold no grudges.*

The young doctor returned with a piece of paper, and said, "This is a free bill that lets you out of the hospital when you get better."

My mom said, "Oh that'sfunny. I knew you were going to do that."

I scowled in anger, and thought, *let me up, my energy is back. I'm going to beat that guy with that very piece of paper, and figure out a few more things while I'm in the process before he hits the floor!*

He left with a dramatic flair, his smug white coat spinning with him like a BMOC who got the big part in the school musical. Actually, it looked more like a white cape. And me, I was the nerd stagehand left there to rot, and pick up electrical cords, or whatever the hell nerd stagehands do.

I must have fallen asleep because I awoke later to find the very same Dr. BMOC looking straight into my face only about a foot away. Up close his features were very pronounced; he had these huge teeth, and began to drool or cry on me. I couldn't tell which fluid type I was receiving, so I looked down with alarm as it hit wherever on my person. He looked upset, and a little more serious than when he first pranced into the room.

It's about time I see your serious side! I thought.

As his face got wetter and wetter I grew more and more concerned, because if this clownish guy is becoming overwhelmed then I was in serious trouble. He stopped what he was doing, stood up, and nonchalantly wiped off whatever fluid had collected around his mouth.

I could only think, *oh sweet unconsciousness please take me away,* and surprisingly it listened and did.

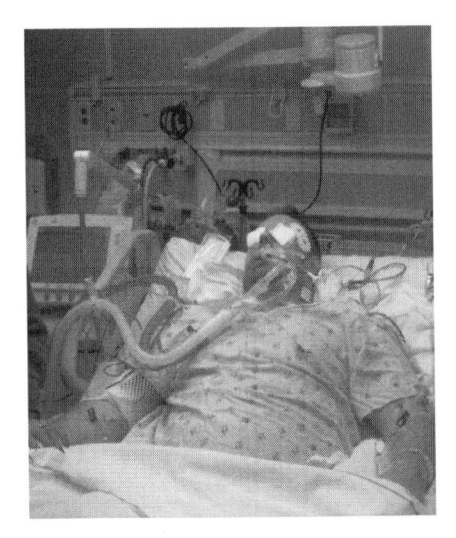

PART II: I'M MILES AWAY[15] - BEARINGS

January 17, 2009

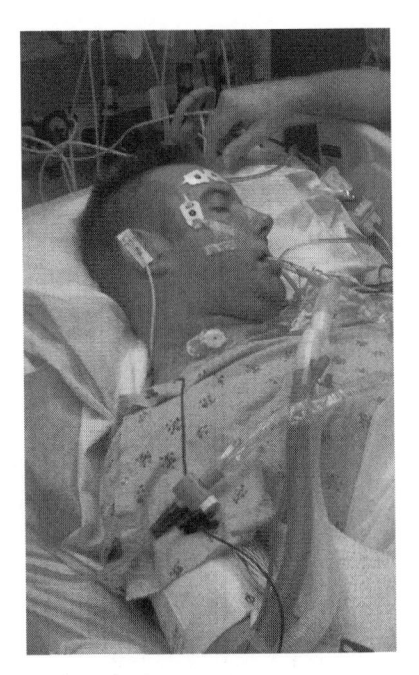

January 17, 2009

CHAPTER 7

Frequent Flyer

Fever is the most common presenting sign, although hypothermia may be present in patients with shock.[21]

THEN I GOT THIS FEELING THAT I NEVER HAD BEFORE[22]

Why, oh why did I have to use my body as a shield to protect that Confederate building from destruction? I had heard that there were many other protesters there that had also been injured. I heard that the workmen that came in and found us could only sweep me up, and put me on a gurney. I was lucky to be alive at this moment. My last memory was lying in a dust-filled room, the sun shining on my face through a hole in the building. There were other prone bodies littering the floor, not moving, not making a noise. I didn't know them, and I really didn't know me at that point. What had befallen us? Whose idea was this? I could remember getting out of the car on a dirt road at the top of a sunny grassy hill in the country, and walking toward what would be one of the last decisions I would make as a healthy able-bodied human being. We were in a jovial mood beforehand, how did this happen? There had been an argument on the way there about who had the better doughnuts that we were about to stop and get before our arrival: Dunkin Donuts or Krispy Kreme. Lighter times.

I could hear, since no one really spoke to me directly, that I was the last one in the hospital. Becky was released, and Lorraine, my sister, was still injured but was also released. She got to use a laptop at home now. So, why was I still here? Did these people know what they were doing? This hospital seemed so dirty, there were these wispy things floating in the air like that colored party string. There it was hanging on the clock, on the wall, floating over my bed. This was just a filthy place. What hospital was this anyway? I could not seem to figure out where I was. This hospital must have been an annex to that Confederate site I tried to save, there was no other explanation.

"What are they serving downstairs in the cafeteria?" I heard a female voice say interrupting my important thoughts.

"Spaghetti." was the reply.

"Oh, I guess I can eat that again, they always serve that. I'll be back again in a little while," came the first voice.

Not only was this hospital dirty they couldn't seem to vary the cafeteria menu. What was this place? How could I get out of here, this place with limited dining options? Why were they holding me here?

My parents walked in. I could not talk, move, nothing. I could not communicate in any way. They stood there looking at me with utter pity in their faces.

My dad finally spoke. "They hardly found anything of you. They had to sweep you out of there. You're lucky they found you when they did," as he pretended to hold a broom and make a sweeping motion.

I wanted to ask when they were released and how they healed so quickly. Why were they able to walk and talk? Was I the only one committed to the cause? What was the cause? Did I follow through like a sucker? Why was I taking so long to heal? Did I shield all of them from harm? I felt like I was fine, that I could get out; I could show them if I had the opportunity. It was useless. No matter how hard I tried to move or initiate a motion in some way I couldn't do it. I didn't know what happened to anyone else, and I was just beside myself with horror trying to tie together the string of events that brought me to this point.

With all the questions in my head, I could only form one thought to try and attempt to say, *please don't leave me! Please don't leave me here! They have you all fooled. I'm still here, I know who you are, please don't go away! Please don't go!......please don't go.*

A male voice said. "Try to turn his head in the other direction. It's not good for his neck and face for it to be facing down like that in one position for too long."

Oh no, my face has fallen off, I thought to myself in a panic. That building must have crushed me when they demolished it all around us. How could they not have known that we were in there? I was deformed, and nothing anybody could do would ever get me back to where I was. I probably had half my skull showing ala Two-Face. There was no sense in anything that was happening.

***

ALL I'VE GOT'S A GHOST OF WHAT COULD BE[23]

There was a film running in my head of me in a wheelchair wearing tan bermuda shorts, an olive-green T-shirt, tennis shoes, and socks. It

PART II: I'M MILES AWAY[15] - FREQUENT FLYER

appeared to be from 1995. I could tell from the haircut and the high ankle socks, the horror. In the film I am in a hospital corridor by a set of glass doors, get up from the wheelchair nonchalantly, and walk whistling out of the hospital. That was my hope, to someday do that. The film kept repeating; it offered me comfort; a target to shoot for. I needed to make that film happen, especially the whistling part since I can't whistle. Even with this recognized infirmity, I knew I would show them all, it would happen, I wasn't always like this.

Word somehow got out that I wanted to be released, and that I should be examined once more so that I could whistle on out of here. I had no memory of putting in this request but somehow it was put through the appropriate channels. There was no reason for me to be here. I should be home, convalescing, and getting stronger. This place was driving me up the wall. It seemed to be more like a narrow ward I was in with an exterior glass door leading to a patio to my left. A wall was to my right with adjacent stairs leading down to what must be the cafeteria. By the way, I wished I could go to the cafeteria and get some spaghetti.

A doctor entered the room and looked me over. For some reason he was wearing a dark robe with a dark shirt with a turned around collar. I couldn't tell if he was a priest moonlighting as a doctor or if it was the other way around. I could only figure that the hospital was so cheap that they could only afford one person that did double duty. He had salt and pepper hair, was in his sixties, and spoke with a southern twang. The doctor/priest finally spoke, "I hear you want to be released. Well, I'm here to see if that's possible."

In less than ten seconds that son of a bitch shook his head and said, "I'm sorry, we need to keep you here longer, and this is going to take some time to heal."

I was absolutely deflated. He turned, sat down in a chair over by the glass door, and began to read a Bible. I tried to attract his attention. I was in such utter pain emotionally and physically. I had been in this physical position for I don't know how long, and I couldn't just lie here anymore. Rudely, he never looked my way again. I tried to shake and shimmy, move the bed, anything. I couldn't move, it was impossible, and it was obvious this person didn't care. I was a prisoner in my own body, and it was hell.

My parents came into the room, unaware of the "checkup" I had just received. The priest/doctor just kept his head down. I was really wondering what I had done at this moment that placed me under the care of this jailer, and why there was still no explanation of who, what, why, where, and to what extent. And "how", that was most important.

An orderly or Nurse's Aide came into the room, perhaps to shake up the inertia that had evidently descended upon the scene. He was tall with braided hair. He reminded me of Larry Fitzgerald, the Arizona Cardinal wide receiver that had just run roughshod over the Carolina Panthers right in front of me at a playoff game. That did happen, didn't it? He was telling my parents about some apparatus to my right but I felt nothing. My mom and a couple of unidentified attendees appeared interested, approached the apparatus, and listened politely.

"This instrument measures the oxygen levels and the amount of air that's getting through to his lungs," Larry said authoritatively. "So right here at this level it's like you're running really hard up a hill. Like sometimes I do when I'm working out and I really red line it," he jabbered on.

I thought presumptively that I could have just given that explanation by looking at the instrument. Of course I couldn't see it, I didn't even know what it was. I could only assume some understanding. So with this questionable debate ammunition, I thought, *excuse me, are we here to talk about your workout routine or is somebody going to get me the hell out of here! This guy doesn't know what the hell he is talking about!* No one heard this silent tirade as I looked away in disgust and continued to feel ignored. I would have been the guy in the Ed Sullivan Theater in the front row with the furrowed brow and crossed arms when the Beatles first played.

Did someone mention emphysema? Why did that pop into my head?

I should say something. This was my moment to shine. I would amaze them with my determination of wanting to leave. As a bonus, I would show that asshole in the robe sitting by the window how wrong he really was.

I put this determination to work, and tried, and tried to get the words out. I was working hard, so hard to get the air in my lungs to get the question out. I worked and worked. I could see the wall facing me, dark figures standing at the foot of my bed, and could feel that unconcerned priest/doctor sitting on his ass, doing nothing. I knew I would amaze and confound them all. They thought I was finished just lying here. I would show them. I would speak. They began to look at me expectantly, waiting for all of this to end, anticipating something. Are they concerned, surprised, horrified? I could tell, they were taking notice. Then I finally said it, I did it, and I screamed the question for the ages: "WHO HAS EMPHYSEMA?!"

But nobody heard, and no one was impressed. There was an empty unfulfilled feeling that passed over me as the darkness came.

***

WHEN I CAN FLY WAY BACK HOME[24]

"We moved to New York," a female voice said. "Oh, you'll have to visit."

I heard the name of the speaker, Clarice Roberts, and realized that it was a good friend of ours. This made me feel much better that someone I knew was around.

Taking her up on her offer I thought, *don't mind if I do*. I was immediately whisked away on a plane, and was flying away; I could see out the window. I still couldn't move. Somehow, I felt the horror was about over now, I could feel it. I was on the move, and moving was good. It made me feel like I was doing something. It was such a beautiful moonlit night on the Atlantic, the light was reflecting peacefully off the water. Was that Long Island Sound I saw? I could stare at this for hours. I was getting out of the grips of what had me. My situation was becoming safer, clearer.

I was now out of the plane and hovering over Manhattan. I came to the apartment building where our friend and her family must live. Something guided me, I had no address, no directions, but I knew where it was. The building was well-lit and pretty modern looking. I found in the vestibule the bell for their intercom. It had their name on it all right, and there was a note that said, "We moved to London, catch you later."

What the hell? I came all the way to New York to visit, and they moved already? I guessed I would have to fly to London. No way were they throwing me off now. I had come too far, might as well go another 5,000 miles.

I could once again see the Atlantic Ocean bathed in moonlight. This was so much better than my hospital room. I was really happy that they let me go on this jaunt. I was lucky to be here and out of there. I was out of the woods of my plight. The plane was hovering over London now, there was British invasion music playing from the mid-60s, such a familiar sound. I now found myself hovering over a plaza on the Thames River.

Clarice interrupted my experience, "We live in an apartment now."

No one seemed to correct her that they are called flats in London or advise her to look to her right when crossing the street.

Another voice said something about strep throat. "Yes, you can get the strep bacteria from anything, there is a wild cherry ice cream that has not been pasteurized that carries the bacteria, you can catch it from there if you aren't careful."

I had a question for the disembodied voice, *Ms. Disembodied Voice, excuse me, but how can I be careful about eating ice cream that I know may or may not have the strep bacteria, wouldn't I just not eat it or do I just eat around the strep parts? Oh, and a follow up question: what might those parts look like?*

The voices didn't listen, and began to get on my nerves so I ignored them, and walked through the plaza. I could see the brick-lined plaza quite clearly, no one seemed to notice me. There were a number of British invasion rockers with dark suits and shaggy hair sitting at all the tables smoking like chimneys. They thought they looked cool, each one thinking they were the next answer to the Beatles when really they weren't even the next answer to the Beau Brummels.

"Smoking can really kill you, especially when you're in this state," another disembodied voice added. The voices seemed to be following me now.

The rockers were eating wild cherry ice cream thus putting their questionable music careers on the line. I must have travelled back through the mists of time to a place called the 60s. It was so obvious they were so ignorant about the hazards of smoking and wild cherry ice cream. As I passed judgment on them my thoughts turned to my appearance, and that I had no idea what I was wearing. I was sure I was not dressed properly for swinging London.

I quickly departed the plaza hoping not to be discovered and mocked by the rockers who would become mockers in their dark suits and mockful hair styles as they mocked my alien presence in their midst. I made my way to the apartment building, excuse me, flat building, where our friends now must live. I found their name, and rang the bell yet no one let me up.

Son of a Bitch! Let me up! I shouted to myself.

As suddenly as I had found the building I found myself hovering backward, over the city lights and back on the plane. It seemed that my time was up in the jolly old Roman outpost, Londinium, and I was now headed back across the Atlantic. The moon was once again offering me company with its reflection off the water. There came the lights of New York to welcome me home to the US, marking the end to my unfulfilled trans-Atlantic journey.

There was a voice talking about Kate and Phoebe which seemed to mark the end of my field trip. I was so excited. The little babies were still around? How old were they? Kate must be four, and Phoebe was two. My thoughts of them could not get them out of this age even though I knew in the back of my mind that they were seven and five. However, I couldn't imagine them at any other age. By the way, how did I come to be back in the hospital? How did I get back here already? The plane was just flying around Manhattan a moment ago.

The voice continued, "We were taking Kate and Phoebe somewhere, and Phoebe claimed she could sing opera. Kate yelled at her that she couldn't, but Phoebe tried anyway. Kate yelled at her to shut up, and Phoebe was really upset."

I was upset hearing that Phoebe was upset and I couldn't do anything for her. The two-year-old version of Phoebe singing opera? What a hoot. I wish I could have been there, she loves to sing.

Before I could finish that thought my journey outside the hospital was on again. I was off, hovering out of the hospital, was I out finally this time? A trip to London and New York was one thing. Was this the final time? Was the journey going to be a lie this time? I felt free, so free, I was out! I must have been out! I was hovering through a rural area, and could see a dark road beneath me. It seemed to be some sort of drop off/pick up point for the girls. Becky's mom was switching the girls with my parents for some reason on this country road that must be near my hospital. They must have brought the entire family here to live now wherever that may be or perhaps we always lived here, I didn't know. As soon as I found a piece to the puzzle, ten more missing ones presented themselves.

I came closer and closer to the car, hovering once again. No one seemed to notice me looking through the open door at Kate and Phoebe in their car seats. They looked two and four, five and seven must not have happened at all. What form had I taken? I felt a part of this gathering like I was supposed to be here, however no one paid any notice to me. If only I could pick them up and take them home. I just wanted to touch them, say hello, and tell them I loved them and that I was OK. I just couldn't.

As soon as I moved into the car, and could see them up close I was hovering away again, over the country road. They didn't even know I was there, that I still cared about them but I couldn't let them know. My journey was over as I could feel my prone body lying on my back where I started, in the hospital. All the hopes that I had of getting out were gone, and I was stuck in this place, wherever it was, again.

Then a voice that I recognized as my dad's spoke in my ear through the darkness, "Love those Babies."

CHAPTER 8

Body of Work

Shock at the time of admission or within four to eight hours is present in virtually all patients with GAS TSS and is due both to capillary leak and vasodilatation. Despite aggressive therapy, the systolic pressure remains depressed in 90 percent of patients after eight hours.[25]

MANHATTAN TAKES HOWARD

Darkness, solitude, emptiness. There was a hopeless and helpless feeling I got, like I had lost something or that I might lose it at any moment and there was nothing I could do about it. That was how I was feeling about my life, my family, Becky. My travels at this time had taken me to God knows where by God knows what means. Understanding whatever force it was that was pushing me to these new places that I had not been before, or I had not been for quite a while, eluded me.

The one thought that kept pushing itself to the surface of the uncertainties I was embroiled in was a dire need to find my life, to find her, to believe that I was still me, and to shield me from whatever world I was now in. Anchor me! Don't let me keep moving! Each place was more horrible than the last! However, my quest to find her was not merely one of location but of understanding because I had been somehow burdened with the knowledge that I did something terrible to drive her away.

As my mind burrowed its way to some unholy corner to find reason in this world it came back with reasons that were ridiculous yet plausible at the same time. Who was I to question what must be fact and empirical? The reasons seemed to be rooted in a weekend trip to Manhattan, yes, Manhattan which was strange in itself since I had only been there once since I graduated from the United States Merchant Marine Academy in 1991. I was hell bent on staying at least 150 miles away when that day of commencement came with a handshake from Dan Quayle. Incredibly, a moment of weakness brought me to a mini-reunion in January 2008 and a stay in the Waldorf Astoria.

However, none of that entered my mind as I considered my current so called trip involving me as the subject of a body re-building exercise. By body re-building, I don't mean working out, and getting on the treadmill. I mean a tear off pieces and start over, as one would do with an ugly house. Of course, that was what I figured must be the root to my current problems, stupid vanity. Bedridden, away from home and family, not sure of my real existence, all these things were my fault. There could be no other explanation. And the root, the root of this troublesome weed lay in a hospital in Manhattan that I somehow knew was the mother of all elective surgery. Unsuspecting patients, patients with no self-esteem, patients conducive to a strong sales pitch or a weak sales pitch go there under their own free will or someone else's free will to have their bodies re-built. Yes, re-built as in limbs, torso, maybe a head, whatever the patient desires, and perhaps a little bonus addition for their trouble from this place of evil.

PART II: I'M MILES AWAY[15] - BODY OF WORK

This seemed logical at the time so why shouldn't I have taken my parents along as well, and my sister and Becky? We would go, and check into the Plaza, and paint the town red before I got my perfectly good body altered in some fashion. I supposed this was necessary to satisfy my over-inflated ego and sense of well-being which I really didn't think I had. The thought of adding luxury to a time of horror puzzled me.

This hospital was somewhere just south of Midtown. It was an imposing building dwarfing everything on the street with its girth. Bats cartoonishly flew around its Gothic features non-stop. We arrived at the hospital before my procedure to take a tour of the facilities. A little meet and greet never hurt anyone. The surprise was that the interior belied its exterior. What I was expecting to be a classic wood-covered interior with a fire cozily crackling in an imposing stone fireplace was instead a fluorescent lit sterile nightmare of nothing but white. Any other color was in stark contrast to the pure white that covered everything. There were large rooms connected to one another with ceilings thirty to forty feet high. Conveyor belts criss–crossed the rooms, exiting through openings in the wall, and re-emerging in other rooms. Body parts were being moved on the conveyor belts, their destination determined by some method to where they were needed for re-construction. The reality of what I had signed up for was hitting me hard at this point. What I thought would be a spa–like atmosphere turned into some grisly butcher shop that would have made Leatherface from *The Texas Chainsaw Massacre* blush. Perhaps it would have forced him to write a strongly worded e-mail to hospital management.

As I took all of this in, my mouth agape, I looked up, and saw two naked fat men running in place in a large glass container of some yellowish liquid. They were suspended ten to fifteen feet in the air.

The official noticed my gaze, and said to us, "Those fat men you see are comprised of purely reconstructed body parts. They were our first reconstruction. The doctor likes to keep them around for posterity."

Their bulbous ass cheeks wiggled as their plump hairy legs churned the liquid for what purpose I had no clue. We kept staring at the horror as we walked under the vat of liquid, and to my chagrin nothing was left to the imagination as every angle of their hoggish appearance was unobstructed. After shaking myself out of watching that train wreck of "success" we followed the official to the next room.

The next room was not as large as the first; it appeared to be a patient ready room. The walls were completely white as was the ceiling, fluorescent lighting found every corner of my environment as it seared the room with its putrid blinding light. I looked down, and noticed that I was in a hospital gown and now suddenly alone. My group, my entourage, my posse, my family had left me. It slowly dawned on me that this wasn't just part of the tour but the procedure itself. Without a word the faceless official shoved me down onto the end of a conveyor belt. Before I could express my shock at the suddenness of this movement, I slowly began to move up the belt as metal bands were placed on my limbs. I couldn't move, and for some reason I offered little resistance, paralysis seemed to be setting in. I looked up, and saw robotic arms with knives attached come down from the ceiling. The contraption appeared to be from some James Bond movie. However I had no secret weaponry or skills to not only remove myself from the situation, but do it with style. The blades continued to swing wildly as they approached my body. Without a glimmer of mercy they took one swipe at each leg. My legs were now off, and scooted off the belt like a worthless piece of meat. Needless to say I was in shock, and was really

PART II: I'M MILES AWAY[15] - BODY OF WORK

unable to comprehend this as I saw my arms go next from another set of blades that had escaped my attention.

"Please! Not the face!" I begged.

Why must I have been my own worst enemy? How had I somehow agreed to become a quadruple amputee without question or even seeing a brochure of the place? How could I have been so duped? Where in the world was the turnip truck that dropped me off? Now that the damage was done there was no question I was now suffering from heavy trauma, and I would need to depend on these evildoers to help me.

The robotic arms came in next with legs that looked nothing like my own. They were skinny and hairless, like a chicken leg. The skin was wrinkled and pale. Whoever these belonged to before must have long departed this life. Next the arms came on and the hands were grotesquely malformed, they looked like feet with short stubby fingers that were immobile. I was losing my mind as I headed down the conveyor belt not knowing if I had signed some sort of extended warranty or service agreement. The conveyor continued into what I presumed was a recovery room of some sort. The same fluorescent light surrounded me as I tried to gather my senses on what was supposed to be a tour yet had become a life changing event of my own doing.

I was dumped onto a gurney. A nurse casually walked over to the foot of it and looked down with amusement at my scrawny parts. She was pale as the fluorescent light. She wore bright red lipstick that threw everything in contrast. Her black hair was up in a tight bun under a vintage nurse's cap. Her white nurse's dress and white shoes reminded me of some stereotypical nurse from a 1930s horror movie and her hair and makeup from the *Addicted to Love* video. This time I was not a drooling nineteen-year-old even though I was still taking the scene in with awe, only for an entirely different reason. She was young. Her expression belied her years. She somehow seemed older, wiser, and I had no idea what her duties entailed. Hopefully, one of them wasn't called "An Unhappy Finish."

She grabbed the stethoscope hanging around her neck, and began to listen for a pulse in my ankles. Each time she checked she exclaimed in horror, "I cannot find a pulse! There's no pulse!" She would check again, and repeat her findings again, "I cannot find a pulse! There's no pulse!" She kept repeating this mantra over and over again until I couldn't stand it anymore. I kept looking down at her as I raised my head slightly thinking she would catch my gaze yet she didn't look up. She kept checking for a pulse repeating, "I can't find a pulse! There's no pulse!"

I'm here! I screamed in my head, *I'm looking right at you, why can't you understand that I'm alive!* No amount of wishing or thoughts of slapping her was going to make her shut up.

***

AS IT'S NOT LIKE IT WAS BEFORE.[26]

Darkness set in at that moment brought on by my frustration. I couldn't hear her anymore, either she stopped or I had passed out or worse. I felt myself being lifted, and moved. At that moment I realized I could not open my eyes. My body felt the tossing and tussling to get me out of the room as I was moved for some distance that I couldn't determine. I heard a heavy metal door open; I felt stale air hit me as I was unceremoniously dumped somewhere inside the hospital. What really was annoying me was that I had no way to defend myself. I was

PART II: I'M MILES AWAY[15] - BODY OF WORK

at the mercy of whoever was "out there." Faint light soaked through my eyelids as a light was turned on. All I could gather was that I was now a failure of the hospital, and could no longer be seen. I must be hidden from view, which was quite remarkable given that this was the place that had two wide bodies running in nasty liquid as an exhibit of its success.

There was silence but someone was there, I could hear water dripping as if I was in a basement. The silence was then broken by an uneducated sounding male voice that said, "A duck says what?"

I had no idea what that meant. The voice kept repeating the question as another light was turned on above me. Was the voice talking to me? I felt completely exposed, whoever it was could see me, had carte blanche to do its bidding in and around any part of my body. I was at a severe disadvantage at this moment. I was at the mercy of someone that would ask a prone body, and hopefully not a naked prone body, "A duck says what?" *Seriously, that just makes no fucking sense! God, I know you're still there, please don't let anything befall me further. Please don't.*

I was unable to utter a response, and continued listening to the movement in the room, and waited for what this person may do with my now malformed body.

As I continued to listen to the dripping of water, and felt the cold air on my face, I waited for this derelict to begin stabbing me or worse. Fear surrounded me along with the darkness as I tried to explain my situation to myself. The only explanation was that I was dead but still alive in my body just unable to interact with my environment. Certainly a hospital wouldn't put a living breathing patient down in this place where some insane person was asking such a nonsensical question.

The operation had obviously gone bad, and it suddenly dawned on me, *Oh Lord! I must be in the morgue. I'm in the morgue! I ruined everything. My life for a spot of vanity in getting my body re-built. It was my body, why did I do that?* It was obvious the derelict was a morgue assistant, maybe a necrophiliac, waiting to have some fun with me.

I tried to wait it out. I was awake, yet I wasn't awake. I couldn't open my eyes, it's as if someone had glued them shut. I couldn't move a muscle. I couldn't let anyone know that I was still in here. I wanted to shake that duck man to within an inch of his life. Fear and pisstation roared through me.

I do still have my mind! I tried to yell. Still, nothing came out.

I sensed movement around me. I had hope and despair fighting it out. Was there a Good Samaritan out there? Was the autopsy to begin? I could give you the results right now. I had my fucking limbs chopped off!

A light flickered on above me. The brightness cut through my eyelids like a knife. I couldn't turn away from it. The light just kept getting brighter and brighter, hotter and hotter. The heat was now miserable. I was so fucking hot and so thirsty, this couldn't be happening. Why in the hell did I have to have my body re-built? I was just a fucking heap of shit that couldn't move. Oh, but the mind was sharp as a tack. This was not supposed to be happening. It's as if there was some greater force at work here. Something guiding this charade and my inability to communicate to let anyone out there know my condition was draining all hope.

Was this it? Was this all I had left? Darkness? Some bright light that stabs me like a knife every now and then with none of the benefits of weightlessness and floating? Where the hell is the floating? If I am dead, then this sucks! I at least want to float! In fact, this is the opposite of floating! Plus I want to haunt that nurse and that damned duck guy!

It felt like whatever the something was that was pulling the strings here had doubled or tripled the amount of gravity. I didn't know how to occupy myself. I brooded, *was I ever really alive? I don't remember dying. Did I have a family? Is there anyone left out there? Are they going to put me in the ground and that's where I will remain for eternity? Just thoughts with no memories?*

There was something going on around me, and as expected my pleas and questions went unanswered.

Mercifully the light was turned off however my thirst was an ongoing torment, and hunger added itself to my list of concerns.

I asked the obvious question, *how in the hell am I hungry if I'm dead or in another world? How in the hell am I going to eat? Will I just suffer in silence, and wither away? Certainly torture like this isn't just at the end of life. Once you're dead you continue to be hungry? Fuck!*

Just then as if on cue to my thought waves I felt something hitting my stomach. It felt so damn good. I couldn't believe that something was going into my stomach, I couldn't taste it but it was there, and I imagined some sort of delicious milk shake. All I could think at this moment was, *Yum Yum Yum Yum*, with the most earnest of gratitude to whatever power was in charge, and for hearing my pleas.

***

YOUR DREAMS WERE YOUR TICKET OUT[27]

Perhaps Providence had mercy on me or I turned a miraculous corner with that fabulous milk shake. I finally awakened in a brightly lit recovery room. There was a conveyor belt next to my bed. It was moving, carrying some unknown body part to some location in this sprawling place for some other ignorant victim. I could not feel my body but I was obviously still in the evil Manhattan hospital with no earthly idea of when or if I would ever get out. At least I was out of the clutches of the uneducated medical examiner's Igor, and amongst the living although it was a form of living that I didn't trust in the least.

A doctor entered the room. He was obviously in charge of this malicious program of withered chicken leg insertion and obviously a quack. How he built such a large practice on the most expensive real estate in the world was anyone's guess. Perhaps the zoning committee had been dispatched, and I was peering at one of their limbs slowly making its way through my room. He was tall and slim and had dark wavy hair parted in the middle that covered his ears. Of course, I would have to pick the doctor with the dated haircut. He had the light reflector strapped on his head for full effect—yes, we know you are a fucking doctor, get over yourself—and he was rather young, and quite full of himself. I hated him immediately, and hate was not a strong enough word for how I felt about this guy.

He wasted no time on a greeting or other niceties but got down to business because who was I? His plaything, his unwilling prey, while he was the king of the jungle, and he was fully aware of it. He said in his smug voice, "There is quite a bit of recovery associated with a procedure like this. The recovery will take some time, and so you'll be in here for quite a while."

I was unable to speak and could only think, *first define "a while." Second, I can't, just can't be in here. I don't want to be in here. It's impossible that I am in here. Besides the reason there has to be recovery is because of what you did to me asshole!*

PART II: I'M MILES AWAY[15] - BODY OF WORK

My parents were standing by the bed, and my sister, Lorraine, was there as well, looking pretty somber. I didn't see Becky anywhere which was very upsetting. The room was all white except for the windows. Somehow I had a corner room on an upper floor with windows from floor to ceiling overlooking a Manhattan street below. This doctor may have been a prick but at least these were top-notch accommodations in spite of that body part conveyance thing occurring all around me. As I peered around the room I could see the top of an escalator leading down the outer edge of the building, out of my room. That escalator was freedom.

If it was possible the doctor turned more serious as his glib face attained a furrowed brow, "You cannot leave until your recovery is complete which will be quite some time and, of course, very expensive."

I was seething, *Boooooo!!!!!* during his high and mighty harangue. He was cocky, arrogant, pompous, and did I mention smug? There appeared to be no law in the hospital except the one he had made up. Did the American Medical Association know about this guy? Performing ghastly procedures on patients that had been duped into thinking that a better life awaited them was not what I think followed the Hippocratic Oath or was it Hippopotamus Oath? My mind was gone! I did know that I was in a dire situation, and must get out before something worse happened.

The doctor left and another nurse came in somehow paler than the nurse that could not read my pulse. Hopefully this one had better hearing, and I wouldn't be visiting the morgue again. She had dark hair pulled into a bun, and she was a little more frightening than the first nurse, and that was no easy feat. She stared down at me with pity like a small child about to squash a bug. Without taking her eyes off me she picked up a giant needle, and held it up in a taunting fashion.

Her perfect white teeth were exposed in her tight grin. Her lips covered with her bright red lipstick appeared dried to her teeth as she asked hypothetically, "Are you ready for your transfusion?" No answer I gave was going to alter this outcome. Ready or not, I was getting this transfusion. Nothing was getting me out of that. I kept staring at her, she didn't move. Was she expecting a response? I continued staring, and from the stress of awaiting the where and how of that giant needle, I blacked out.

***

When I opened my eyes only my sister Lorraine was by the bed. I assumed the transfusion had occurred, and I was out of the woods for the time being. Lorraine crouched down close to my head, and whispered in my ear, "I'm getting you the hell out of here."

I was helpless to help myself so someone else was going to take charge. I guess she had also had enough of the nonsense that was taking place which was due to me and due to this freak show. How was she going to get me out of here without one of the hospital thugs stopping us? The escalator was the key to my freedom plus she had been around doctors for most of her adult life. Perhaps the medical lingo she had overheard at cocktail parties had rubbed off on her, and her hastily obtained knowledge would save the day.

By this time I was in darkness once again, and I could hear a different doctor come in. He greeted her, and it sounded like he assumed she was with the hospital, and began talking to her about her weekend. He seemed nicer and more down to earth, unlike Dr. High and Mighty but anyone and anything would be more down to earth than that demi-god. Lorraine described her plans of visiting a lake or

PART II: I'M MILES AWAY[15] - BODY OF WORK

something, and wasted no time in proceeding with an explanation of why I needed to be moved. It was an explanation loaded with medical jargon that I was unable to decipher. I trusted in whatever she said to get me out. Her cocktail party knowledge was above reproach, and it sounded as if she had sat in on a few seminars in her free time. The doctor seemed to buy this explanation of course without consulting a chart or orders, and left the room. Apparently in this world the power of persuasion and acting like you knew what you were doing trumped actually knowing what you were doing.

I could hear Lorraine's footsteps return to my bed hurriedly, and she said, "Here we go."

The bed moved slowly as she put her weight behind it. I suspected the escalator was our destination. Somehow we got down the escalator without tumbling at all. As I opened my eyes I could see that luckily the front desk in the lobby was unattended. We slipped out of the lobby and through the glass doors onto the sidewalk. We were free for the time being in the night air on some street in Manhattan. The air had a crisp fall-like feel to it, and I was no longer in that damn place. My spirits were up.

As the bed was pushed toward the curb I could see my parents outside on the sidewalk as if they were in on the plan. A high school friend of my dad's, Ned Quaker, was somehow on hand. The coincidences kept piling up on our little adventure now with my dad running into his oldest friend.

"Hey," my dad said excitedly, "Uncle Ned is here," not really acknowledging my hospital break or bringing up any further steps to this plan.

Uncle Ned just raised a bottle of Grolsch with the flip bottle top, and nodded with approval in my direction but did not come over.

Strangely, there was no one else on the street except the five of us. This was Manhattan correct? Was the knowledge of what went on in this place enough to keep locals away? Why the hell didn't I notice that? Where was Becky? I kept wondering whether she did not approve of my ghastly procedure. Of course she did not approve, she was sensible. That was why I called her "Wife Sensible."

The ringing sound of a tiny bell broke the silence and my thoughts. I could see it was coming from an old man pushing a Grolsch cart onto the sidewalk from a plaza in front of the hospital.

A street vendor selling Grolsch? I asked myself, *now I have seen everything.*

A Grolsch was handed to me in celebration of getting out of the hospital. However, I realized I could not hold anything nor speak nor drink so the gesture was purely symbolic. Wait, we were still in front of the hospital, had anyone thought of leaving this spot before they noticed I had disappeared, and I got hauled back into that hell? There seemed to be no concern as the celebration continued unabated.

Soon an ambulance pulled up to the curb adorned with the hospital emblem. Lorraine walked over to the driver's side, and talked to the driver. The result was that she somehow convinced him to drive me back to the Plaza. The guy didn't seem to be evil so how could he work for such a butcher shop? I thought this was such a bad idea, but then again a cab couldn't haul around this bed. The driver and his assistant placed me and the bed in the ambulance; somehow the ambulance driver had bought whatever story he had heard.

Once I was in the ambulance there seemed to still not be any urgency in our situation. I was just waiting for someone to come running out of the hospital, and put a stop to this entire caper.

My dad appeared in the side door of the ambulance, and said, "I have another visitor for you."

It was someone he knew, a lady doctor from a real hospital in Manhattan who stopped by to offer me comfort, and deliver news that I had no idea I would receive in a million years. She had dark hair, was perhaps in her late forties, had olive skin, thick eyebrows, and appeared to be of Italian descent.

She said reassuringly, "The baby is fine."

Lady, you must have me confused with another body in a bed on a street in Manhattan because there is no way that Becky and I are expecting a baby, I thought.

Of course, I was unable to say this; however, no one seemed to correct her. Was this the reason Becky was not with me? She just continued to stare at me, and touch my hand affectionately to offer me comfort. I lay there staring back awkwardly. Was I supposed to smile? I was more confused than anything. If I could talk I wouldn't know what to say anyway. I would disagree with her but would that make me an uncaring father? There were so many conflicting emotions with this news. I just got used to whatever number of babies I might have, now this. Well, this was a real busy day for me: my body ripped apart, an escape from a hospital, and now a new baby. I had somehow lost count of my children and my body parts.

Is this four? I thought to myself.

As I was mulling this over in my head trying to dodge the doctor's awkward gaze, I noticed a spider come into my field of vision. It lowered itself down its web from the ceiling of the ambulance, and hung in the lady's face. She didn't swat it away. She wasn't affected at all by it. She just kept holding my hand expecting some response from me in return.

I thought, *Lady, I cannot talk, and I feel quite uncomfortable right now. I am OK, please leave.*

How could I tell her about this spider that was having its way with her dignity? It was really bugging me because if it got on me with me being unable to move then I was going to freak out. To my horror another spider lowered itself, and another. This was horrible and embarrassing. One spider was enough, but two? Now three? If I said something now she might get angry wondering why I didn't say anything about the first two spiders. Before I could think about this issue any further two more spiders lowered themselves, and they proceeded to make webs in her hair. Now not only was her creepy stare making me want to jump out of my skin, her complete lack of awareness over these spiders was doubling my discomfort.

Finally feeling that the moment was getting awkward herself she abruptly stood up, and nonchalantly brushed the webs from her face as if they were just one fly.

Lady, you have no idea, I thought.

As the lady doctor talked to my dad, Lorraine sat down by my side, and the spiders not discouraged by the lady doctor's reaction started lowering themselves onto her. She noticed right away, and seemed irritated with me that I had not notified her of the ambulance's unwanted guests as if these things were doing my bidding. Or perhaps they were wanted. There was no telling with this damn hospital.

The ambulance finally pulled away from the curb, and took me and my dad to the Plaza. I hoped the entire way there that the driver was not asked of his whereabouts or his passengers. It seemed that my mom and Lorraine wanted to stick around the area and do some shopping so they stayed behind. Shopping? I could not believe they were shopping at this hour after my grotesque body had just been sprung against policy from the hospital and the recent discovery of a new grandchild/nephew or niece revealed somewhere in Manhattan. What the hell?

***

UNDERSTAND WHAT I'VE BECOME, IT WASN'T MY DESIGN[28]

We returned to the Plaza where we had reserved a suite in one of the penthouses. Where I got the money to afford such a self-destructive procedure as well as a suite in one of the nicer hotels on the planet was anyone's guess. The room was gorgeous. The windows had lace curtains, a sign of a real fancy place, and the lights from the city peering through the thin fabric made for a beautiful scene. A bathroom light and a bedside lamp on the low setting were the only lights on in the room.

Becky appeared suddenly in the suite, and no mention was made of a baby. There was no discussion of our escape or my body being "rebuilt." She must have been rightly not on board with my scheme.

As she and I settled into bed I looked up to see that a glass canopy covered it. I thought nothing of it until during the middle of the night the damn thing dropped on us. It may have been the stress of the day before or my body rejecting the body parts like in that movie *Body Parts* but I absolutely started freaking out over the situation. It seemed that with my newly reconstructed body I had also in the process lost my mind. I began to verbally berate Becky. I somehow was able to speak, my voice sounded familiar much like it would have in high school. Something, however, didn't seem right. Young and obnoxious was how it sounded. I couldn't get over the sound. I kept talking abusive gibberish. I glanced at myself in the mirror, and I was shocked to see my seventeen-year-old self looking back at me. However, the reflection in the mirror looked away while I was still looking at it, and the prick reflection continued its abusive harangue. I couldn't believe that I was outside of my body witnessing me abuse someone I loved. I couldn't believe it was happening. I was speaking nonsense and in a very arrogant manner about how I could do this and that. Why was I suddenly able to move now?

This diatribe awakened my parents who were in the next room. My dad started getting on me about my behavior, "Stop it, what are you doing?"

My evil self did not listen to my dad which really bothered the sane part of me that was watching this madness.

My evil self suddenly screamed, "Why won't someone please kick my ass? I got my body rebuilt, and now I'm an asshole!"

Please, won't someone, my sane self replied.

To my horror my evil self reached down, picked up some of the broken glass, and threw it at Becky. Suddenly appeased, the beast that was my evil self went back to bed as did my sane self.

Later I was awakened by Lorraine, "Becky's gone."

I was shocked and said nothing. At that moment, I suddenly remembered what happened. *What the hell did you do rebuilt self?* I thought reproachfully. I got up, entered the bathroom, and saw blood in the sink. The glass must have cut her face badly, and may have gotten in her eyes. Distraught, I leaned on the counter, dropped my head down, and yelled, "Why is this happening? Where did she go?" Then there was darkness.

***

DON'T LEAVE ME HERE ALONE[29]

I could not find Becky anywhere, we had a new baby, I was now some rebuilt asshole, and I lost my wife because of me. What do I do now? I felt abandoned. My parents and Lorraine rightfully left me, and went back home since this new Howard just sucked. I was still here, I was still the same guy, I'll get out, I'll show you all that I can do it, and beat this. So if it was me and the new Howard, did I have to depend on him to get me home? No cab was going to take that asshole to the airport.

As I walked through the dimly lit hotel lobby, I had a feeling that I was going to find Becky. I remembered Lorraine somehow passing on to me before she left that Becky would meet me in a dining room on the second floor of the Plaza. I went to the dining room at the appointed time, and she was there at a table for two looking at me. The table was situated against floor to ceiling windows that overlooked the street. Somehow things had changed. I could cut the tension with a knife. She was rougher, harsher, and quite standoffish. My asshole self had run away, and left me holding the bag of the situation he created.

I sat down at the table looking out on the city, and could say nothing. There was no excuse for my actions.

Becky said, "You hurt me Howard. You hurt me so much. I cannot be with you, and I won't."

I just sat there speechless, and she said, "I'm leaving." And with that she got up, and walked away. I had lost her, and I couldn't get her back.

I got up to go after her but I didn't see her anywhere. I came to the end of a long hallway, and there was a movie poster in a gilded frame covered in glass with a picture light accenting it beautifully. I had never heard of this movie. It appeared to have me and Becky starring in it. As I looked at it in wonder I asked myself, *how do I consider myself in the same league as her? Why would she have me? I'm in too deep with her, and now I turned her against me. The evil rebuilt me with the smart ass teenage voice has fucked everything up. Her attitude is different, and I have hardened her and made her get mean. I have to fix this.*

Obviously seeing this movie poster had piqued my interest, and I decided to go to the nearest theater to see how we looked. Luckily it was playing in a theater around the corner. I kept saying to myself or anyone that would listen as I walked down the dark abandoned street glistening from a recent storm, "If this is a dream make me wake up, please."

***

AND YOU WILL SEE WHAT I MEAN, IT ISN'T A DREAM[30]

I did wake up, I felt much better now since this was the real world and no longer a dream. Whoever had listened to my plea got me out of that mad world, and now I found myself in the darkened theater waiting to see the movie starring me and Becky. It was stadium-style seating, the aisle lights dimmed, and the narrator warned that it was intense, and should not be seen by smaller children.

Good grief what do they have us doing in this thing? I asked myself.

I saw her. Becky was sitting in the row in front of me. I immediately got up, and sat next to her very tentatively. She didn't look over at me so I wasn't sure if she didn't notice me or if she was angry about that horror at the Plaza. I wasn't sure if that really happened, so to play it safe I thought that I would play it humble.

"I'm sorry," I said trying not to sound like a spoiled five-year-old.

She didn't say a word, just kept staring straight ahead. After a moment of awkward silence I made the first move, and we started kissing.

I thought to myself, *we're alone in the theater, and this is just great. What a make-up make out!* This was real. I was out of the nightmare world, and now I was awake. Everything would be fine.

Soon, I realized that we were not alone, and that unwanted eyes were watching us. A frumpy lady wearing a frumpy flower-print dress, who had escaped my notice earlier, was sitting in front of us. I didn't know where the hell she came from. It was obvious she heard us since she looked at us with a pinched face, and stormed off out of the theater with her frumpy dress, and her frumpy face, and her frumpy-ass hair tagging along. She returned a couple of minutes later with the manager who was also frumpy.

"OK, out!" he said to us as the light from his flashlight blared in our faces.

The frumpy lady added, "What kind of theater is this? I paid my fifteen dollars, and I want to see the movie not experience it!"

We stood in front of the screen, and I could only say, "You're really fucking this up for me lady, we weren't doing anything! Wait, are you saying I paid fifteen dollars to see a movie?" Maybe I had learned something from the evil Howard.

"Yes you were! I know what I heard and saw!" she said in a disgusted tone.

Becky was quiet, and seemed to be resigned to being ejected. The manager finally said, "You have to leave! Out!"

We were whisked outside into the night through a door next to the screen, and I found myself on the street corner outside the theater. I looked around frantically. Becky was nowhere to be seen.

I exclaimed in horror, "She's gone again! I'm still in this nightmare world. Oh God! Where am I? I want to get out of here! What is real, and what is fake? I can't do this anymore!"

I collapsed on the street on my knees looking up at the movie marquee. I saw our names up in lights, I felt total emptiness, and then there came the darkness.

CHAPTER 9

Uncertainty of the Past

Initial management is aimed at securing the airway and correcting hypoxemia. Intubation and mechanical ventilation may be required to support the increased work of breathing that typically accompanies sepsis, or for airway protection since encephalopathy and a depressed level of consciousness frequently complicate sepsis.

IT'S LIKE A DREAM, TO BE WITH YOU AGAIN[31]

The 1967 Pontiac Firebird made its way down the highway, the engine rumbled loudly, the rural scenery passed by in a blur. I didn't know how I knew it was a Firebird, I could only see the black dash. Perhaps it was the round gauges which had always been a Pontiac trademark. I looked out the corner of my eye and saw Becky. She was there looking at the road with a determined look on her face.

Whatever the method was that we came to having this car I had no idea, my more immediate reaction was the utter joy I felt to be back with Becky. I assumed this trip was much more than a joyride, there was urgency not only in my condition but in the unfinished business we had at that damn hospital. We were now on the lam. It seemed the nasty business that occurred at the Plaza was still in the air. It seemed she was willing to forget it for the time being in order to get me help. I still felt an overwhelming sense of guilt over it, it was something that I never thought I was capable of doing. She disappeared from me and we were now back together. I don't know how, but we were, and I was not questioning it.

My joy was tempered however, when I discovered that for some inexplicable reason I couldn't move again. It was as if my situation had improved yet hadn't. I was as stiff as a board, and just sat on the seat strapped in place like a small child. We were on a long trip though I had no idea where we were going, and Becky wasn't speaking to me. She was communicating through her silence that she was in charge, and we were going to get through whatever this awful situation was since it had not really manifested itself in a way that I could understand.

We were out in the country on a two-lane road, daylight was growing short, and the shadows were growing long. I thought about the car. How did Becky know that the 1967 Pontiac Firebird was a car that I had always wanted in whatever life I had led to this point since high school? I was not only born that year but of the muscle cars from that era I thought the Firebird had the more appealing body style. However, the chances of finding one in acceptable condition at an acceptable price were small, and the chances of me gaining the mechanical inclination to get one in poor condition up and running were even smaller. So I had sat on that desire, and decided that wanting was better than having.

I looked out at the countryside passing by the window. It was dark by the time we pulled up to a place that looked oddly familiar. The long gravel driveway, the old mature trees, the old white house, all of it looked very familiar. Then we pulled around to the back of the house,

PART II: I'M MILES AWAY[15] - UNCERTAINTY OF THE PAST

and I knew instantly where we were. Why had Becky brought me here? Did she know this was my great grandparents' home in Fuquay-Varina, North Carolina where my great aunt lived until her death in 1992?

It was built in 1917 across from the Varina Depot where my grandfather worked. I still had the Duncan Phyfe table, sideboard, and mirror that occupied the dining room for all of those years. I would visit there every summer during the late 1970s and early 1980s on the annual two-week odyssey down memory lane as the entire family would slowly make its way up Interstate 95 at a blistering 55 mph. Twelve hours from Tampa to Raleigh in a 1977 wood-paneled Ford Country Squire in one day with nothing except your thoughts, and some elevator music was certainly traveling in style. After my great aunt's death the lumber yard next door purchased the land that the outbuildings stood on, and retained the house as a rental property. It ultimately suffered the indignity of becoming a haunted house for Halloween. This went to show that sometimes it was better to have a favorite memory torn down than fade away slowly through neglect and abuse.

As we drove up it felt like the past, it had to be since it was torn down in 2008. It was as if none of my memories had happened yet. I had no idea what year this even was. The familiar sound of the gravel crackling under the tires as we pulled up to the back door made me feel like a youngster looking forward to a week-long visit with elderly relatives unaccustomed to children and quiet rooms with stuck together ribbon candy, and of course, ticking clocks. Ticking…..clocks.

My door was opened, and someone that looked familiar but I couldn't quite place stood there. He looked to be in his mid-forties, kind of a crusty fellow with a dark beard, long dark hair, wearing overalls and a T-shirt underneath. He appeared to have the run of the place, and I knew I had met him in the past because I really was not questioning his presence. Of course, I was as usual, unable to move. I sat there, and stared at him letting the awkward silence envelop us.

"Welcome!" he said in a gruff Southern drawl. "Good to see you again after all these years! Why don't you get out of the car, and come inside?"

I just sat there, and I sensed no movement coming from Becky's side of the car. There was just silence. I was unable to turn in her direction to see her expression or if she was miming something to the gruff man.

"OK," he said looking a little forlorn, "That's fine, I'll just sit out here on the driveway, and join you."

He pulled a beer out of a pocket in his overalls, and sat on the driveway staring at me waiting for me to say something. I thought it was quite rude that he didn't offer me one, at least splash some in my face. I noticed my Aunt Grace, my mom's sister, and her husband, Barry, were standing in the garage staring at me. There was a blinding light behind them. I couldn't see the source of it, it was just pure light. I turned away and stared straight ahead. I felt very rude not saying anything, just sitting there but I couldn't really move at all. In addition, I had this uneasy feeling there was something in my mouth. I was in poor condition so I just kept staring, being the impolite guest.

"Your cousins Shelly and Janet are here," someone said. They are Aunt Grace's daughters about four years younger than me. I didn't see them. I assumed they must be inside somewhere. However, that still wasn't enough to get me out of the car so I just kept sitting, and so did Becky.

I kept thinking, *this is awfully rude but I'm unable to change the awkwardness here.*

Then it happened. An alarm started going off that sounded like a high-pitched squeal. I felt a tightening in my chest, and sides that wouldn't stop. I found it hard to catch my breath as this continued. My body tensed up almost like it was pitching into the air. I heard other voices. There were others around me, around the car. I just couldn't see who they were. The scene outside the garage, and the awkwardness that went along with it, dissolved into darkness.

***

GHOSTS APPEAR AND FADE AWAY[32]

I finally felt myself floating out of the car and into the house, I saw no sign of the gruff guy whose presence so puzzled me. As I passed through the house I could hear my cousins Shelly and Janet, Aunt Grace, and my mom speaking in an argumentative tone. I continued floating through the house when I came to the foot of the stairs. I ascended the stairs looking at framed photographs on the wall of the staircase. I had never really been upstairs in the house for any extended period, certainly not when it was being used on a regular basis. It felt more like an attic but it was a full second floor. Whenever I did visit I viewed my trips upstairs as more of a tour through a museum.

I could hear Shelly say, "I cannot get my kids to eat any vegetables except for potatoes and maybe corn."

My mom then chimed in, "Corn is not really a vegetable and potatoes certainly aren't either."

I could feel a big argument brewing about the merits of the two food stuffs, and wanted to get into a bedroom, and close the door before the storm came. This argument may be talked about for years to come.

I finally found myself in the bed of one of the upstairs bedrooms. Mala, my great grandmother, who died in 1968 when I was barely one-year-old, entered the room. She said as if she were expecting me, "Now you just lie there and rest, I'll get this room all fixed up."

I continued lying there looking at her thinking how amazing it was to see someone that I had only seen in photographs here in front of me putting pillow cases on pillows. She was as nice as I had been told. She had a look of determination on her face that she was going to make me as comfortable as she could. I realized that Becky was lying by my side at that moment.

Although this was my family's home, I still felt like an interloper even with Mala's graciousness.

What year's this? I again wondered.

As time went on I was able to forget about the problems with the hospital that was still in hot pursuit. I heard no more alarms, and I began to relax. Suddenly Pa, Mala's husband and my great grandfather, burst into the room acting belligerent as hell. Pa died in 1974, and I still remembered visiting him, and him sitting in that chair in the sitting room downstairs, saying hello. I didn't really have any idea who he was at the time except that he was some old man in my life I was required to visit. He was always very nice, which was why I was surprised by his demeanor.

He stomped into the room, and said very angrily, "I don't want any unmarried couples sleeping under my roof!"

Mala then said in a soothing tone, "Of course they're married."

I was beginning to think that Mala's positive soothing attitude would not win the day.

"As Baptists!?" Pa yelled.

"No, Episcopal!" Becky replied with an air of disgust. Oh, she sounded pissed. Those were the first words I had heard her say in a while.

"Get the hell out of my house until you're married as Baptists!" he yelled.

This was shocking. According to his tirade we had been living in sin for the past thirteen years. Why was he being such an asshole, and how the hell was I going to get out of here? Then the scene suddenly went dark.

***

AND I FEEL LIKE I'M SWIMMING OUT TO HER[33]

I woke up in the front seat of the car in the driveway with the alarms going off once again. I could only surmise that the hospital knew that I was here, and they were tracing me. They must have planted a chip or something in me that traced my every movement, and told them my geographic location. Escape was hopeless. They were going to send me back, and I didn't want to go back. Don't let them send me back. My thoughts went back to the movie poster that I saw of me and Becky in the Plaza. This must be the adventure that it foretold that we were going to be having together. She had turned into a bad girl, but I could not think of anyone better to have my back. I still thought I was in way over my head with her. I was just a hopeless nerd from high school that couldn't get a date. What did she see in me? My feelings for her ran deeper than I could have imagined.

Becky started the car to cut our awkward visit short, the car rolled about fifty feet down the driveway and stopped. I could not believe this beautiful car wouldn't start again just when we needed it.

The bearded familiar-looking gent got up off the driveway, and walked to the car. He was followed by a couple of other men that were faceless to me. He said, "You got car problems? We hate to see you go without saying good-bye."

Calling attention to our rudeness just when we were in trouble made me feel worse. Becky said nothing. He then walked over to the car, and looked in the backseat.

He said incredulously, "What's this? Did you build yourself a car?"

I had no idea what he was talking about until I began to inspect the vehicle in some disembodied fashion. It was then that I noticed I was sitting on a hay bale with some very rudimentary seat belts made of rope holding me in. I looked in the back, and it was devoid of any seats, and only had loose hay covering the floor. I knew Becky had this persona we call "Blue Collar Becky" that we laughed about. At times I am Mr. Fix It where I do have successes but can have little patience so "Blue Collar Becky" will step in, and in a few seconds will have fixed the problem. She would also jokingly use a gruff voice, and preface every sentence with "Howard." It is very endearing when she blushes since she knows she has taken yours truly in the blue collar arena, but building a car that actually runs? This was ridiculous especially with her overlooking basic safety measures.

"Let's see, I have a charger in the garage I can get to see if it's the battery," he said. He was gone for a moment, and returned rolling a charger behind him. He popped the hood.

Just then I heard Becky's voice except I couldn't see her, her voice sounded distant and far away. "Something's wrong, it keeps going off."

***

BABY YOU'RE THE BEST[34]

I could feel Becky lean over the seat, and whisper in my ear, "Come on Super Hoov, you can do it." I didn't know exactly what I could do at that moment to help, and then a crazy far-fetched theory dawned on me that would make MacGyver roll his eyes. As part of the body-building process, and to turn the tables on the hospital, I could use the alarm to internalize my desperation into an intense energy that would start the car, and send us on our merry way. This was going to be incredible and a little preposterous.

The unkempt fellow closed the hood, and said, "Can't get it to work. I'm surprised you got this far in this thing."

I decided to take the lead, and to stop sitting there like a lump of shit. The hospital would be here soon to take me away. Sitting still was not an option. I tensed my body, and concentrated to try to start the car. Becky was still whispering in my ear, encouraging me in a sultry manner, "Come on SuperHoov you can do it." The pain was excruciating, I couldn't seem to breathe. It felt like there was someone sitting on my chest, and I needed to just shove them off. The alarm sounded again. I felt the discomfort and pressure reach a peak then relief as the car immediately started. I had now found my super power. Becky hit the gas that left behind flaming tire tracks in the driveway. I could only assume that the bearded gent was left scratching his head.

***

CHURCH ON TIME, TERRIFIES ME[35]

I awakened outside somewhere staring down at grass. My wrists were tied to a railing to what must have been the front porch area of a building. I could see steps to my right leading down to a walkway that led to a sidewalk. The steps, the railing, the columns at the top of the steps made me think that I must be at a church. I thought we were still in Fuquay-Varina, and I just knew that this must be the church my parents were married in. I couldn't move once again but I could sense that Becky was tied up next to me.

A girlish screech broke the silence as I tried to verify my surroundings.

"You're the product of hell fire, and the demons will come screeching from your bones!" the screeching voice said.

I looked up in astonishment to see if that comment was directed at anyone else that might be tied up around here. I saw a girl in her early twenties wearing glasses, with brown hair pulled back in a ponytail. She was skinny, dressed in a long black skirt, a brown top with a hood and black boots. She had a very passionate look about her. The look said that this was what she believed, and no amount of reasoning with her would change that.

There were candles set along the front walk from the sidewalk to the church steps. She was unhinged as she spouted her sayings to us. It appeared that we were involved in some sort of conversion to become Baptists. I guess being Episcopal wasn't good enough, and now we were admitting our marriage was null and void, and we would need to get married as Baptists or we wouldn't be recognized in the eyes of God. Or for more material reasons we wouldn't have a room for the night at my great grandparents'. I just could not believe that we had signed up for this though, certainly we wouldn't have agreed to this ceremony in the middle of the night. I had no way of conveying my unease as I was defenseless and soon realized that my entire body was draped over the railing with my ankles tied to it as well.

As the young girl's shriek continued she started screaming at us, "Hellfire! Hellfire!" Just then she began to throw some sort of ash at us that burned my skin on contact. It was not comfortable by any means.

Dammitt!! That hurts! Perhaps the devil is in me, I thought.

"The devil must come out of you!" she screeched again.

At that moment I realized that Becky had somehow gotten loose from her restraints. It seemed she had tired of all of these ceremonial trappings. I was relieved yet disappointed. I was willing to become a Baptist if that is what someone in my family wanted no matter how crazy the demands were. I was hoping she would make that commitment yet on the other hand somebody had to stop that crazy bitch from throwing ash at us.

Becky ran across the lawn, picked up a candle, and threw it at the Church girl who then screamed and cowered as she ran across the lawn shielding herself with her arms. Becky then kicked her in the ass and chased her out of view. My, Becky had turned bad, and was taking no shit.

Becky yelled after her, "I've had enough of your crazy shit, get the hell out of here."

Oh, how I love her.

For a moment she was still out of my field of vision, when suddenly a large needle was before my face as someone got me in a headlock.

"I owe you something, you know." It was Becky's voice. "You hurt me back in New York, when all I did was care for you, and you stabbed me in the eyes."

I was silent.

"Now I'm going to do the same to you, are you going to beg for mercy? Are you going to have me do it?"

I didn't argue but I knew she was faking it, she couldn't hurt me no matter how bad she was acting, no matter how sharp her edge had become at the Plaza. Something had possessed her, this wasn't her. I decided I was going to remain silent on this one which was the right decision since I couldn't speak anyway. I love her so much I was willing to let her do anything to me if it made her feel better. It didn't matter to me, I hurt her, and I deserved what I got. So, I just remained still.

A female voice then broke the silence, "Put it down!"

I looked over and saw a short female police officer walking up with her hand on her pistol which remained in her holster. Becky released my head but I couldn't see where she had gone. The police officer came over to check on me and radioed in that a perfectly sensible person with some strange tendencies was on the loose.

Goddammitt! I lost her again! I got her into trouble, and now she's gone. She's trying to help me, and now she's on the run from the law, I thought in a panic, *I just hope she remembered where she parked the car.*

***

PART II: I'M MILES AWAY[15] - UNCERTAINTY OF THE PAST

WHAT AM I DOIN' HANGIN' ROUND?[36]

I awakened in some sort of strange garage. I could see out to the street. I seemed to be in the prisoner booking station at the Fuquay-Varina police station. The garage was narrow, perhaps only wide enough for a paddy wagon to access. The walls were painted urine yellow. To my left I could see a control room with two officers that jutted into the garage about two feet. Flystrips were hung all over the walls with dozens of flies on each one, the air was filled with them, and with my inability to close my mouth I was certain I would end up choking to death. Then I realized I was hanging from the wall. Just hanging there. I lost Becky again and now I was being transferred somewhere. Why was I being arrested? I was the one getting shit thrown on him.

    A paddy wagon backed into the garage, and stopped in front of me, its engine running and the noxious fumes began to make me gag. Below me was a prisoner, a short bald man with a goatee who appeared to be drunk and out of his mind, walking around hugging the ankles of other prisoners hanging on the wall. At least it appeared to be other prisoners, I couldn't be sure. He got to me, and he started hanging on my ankles. He just wouldn't let me go. The two officers in the booth paid him no mind. Was he like some sort of mascot? I couldn't kick him off, I couldn't move, I couldn't yell at him, I just had to take it. I had no idea what the hell he was doing down there. Then I heard someone yell something unintelligible. The man must have been called and released my ankles. He climbed inside the paddy wagon staring at me with a blank look. The doors shut and the paddy wagon left. I remained, hanging there. Then darkness.

***

SOME DAY GIRL WE'RE GONNA GET IN THAT CAR AND GET OUT OF HERE[37]

I woke up in a car that looked familiar, I realized it was the 1967 Firebird except something seemed different. I was in the front passenger seat, and I could feel the warm air in my hair as it made its way down the highway. I looked out of the corner of my eye, and saw Becky driving. She came back for me, I couldn't believe it, and she risked everything to get me out.

She noticed my stare out of the corner of her eye then said with her eyes still on the road, "You like it? I made it into a convertible." I nodded, unable to speak still, and looked back at the road. We were definitely further south, I could tell by the thickness of the air.

"I had to get you, we need to get you better," she said sounding very concerned.

I was so relieved right now that we were back together. I couldn't get over it. It seemed that my recent adventures had done little to improve my health. I didn't want to bring up the church and what happened, and she didn't mention it. I guessed it was forgotten.

We arrived at a beachfront strip, the ocean was on our left, and there were condos and beach houses lining the road. Everything seemed dated like we were back in the 1970s. The scenery looked like it had a yellow sheen to it. We pulled up to a McDonald's that was of a vintage style across the street from the beach. I stayed in the car as Becky went inside. Still unable to move I looked straight ahead, and noticed some teenagers sitting on the concrete picnic tables just outside the store. They were listening to some early Beatles on an old tape player. The air was hot and humid. I could only imagine that we were somewhere in the Florida panhandle, perhaps near Becky's hometown of Tallahassee.

My eyes then fell on the newspaper machine, and I saw the headlines that read, "Redhead and Super Hoov Still on Run." Fear spread across me as I saw the pictures of me and Becky from the movie poster on the front page. It seemed like our movie was going to get a little more interesting. I didn't understand if we were in the movie now or not. Becky quickly walked out of the McDonald's, got into the car, and didn't say a word as we drove away. She acted nervous as if she had been spotted.

I had no idea how to tell her about the newspaper, it was probably best that she not know. I dozed off and awakened to see that we were now on a straight country highway with farmland on either side. The flat farmland slowly gave way to foothills and then to mountains. We were headed up and up and up into them, and in no way was I able to ask where we were going. All I knew was that it felt like time was running out for me. I now found myself lying on my back behind the front seat in the straw. I must have been a nuisance falling over all the time.

Becky then said to me, "I found a childhood friend of yours. He says that you guys know each other from back in the 1970s in Brandon. His name's Ralph." I didn't catch the last name. I listened intently thinking I knew who it might be although what was coming to me wasn't a good memory.

She continued, "He says he's going to help you, and will work to solve your problem and condition. He's researching it now." From what I gathered it sounded like he was some sort of doctor/lawyer super person. I do recall him as a bully, but really fifty percent of the kid population in the 1970s was bully and the other fifty percent were the picked on, so that didn't shed much light on who it might be. I gave no response as I just lay there in a heap in the back of the car as we went up into the mountains.

CHAPTER 10

Lessons

Streptococcus suis has emerged as a cause of streptococcal toxic shock like syndrome. Although this pathogen is traditionally associated with bacterial meningitis, a highly pathogenic strain has emerged with the ability to produce massive quantities of proinflammmatory cytokines.[38]

I MISS YOU/DON'T LET ME WAIT TOO LONG[39]

I awakened in another hospital. I figured I was up in the mountains somewhere, perhaps Becky felt I needed to get back under professional medical care before we carried on with our fugitive ways in outrunning that evil place. She must have dropped me off at the front door. I knew she would be arrested if she kept hanging around. Thank God she came back to get me, she was still in my camp, now if I could only get the power of speech back I could apologize properly.

As I would come in and out of consciousness, it seemed from listening to the staff and looking around that I was in a small metropolitan area that I had never been before. Still, the doctors were trying to correct the mistake that I had made in getting my body rebuilt. I didn't see Becky anywhere, all I could see was a gate agent sitting in my room. She was processing what appeared to be boarding passes.

Dammitt! I thought, *Am I in another hospital/airport hybrid facility again? Why can't the two exist separately?*

I tried to get my bearings on where I was since no one seemed to want to fill me in. I was in a large room, and I could see people coming, and going not paying me any mind. I had two issues: I didn't think I was in the best hands being in a small no name hospital plus I was still on the lam from that quack in Manhattan. The fight in me was almost gone, I was resolved to the thought that my body was the quack doctor's, and he had to complete what we started. A doctor came trouncing in talking with my parents.

How the hell did they know I was here in the mountains? I wondered.

I overheard someone say that the doctor with my parents was the best doctor in the area.

I thought reproachfully, *I hope this mountain backwater's best is good enough and can get me out of this.*

As my mind relaxed I could still see people coming and going, and I felt like my inquiring mind was getting me nowhere. It was very similar to what that other hospital was like. I grew very tired knowing that all of that travel and effort got me nowhere, and my eyes shut.

***

WE COULD LEAVE TONIGHT/YOU CAN SLEEP ALONG THE WAY/DREAM IN BLACK AND WHITE[40]

I awakened in the back of the 1967 Firebird once again. I was becoming quite familiar with the ride and feel of the car, and the straw that was getting all over me, especially in my mouth. Somehow I had been released or had escaped from the hospital. I didn't know which to think anymore, this pattern was very abnormal. I guessed they were tired of dealing with the mess someone else had made or perhaps Becky took me away from their incompetent hands. Perhaps they were not equipped to handle the level of heat that the quack in Manhattan was putting on them to get me released. I must be a real hot potato patient for a hospital to release me in this condition. I had no idea of the level of care or the level of their abilities but I did know that what it got me was me just lying in the back of the Firebird as we made our way on what must have been a twisting turning mountain road.

I heard Becky in the front seat say to me, "They couldn't handle you anymore, and released you. One doctor convinced me that you need continued care and he has offered us a place to stay at his home in the mountains. Nobody knows about this, and our whereabouts will hopefully remain a secret. He says he can do something with you that he was not allowed to do in the hospital. It's our only hope."

Except I was devoid of all hope. I felt weighted, used up, my body rolled with each twist and turn of the road. However, I was quite puzzled how an old cabin, I assumed, was a healthier alternative to a real hospital. I didn't know if he lived in this cabin or this was his property, and his real house was elsewhere. Unfortunately, my assumption would be proven correct since what I was about to see made the cabin from *The Evil Dead*, the Sam Raimi version of course, look like Buckingham Palace. We pulled up alongside the dirt road in front of the cabin. By this time my vision was coming and going. I could hear the car door open and the cold air hit me.

I heard the doctor's reassuring voice, "We can carry him inside. I have a place in the basement where I can examine him."

They struggled to get me out of the car as I felt myself being lifted and carried. Becky and the doctor somehow got me down the exterior stairs into the basement. I looked up and could see a ratty old screen door at the foot of the stairs that opened into the basement. Five-star treatment here. Nonetheless, we were on the lam, and they would never find me here. I just hoped I could hold on. I didn't really know the plan at this stage. I was just a piece of furniture. They carried me through the dark, dank basement and lowered me onto a wood plank table held up with saw horses. Becky left me in the hopefully capable hands of the doctor while she stepped out without a word. I just lay there with my thoughts thinking if there would be a time in the future when I wouldn't be so helpless. I fell asleep with the strong feeling that I was going to have to go back to that asshole doctor in Manhattan with my hat in my hands to get out of this predicament.

I awakened to the sound of a car door opening and closing, and I heard Becky say, "Thanks Ralph." The car peeled off down the road.

I was afraid this might happen. That Ralph guy was putting the moves on my wife since I was in this weakened condition. Help me out indeed. She was putting her emotional well-being into this guy that tormented me as a youngster. Ralph, rat bastard that you are, you sure as hell have found a way to fucking get at me in adulthood aside from memories of the childhood physical torment. I was just resigned

PART II: I'M MILES AWAY[15] - LESSONS

to the fact that my marriage was ending because of my severely infirm nature. How do I broach the subject with Becky? I was a total dependent with nothing to offer. She was out with another guy while I was in here. Were they just having coffee or what? Perhaps I should keep silent. That was really all I could do at this point anyway. So I lay there silently.

Becky entered the basement and said, "We have to leave now!"

"You're kidding me, you can't leave; he needs to be here. Besides, it's the middle of the night, and a snow storm's blowing in soon," the doctor objected.

"We have to go now, it's not safe. They know we're here already. Our location has been compromised!"

Oh God, how can that chip work up here? I thought.

"It's not going to get better until you stop running but I can't stop you. If you feel you need to go then go. Just promise you'll seek help as soon as possible when you feel safe," the doctor said.

I could see him, finally. He was a tall man with sandy blonde hair and glasses. He was skinny and spoke in a deep voice.

With obvious doubt in his voice he said, "OK, let me help you get him out of here."

They struggled with me once again and got me into the car. The door closed.

"Please be careful, the roads are terrible up here when this stuff hits," the doctor said.

Becky made her way down the road very cautiously. I still didn't know what she had found out or what had transpired with Ralph. Was Ralph a mole? Did Ralph plan on getting me in the middle of the night or was he warning us?

Good Lord, I thought, *we're playing right into his hands.*

As we headed down the road only ten minutes from the cabin the alarms started going off again, except there was something different about them this time. I felt darkness around me, and knew that it wasn't just the hospital that was checking on my location. There was something medically wrong, and this was it. I tried to do my patented "SuperHoov" move this time but it didn't work. I compressed my chest, and tried to let it out, make this car shoot flames again, get me off this mountain; it didn't happen at all.

I could feel and hear activity around me. It felt like I was out of my body, beginning to float. There seemed to be nothing left in me, I felt empty, at the end of the road. I put up a good fight but I couldn't do this anymore.

I heard the car door shut and hurried footsteps outside. I heard Becky talking to the doctor in a very urgent tone of voice. I couldn't make out what she was saying. I assumed we were back at his place. All I could hear was, "Please help him! He's really bad!"

The doctor's voice sounded very grave. He replied almost like he was reluctant with continuing care outside the hospital. It was unclear exactly what he was saying.

I thought, *What the fuck has changed since we left here a few minutes ago? Who got to you? I fucking hate it when people suddenly get wishy washy, and don't explain themselves.*

He finally said, "I'll see what I can do."

I felt my body being removed from the car, and I was still in total darkness. The crunching of the branches under his and Becky's feet could be heard as I was taken to the house. I could hear the same cellar doors opening, and I was lowered down again on the wood plank. There was low talking. I had no capacity to make any sense of it.

Once I was on the table his voice grew more urgent, "I have to do something now!"

The alarms kept going off, they just wouldn't stop. No "Super Hoov" was going to work this time, I felt myself going as I kept hearing him say, "Come on Howard. Stay with me." I couldn't hear Becky anymore. I didn't know if she had left or not, I just didn't know anymore.

***

ONE STEP CLOSER TO KNOWING[41]

The house stood there looking back at me with mischief on its mind. It was a simple wood frame house with rough-hewn wood siding. The windows stared at me like eyes half shut with drapes partially drawn. The door stood wide open with a straight dirt path leading to the covered porch. I looked around, and saw only farmland and some woods off to the left. There was no color, I was in a black and white world. If possible, it was even stranger than that, it felt like it was the late nineteenth century. The house was more a farm house with two or three rooms, the kind I would have driven by countless times on a country road and paid no mind to.

I stood there staring at this house for the longest time. I was definitely on a farm and there was no one around, there was no wind, no noise, nothing. I felt small, I looked down at my feet, they were small, I had no shoes on, I was wearing overalls. I was definitely someone else, except the house looked so familiar to me. I was a little boy, and I was home. The house looked empty with no lights on, nothing, just darkness emanating from it. I just kept staring at it waiting for it to do something, to speak, to move, anything. I was on a tightrope of indecision. Should I walk toward it? Wait for it to do something? Run away? Where?

All of a sudden out of the corner of my left eye I saw this spindly woman with a gingham dress approach me. She wore round granny glasses, had dark hair pulled back in a tight bun, and her face was pinched. She looked strangely familiar as if she had popped out of one of the ancient family photos that my mom liked to have around for obvious shock value. She looked pissed off and it was obvious that she knew me. This was not a nice welcome to this strange world. She was the ideal character for the setting that I now found myself. I was so shocked by her sudden appearance that I said nothing to her. She was serious, and she was angry with me. From what she said it sounded as if I had found trouble somewhere, and now it was time to pay.

She yelled "You're coming with me!" as she pulled me by the ear with her bony fingers. I was really upset, and it was quite painful so I followed dutifully along whimpering. "Your father will know what to do!" she said adamantly.

"Oh, he'll be ashamed! Don't tell him!" I screamed with a power of a voice that was not my own, knowing yet not knowing what the fuss was about.

She led me behind the house, and suddenly I collapsed. I began to turn to her to beg her not to tell father. As I did something in the trees grabbed my attention. The leaves were moving rhythmically but there was still no wind. The leaves had no color, and I couldn't stop looking at them. The lady was quiet as she stood there looking up as if this was where she meant to bring me, to show me. Surprisingly, she made no move toward me. She seemed just as hypnotized by the branches as I was. She was waiting for something to happen.

I found that I had collapsed at the base of a large oak tree. As I continued to stare upward I forgot about the lady. I didn't know if she was still there or not. I felt lifeless, and a floating sensation came over me.

Is this it? Is this it? I kept asking myself. *Is this what it feels like to die? This must be the end.*

It all seemed so final, I felt very anxious, nervous, depressed but accepting that I was going to experience death, and it was going to happen. I began to float up into the tree. There was a feeling of finality to it all then a sudden feeling of sadness overwhelmed me as I thought of my family and not being there for them. My eyes closed as I surrendered to the feeling and let it envelop me.

CHAPTER 11
South Dakota

The demographics of invasive GAS infections have changed over the last 40 years. Persons of all ages may be affected with GAS TSS and most are not immunosuppressed……This is a sharp contrast to earlier reports of invasive GAS infections associated with bacteremia in which most patients were either less than 10 or greater than 60 years of age, had underlying diseases such as cancer, renal failure, leukemia, and severe burns…[42]

YOU ARE FORGIVEN[43]

I opened my eyes, once again I was in bed at an airport or was it a hospital. I still had not determined which had come first. It seemed familiar, where was I now? Was I dead? Was I awake? Had I survived? The gate to the jet way was once again to my left, there were people coming and going, and the place was once again bustling with activity. As usual, there was a ticket agent standing right in front of me, busying herself with boarding passes at a podium. She was focused on stamping pass after pass, giving them to people who disappeared through the open door. Was I waiting for someone to get off the plane or was I going somewhere?

Becky was sitting by my bed looking at her Blackberry, she did not look up. Was this a memory of her that I was now seeing? Somehow I knew that she was pregnant again. There had been news, someone told me, I just didn't remember who it was. I didn't think that we were once again expecting. The confusion took ahold of me further as my mind brought forward some memory of her OB/GYN, Dr. McCardy, having his office call to relay a simple message: No Air Travel. It seemed that he had gotten a little more restrictive with mothers to be and their traveling by air. Previously, before our other children were born, if such a thing had happened, Becky was able to travel up to only a couple of months before the due date. Not now, and they seemed to want to make the point that in no uncertain terms was she to travel by air.

Since I had to continue the treatment for my broken body, it was obvious that Becky was not going to let this news stop our departure. I was unable to speak, and I looked over at her hopefully thinking she would change her mind and not go on the flight. She looked disinterested when she looked over at me with an expression of, *don't tell, because I'm not telling*. The gate agent issued her our boarding passes. Without being able to speak I looked at her hopefully, and wiggled the pinkie on my right hand to symbolize our baby. I had already picked out a name and it was Beatrice, because I just knew it was going to be a girl. I could see a picture of her, framed, right in front of me, and she was going to get away from us if this simple message was not heeded. The photograph that I could see was an old fashioned photograph, a little brown, with Baby Beatrice smiling and waiting to be here. I had a feeling that she wouldn't have a chance to be around, and I didn't know what to do because no one could understand me.

It was time to board the plane, and Becky got up. While I thought Dr. McCardy was being ridiculous, there must be some health concern for her not to board the plane that we should not be questioning. Where my crippled self was being taken I had no idea. I was at the mercy of some plan concocted by some unseen force that I still had not identified. It appeared to be some specialized medical flight with all the first class seats having been removed to allow for rolling beds to be moved on board. This explained the hospital as terminal area which kind of made sense. Operationally I still could not see that as being very efficient.

My bed was hauled into place. The overhead compartments, the labels marking the seat numbers gave every indication to the familiarity that it had once been a normal passenger plane with the exception of all of the medical equipment.

My thoughts turned to Beatrice, how could Becky be so cavalier? Then on instinct I knew that I was the only hope that Beatrice had. So I did the only thing I knew to do, I acted like a hard ass on the no-flying orders. I couldn't take it anymore, I had to say something. Becky was going to be pissed but I couldn't live with myself.

The plane began to taxi, and as it began its take-off approach the words just came out of me so abruptly that I surprised myself, "She's pregnant! She can't be on the plane!" The thought hadn't dawned on me that I was only able to speak when I was ratting out my wife.

As the plane was moving a hatch that must have been in the rear of the aircraft began to open, and sent a strong vibration through the plane. I could see out of the corner of my eye Becky give me a withering look. The wind began whipping everything around us as I continued yelling at the flight attendant, "Don't throw her off!" I could barely hear myself over the wind.

The flight attendant in her blue suit and eighties blonde perm hair yelled down at me, "She has to get off the plane! No exceptions! I have got to close the hatch now!"

I could see myself as if I was outside my body looking in. I looked like the seventeen-year-old Howard with the big bulbous jaw that had yet to develop and Peter Tork of the Monkees hair, just like I did when I turned into an asshole at the Plaza. What kind of cruel twist of fate would give me Peter Tork hair? *Auntie Grizelda* was the only song he sang and that sucked. I screamed as the cold air rushed past me, and I lay there in my hospital gown, helpless. I thought at least they would turn around and head back to the gate. Becky got up, looked down at me, and begrudgingly exited the plane on the tarmac in the middle of the night. She was gone again, because of my big mouth. I felt sick. I had good intentions. I didn't want her to be angry with me. I was not going to live this one down. She had to know something I didn't, that she couldn't say, and I betrayed her. I felt sick, and we were taking off to God knows where from God knows where.

Once the plane was up in the air at a comfortable cruising altitude my thoughts of Becky were interrupted by the assignment of some sort of therapist to look after me on the flight. He was very boisterous, had a receding hairline and glasses, and was wearing this putrid yellow smock. He began to stuff what appeared to be bottles of some sort of orange drink alongside my body under the sheets. The damn things were freezing, and they had the same color of an Orange Julius. Orange and foamy looking. I bit my lip as I suffered from the cold with a look on my face of, *what the hell's this?*

"These will prop your body up so it doesn't collapse," he said

Collapse? Like gravity was so harsh on my body now that I would virtually implode or was the pressure on this plane not regulated properly? If that were the case I knew I would need more than a propping from some Orange Julius bottles. And from the looks of it, it appeared that everyone was hooked on the stuff. They were serving it in the cabin, all around. It must have been some sort of local thing.

The plane landed, and the therapist who had really done nothing for me by this point was now going to let me disembark as he told me quite emphatically, "You need to drink these bottles to get stronger, and work out with them so your body doesn't atrophy further. Remember, use the bottles and the exercises I taught you."

Taught me? He didn't teach me anything, and besides I couldn't even move. It seemed my sudden burst of the power of speech had disappeared. How could I do anything he taught me without moving? I gave an understanding look so he would leave me alone as someone pushed me off the plane. I just hoped whoever it was pushing knew where to take me.

***

DON'T SIT SO CLOSE TO ME[44]

When I awoke I found myself in a strange room with a haze that I couldn't quite see through. There were two ladies in short dresses sitting by my bed. A Caucasian brunette sat closest to my bed, an African American lady about ten feet behind her. At first I thought it was Becky but as I regained my focus, I was so disappointed when I figured out it wasn't. They smiled, and looked at me, and waved. Did the guy pushing me off the plane have orders to take me to a house of ill repute? Buddy you got the wrong guy. As I registered their friendliness as anything other than earnest I decided I wouldn't, and couldn't encourage their behavior or I would consider myself to be cheating, and besides, where the hell was Becky? What happened to her? Why when darkness comes do I awaken in a different place? This could not be the best method of recuperation.

The two ladies never said anything to me, just sat there. I kept looking over at them thinking they would do something else. They kept looking at me, smiling. I didn't know what to do so I acted disinterested and ignored them. I should have been a little more receptive to those around me but I was just deeply sad. I had no idea where I was, I knew no one around me, I had no clue why I was in the state I was in, I had nothing...

As I pondered the thoughts that kept me from losing my mind, I realized that perhaps it was not a house of ill repute. I had been shipped to some sort of beauty salon, and here were the two beauticians that were to care for me. So I supposed a beauty salon/hospital was now a licensed medical reality. An illness such as mine, or a horror perm, or ungodly Peter Tork hair could be dealt with in just one stop. I had no idea what shape I was in, and I had had enough so I forced myself to go back to sleep hoping I would wake up and find myself someplace more familiar. My life had become a slot machine, might as well pull that lever one more time for a better outcome, it had to get better, right?

***

I WOULD BREAK DOWN AT YOUR FEET AND BEG FORGIVENESS[45]

Once again the slot machine did not disappoint as I kept getting moved every time the darkness came. For once I would like to wake up in the same place. I had only one request and that was: Please stop moving me!

This time the place could not be mistaken for anything other than a beauty salon. As I looked around I discovered it was not only a beauty salon but also an auto parts store. It had a glass wall running down the center of it separating the two. I seemed to have fallen into some place that one of my nurses co-owns. I didn't know how the hospital felt about moonlighting. That was the least of my concerns, one being that it must be hospital policy for staff to take patients home with them as "homework." Fear was coming over me as I again had no idea where I was. I was away from those I loved with no hope of returning, and I felt a great discomfort all over my body. It appeared I had been deposited in some display bin in the auto parts side of the store. There was a neon sign showing a hubcap directly above me with the name of the auto parts store on it. The bin was located in front of the counter, and there was no one around. The place was dimly lit, and I felt very depressed. I was alone, and I knew no one, and I didn't know where I was at all, and no one was going to come and get me.

Suddenly a lady walked in and looked down at me as she walked quickly past. "Hello! How are you doing?"

I realized it was the same brunette that had been sitting next to my bed when I woke up after getting off the plane. She was dressed up for going out with a leather mini skirt, fish net stockings, high heels and a blouse with spaghetti straps. It seemed my expectations of having top notch care were being lowered, and lowered each time I woke up. *No hospital will have me now?* I wondered.

After thinking awhile the same thought was with me. After seeing how helpless I was, this lady or nurse or beautician as it were took me from the hospital, and brought me here to this beauty salon which she must co-own with that other nurse.

PART II: I'M MILES AWAY[15] - SOUTH DAKOTA

I was a little embarrassed about how rude I had been initially to her friendly waving when I first woke up. Somehow I communicated to her that I wanted to know where Becky was. "She's not here. She must be out wandering the streets," she said.

Lord, she's still on the run from the law! It's not safe out there! We need to be together! I thought deliriously.

I was then picked up by some unseen force, and put in a chair under one of the hair dryers. The sound was deafening. *Do I really need my hair dried right now?* I thought, *I don't remember it getting wet at all. Besides, there is no time for this nonsense.*

As I sat there I could see a white board on the wall. An athletically built tall man with braids came into the room wearing a blue outfit. Why, it was Larry Fizgerald from the Confederate hospital. He picked up a marker and began to write on the whiteboard. He wrote "How to Win with the Ladies," underlined it, put down the marker, and began to speak without introducing himself. "I'll teach you the many ways you can win many a lady by following my lessons."

I saw out of the corner of my eye that I had classmates to my left who were also in my condition. Were they trying to give us skills so that when we returned to the dating world we would at least have a fighting chance? I still couldn't speak. I knew that I didn't want to be here. Didn't they know that I was married? How could I communicate this to this guy so I could stop feigning interest? What if Becky knew I was in such a class? I swear I didn't enroll in this, I'm not even auditing it!

Larry continued, "First, you have to carry yourself a certain way," as he struck a pose with his upper arms out parallel to the ground, and his lower arms hanging with his hands swinging slightly. He continued, "The key to making it with the ladies is upper body strength."

Where the hell was I again? I don't want to be here! I don't belong here! How are these lessons helpful? As suddenly as he had entered the room he mercifully left. The brunette lady immediately came back in to tend to something around me, I knew not what. As I wondered what she was doing, I looked to my right, and saw out of the corner of my eye a figure on the street looking in the window at me as the brunette continued to mess with something around my bed. The figure wore some putrid yellow smock that I had been seeing quite a bit of lately. As the figure looked in the window it walked toward the door with a determined stride. I realized as the figure burst into the room that it was Becky. She had a very aggravated look on her face.

Oh thank goodness she's safe! I thought.

Upon further examination I realized the putrid yellow smock was some sort of barricade fabric similar to something used as a warning in a construction zone. Then as I looked at her face and arms I discovered to my horror that they were covered in blood and dirt. Seeing my eyes glancing over her disheveled form she shouted, "You left me stranded in Sioux Falls!" No one noticed her; it was as if she was invisible to them.

Sioux Falls? What in the world would bring us to Sioux Falls? And what form had she taken? Hologram? Invisible Woman? Ghost? Was this her spirit standing before me tormenting me over something I did with only the best of intentions at the time? How was I to know that the airline had such a poor customer service record? I was beside myself with grief over having left her and upset that she was so upset. Why did I have to be such a goody goody and bust her?

"I was worried about the baby," I somehow communicated to her. "I'm so sorry."

PART II: I'M MILES AWAY[15] - SOUTH DAKOTA

Or perhaps there was no baby. So based on a hunch I unwittingly sent my wife to her death. This day was getting fucking worse and worse.

"I didn't think they'd toss you off the plane like that on the runway," I communicated to her. The brunette lady didn't seem to hear me, and it was obvious that only I could see Becky.

The brunette lady was joined by someone else. They began to fluff up my pillows, and made me feel comfortable, speaking to me in a soothing tone. I felt so guilty having such a fuss made over me. I felt like a Class A wilted flower while Becky was sitting over on a couch against the wall looking rather uncomfortable even though she was in some otherworldly form. She looked agitated over the scene of me being fussed over when she had to fight her way from Sioux Falls on foot in the dead of winter to get here all because of my big mouth. There was beginning to be an inverse relationship between my comfort level and the effort the ladies were making to make me comfortable.

Becky continued to sit there with that awful putrid yellow fabric on her, staring at me being tended to like I was a spoiled child with an expression that I could only imagine was disgust. "I'm so sorry," I kept communicating, "if I could take it back I would. I have been looking for you everywhere, I just cannot move." Although it was not my intent it sounded like a hollow sentiment like OJ saying he is still looking for the real killers. I would have told the ladies to back off, be a martyr, but I couldn't, and to my chagrin it seemed my comfort was a top priority.

When the two ladies were finished, they left the room. Becky slowly stood and walked over to me. She got close to my face as she said in a sarcastic tone, "Are you comfortable?" I blacked out.

ALL MY LITTLE PLANS AND SCHEMES JUST LIKE SOME FORGOTTEN DREAM[46]

With all of the talk about babies and whether Becky was indeed expecting, a bizarre concept found its way into this world that had to have its origins in bad cinema. Of course, that's only an assumption since I never have seen the movie *Junior*. So why did the implausible plot enter my mind and seem to have a hold on me here? The movie with Ahnold and Danny Devito appeared unwatchable, and I have never seen it due to that strong feeling. Beatrice may still have been coming. I needed to ensure that we were indeed a family of three, four, five, perhaps two, I didn't really know, I lost count. If the concept of *Junior* had taught me anything, without actually seeing it, was that a male could bear a child. The science must be there, Hollywood said so.

I may have gotten the procedure done at the freakish hospital where I had my body rebuilt. I think they were having a two for one sale there, and I may have decided to have it done. Nothing was beyond my questionable decision making. The good news I found was that males didn't carry the baby for nine months like suckers. The baby could come out after three weeks. My journey had somehow deposited me in upper Manhattan ready for this to happen, I was about to give birth to it. It was happening, and the best thing was that it would grow in some incubator after it was delivered. I was just giving it a jump start. I call it an "it" not because I have an iceberg heart but because truthfully this was too crazy to lend credence to even in this world. A horrible mistake, I just needed time to adjust to this news.

PART II: I'M MILES AWAY[15] - SOUTH DAKOTA

I was lying there in some dark maternity ward with other mothers or fathers, there were other babies being cared for, and I was shown my baby and, wow, there it was. It appeared to be a small baked bean on a towel. That was it. It had all the qualities of any male birth: fantastic and freakish. Was the towel part of the baby or was it just the baked bean? What the hell had I done? That wasn't a baby! What was that? I was wondering whether I should have some sort of intervention on my elective medical procedures.

So now I had five kids, three that may or not exist, Beatrice, which Becky was carrying, and my new baked bean which I had not named as of yet. Our family was a little sloppier than Brangelina's. We're dropping new kids around here like new Raisin Bran from the box over the soggy stuff in the bowl.

I was lying there full of thought over this newest development when Becky decided to go to the grocery store to get beer and diapers. A purchase she made when Kate was only a couple of months old that in hindsight was very funny to both of us. She must have needed a beer lugging my ass all over the country undoing all these unwise decisions that I had made. What the hell had gotten into me?

One of the post-partum nurses, come to think of it, I didn't know if she was a nurse at all. She wore a hoodie and jeans and her black hair was pulled back in a bun. From the looks of her surly demeanor she may have just been there for community service hours or a disgruntled visitor. In any event, she seemed bothered by Becky's indifference toward the baked-bean baby, and her refusal to even look at it. She got up and followed Becky across the street. It's as if I was following them except I was still in the hospital. I had a bad feeling about what this person might be up to. I could hear the conversation as Becky left the grocery store.

Surly girl confronted Becky over her non-caring attitude, "Why aren't you back in the hospital looking after your new baby. Don't you even care?"

Becky yelled at Surly Girl, "Get the hell out of my way; it's none of your damn business!"

Three gunshots rang out, and the nurse ran off leaving Becky lying there in the parking lot.

Someone came in the room and announced to me that Becky was dead. I began to bawl, I couldn't believe this had happened all because I was trying to get fancy with my body. I didn't know what to do; this was utterly the worst thing that I could have ever imagined. All the times we had been apart and gotten together just to have it ripped away from me. I could not take much more. I screamed, "You have to save them! You have to save her and Beatrice! They can't die! You have to save them!"

I couldn't get anyone to listen to me, they were not hearing me. All I could do was wallow in my sorrow over having lost the love of my life and the daughter I never knew. I just wanted to die. This had to not be happening. This was too damn cruel. Now I was alone, with an unspecified number of kids, I thought, and a baked bean and to be honest I didn't really know how the hell that was going to work out.

***

SEEMS LIKE ALL I REALLY WAS DOING WAS LOOKING FOR YOU[47]

After the disaster at the maternity ward I was transported elsewhere via ambulance. I knew I had to do something to get Becky back to me,

PART II: I'M MILES AWAY[15] - SOUTH DAKOTA

and I knew who to call even if it was against every fiber of my being. I had to swallow a lot of pride to do it. I needed to get her back. I somehow got in contact with the most hated voice I knew. I knew he would be able to help. I needed to give myself up to the man and the hospital that had been hunting us like dogs.

A call came in over the ambulance loudspeaker, and I heard that fucking voice that I wanted to strangle. "Hello, Howard" the voice said in a self-satisfied tone. "This is your doctor from the hospital where you got your body rebuilt, nice of you to get in touch with me. I need to let you know that I can help your wife through the same process that helped you but you're going to have to come in for your transfusion. As you can see I'll be getting you back. After you sign a few papers we'll do what needs to be done."

I nodded a quick agreement to the attendant that was sitting next to me in the ambulance, and we headed over to the evil hospital that I tried so hard to get away from. It was time to pay my bill.

***

DON'T WORRY BABY, IT'S GONNA BE ALRIGHT[48]

Utter confusion gripped me. While I thought I was going back to the evil hospital I seemed to have ended up somewhere else. Did Doctor High and Mighty really talk to me? Was I ever going to pay my bill or was I just putting off the inevitable of that transfusion? Somehow Becky was with me again, and did not end up running in a vat of grotesque liquid like those fat guys. I had no idea if she had really died, and been re-animated or if I had satisfied my bill or I was getting away with something. I wasn't going to question having her back. I just hoped she was the same person and not some awful *Pet Sematary* zombie that would ultimately maul me.

We were in a mountainous rocky area void of any trees. Were we still in South Dakota? We stood outside some type of tourist attraction that had a visitors' center carved into the side of a mountain. The cave was rather spacious and clean. We entered a long corridor, and as we turned to our left there was a ledge overlooking a large room. There was a drop off of about twenty feet from the ledge to the rocky surface below. The room was approximately fifty by one hundred feet in size, and about fifty feet high. There was a sitting area in the middle of this space with plush leather furniture and a nice oriental rug. Torches placed on the cave wall added to the rustic quality of the location that lent an eerie light to the room. I peered in, the place looked very familiar. I knew I had been here before but could not remember when. It was obvious that some sort of show was about to take place.

A bespectacled American Indian gentleman with short hair and a slender build wearing Western style clothing walked to the center of the room, looked up at us and spoke in a calm voice, "Welcome, to our show. You'll be introduced to many primates that few have ever seen."

And with that eerie yet promising introduction a few of these primates entered the room from an opening in the cave wall, and others scurried from an opening in the ceiling down a large chandelier that I had just noticed. The room had a warm glow about it. Becky and I still stood there wondering how or if we were supposed to get down there. The primates were like none I had never seen before, half the size of a human with grey fur and muscular bodies. The trainer seemed unconcerned with being around them. He seemed to be the only line between them and us.

"Come, come down," he beckoned.

I just kept staring down at him. Encouraging us he said, "You'll need to swing down from those vines that are by your head."

Swing down? Was he crazy? A twenty foot drop onto a hard cave floor? And I didn't even know if I was able to walk.

The primates seemed calm, and the show looked interesting. I wondered what they were going to do. Just as I got that thought out I noticed some Korean guy in his thirties standing next to us. He was wearing a Bluetooth cell phone apparatus of some sort that began to make this high pitched squeal. The trainer quickly said, "Please turn off all cell phones and other electronics. They emit a high pitched sound that drives the primates crazy."

As I was mulling how I was supposed to get the hell down there, I watched the man trying to turn off his cell phone as two primates made their way up to the ledge with the most vicious expressions on their faces, and begin to attack him. He struggled with his phone which did not seem to want to turn off as he fended off the savage creatures. The more he struggled, the more they attacked yet the furry monsters paid us no mind. As for me I was not only paralyzed with fear, I was just plain paralyzed. There was no hope of getting my body out of the way if one of those fluffy demons made a move toward me. The claws or gravity or choking by fur, either way it would be the end of me.

The trainer was incredulous, calling them by some Indian name that I couldn't make out. "Agave, Tatanka! Why are you acting so crazy! Calm down! Get that man out of here!"

The Korean guy eventually gave up, and under repeated gnashing he left the cave altogether with his arms covering his head. It was just me and Becky, or was it? I couldn't see to my right or left at all so I assumed she was there. I still couldn't move but found myself sitting on the ledge, and hoped the primates would leave us be. After a while they lost interest, once sweet silence returned, and went back down into the cave.

I sat there awhile not knowing if I should go into the cave with such beasts, if the vine didn't kill me then the primates certainly would. As I thought about it, I noticed we had company. Two American Indian boys were crouched down in front of me. They wore loin skins, were shirtless and barefoot, and had long unkempt hair that came to their shoulders. They spoke to each other in a language I could not understand. One of them held a bowl, and the other began to pick up pieces of broken glass that seemed to litter the cave ledge. With the broken glass the one boy slashed my arms repeatedly then examined the blood on the piece of glass. He would then hold the glass over the wood bowl letting it drip inside looking at it with grim satisfaction. He seemed interested in the outcome with each swipe of the glass, and would examine it like it was magic. They kept talking to each other as if they were accomplishing something. They were pleased and from their visible curiosity more needed to be done. What it was, I had no idea. I could say that I was getting pretty pissed off. This whole not being able to move posture that I could not seem to break was not really coming in handy right now. My biggest wish was the ability to kick their asses off this ledge down to the rock floor below. I sat there motionless and took it. The pain was immense and would not stop.

After what seemed like hours of this, Becky returned from wherever she had been, she couldn't have been beside me with this occurring. She quickly shooed the little parasite bloodsuckers away as if they were roaches. I was helped up, and was in the process of leaving the ledge area when I noticed a sort of exhibit space that had been cut into the tunnel walls. There was a half wall there and a large opening.

Inside I noticed a bevy of activity going on but it was dark, and I could only make out shapes.

Then I realized what I was seeing were figures as they came into focus and into the light of the cave. They were ugly creatures, uglier than the primates I had seen earlier, if that was possible. They looked like dogs. They walked like humans and wore jewelry and crowns on their heads. They were making this high-pitched chattering sound as they entered the tunnel and came right toward us. They had a human quality to them and they just would not be quiet.

Suddenly the trainer from the cave below appeared and tried to apologize, "I'm so sorry for their behavior, they usually don't act like this."

With these "Dog People" just feet away I did not want to hear it. I wanted these fucking things to get away from me. The terror within me felt like it was going to bust out at any moment. They kept coming at us, opening and closing their mouths in rapid succession as they spoke their grotesque language. They then started to claw at me. They had five claws on each paw that were circular in shape and about five inches in length. My God it hurt. Compared to this, the Indian kids were nothing.

I couldn't take much more of this when I was somehow pulled out of the cave, and suddenly found myself by the entrance. The Dog People were not following us by now. However, they did look plenty pissed at our presence still, since I could see their snarling faces flitting in and out of the darkness.

What kind of damn tourist attraction is this and I want my damn money back, I thought. If we were able to get our money back after a lame bus tour Becky and I took in San Francisco back in 2000 then I think there was a great possibility here.

As an apology the trainer and a couple of assistants who might have been the Indian Boy cutters allowed us to bathe and clean up outside the cave. This was not really what we had in mind. With the realization that we probably had some sort of diseased animal/creature germs on us it was probably wise to do so. They brought out a bowl of some sort of porridge substance that appeared to be what we would clean with. Becky knelt down in front of the bowl and stuck her entire head in it.

She looked up at me with a disgusted look on her face, and said, "Don't do this, and hand me a towel." Of course I could not move or speak so I stood there somehow staring, and knew my cleaning would have to come later.

***

THERE'S ROOM ENOUGH HERE FOR TWO[49]

We were in the same town that evening or at least I thought we were. We had cleaned up, and were asleep in what appeared to be an older house that must have been a bed and breakfast. We were in an upstairs room, and strangely enough there was another two or three people sleeping in the same room in a bed next to us. Either we were chintzy or the proprietors had totally screwed up our reservations. Becky was lying next to me looking as beautiful as ever. If there was one thing she could do was fall asleep in an instant although I have been faulted with being Homer Simpson, turning off the light and immediately begin snoring.

The wood in the room on the floor, the door frames, the window casings was well finished in a dark color, and had that aged smell. The door leading to the stair landing was about six feet from the foot of our bed. There was a closet door to the right of the bedroom door and between the two doors was a small hatch door that led me to believe that this room was settled into the eaves of the house. It was winter, the room was cold and I could feel the dryness of the furnace heat fighting a losing battle. A small lamp behind me bathed the room in a dim glow. There was a stillness outside the window like snow had just fallen and we were tucked away safely.

I was contemplating how I got into the bed, and what we had done since being attacked by the Dog People when the window latch began to wiggle. All I could do was move my eyes and when I looked over there was a young Native American male hanging half in the room and half out. I grew more panicked once I recognized the son of a bitch. He was one of the loin-skin-clad youths that was cutting me back in the cave. Hell, I could not take any more of that, I would find a way to kick his ass, I swear, or at least give him the scowling of a lifetime. He didn't even look at me; he just stared down at Becky. I thought she would wake up at any moment with the sudden blast of cold air coming in but she didn't. She was lying there and he still looked at her just inches from her face, caressing her hair. I supposed he had never seen red hair before or like I like to tease her, orange hair.

Wake up! I thought.

My ass was useless here. I could not move. I could not make a sound. All I could do was watch this weirdo looking down at my wife in utter amazement. He was acting like Chucka from the Sid and Marty Krofft time drain *Land of the Lost* would while looking at some shiny object. Nobody in the room would wake up. I could not believe this. I was convinced if I was to walk across the floor to the bathroom and a floorboard creaked the lights would go on accompanied by scowls.

The young male proceeded to come into the room and closed the window. He had not noticed that I was looking right at him. He proceeded to go through the drawers and he proceeded to the hatch. I thought, *Oh no, our valuable valuables are in there! What do we have in there? A necklace or something that's irreplaceable?* I blacked out from anger, fear, and frustration. I might as well have been unconscious with how much help I was being in this situation.

I awoke sometime later in the pre-dawn hours. A purple glow was beginning to compete with the light from the small lamp. The closet door was open, some of the drawers were open, and I could hear a chirping sound like something wanted us to wake up and find that we had been robbed. It must have been that guy's calling card, boasting of the fast one he just pulled on us. The sound went on forever, and everyone still just slept. This kid was in trouble. I was going to finger him big time in this escapade of theft, and for coveting thy neighbor's wife!

There was finally a stirring to my left. One of the other guests awoke and the middle-of-the-night heist had finally been discovered.

"We were robbed!" I heard a lady shriek.

"Duh, Yah think so?" I would have chimed in if I could have. At this point that was not possible.

I was wheeled out of the room and onto the stair landing. It was quickly discovered that the perpetrator was the son of the proprietor. I could hear the mother screaming in disgust at this crime, and her disbelief at who had committed it. What about inappropriately coveting guests? You don't know about that do you?

***

THERE'S A PLACE[50]

With all of the excitement of Dog People attacks, blood-letting, and bed-and-breakfast room invasions, we needed some recreation. We heard of a massage parlor down the street. It was an older tree-lined street with modest bungalows. The owner was an older Chinese lady, who allowed guests to relax in her living room after their massage.

That seemed fine with me since at that moment I couldn't move so I guess relaxation was all I would be able to do. Whether I could feel a massage was another matter.

As expected, after the massage I tried to relax but that just couldn't be accomplished in my immobile state. Relaxation was not what I was about at the moment. It soon became apparent that the older Chinese lady had a surprise on her menu. Something called "A Happy Finish" was offered, and she had a staff of people that could take care of couples with this need for a small fee. I didn't know how I was coming out on top on this deal with my body being as it was, and me having the honor of footing the bill so I politely declined. The older Chinese lady guaranteed that it was all quite impersonal. Her two staff members would wear giant sumo wrestler outfits like fans do at sporting events at halftime to wrestle each other. They will also don large fake phalluses so everything's on the up and up.

How was that "A Happy Finish" for me, and how was this on the up and up? The Chinese lady must have brought a bunch of "yes" men to the last massage parlor strategic retreat to have everyone agree that this was legitimate. It then dawned on me that Becky was the one who this "Finish" was intended for. Not only could I not move or talk but I obviously didn't have the street smarts to survive South Dakota.

So I shook my head, and much to my relief I had correctly assumed Becky's stance on the issue as two men in sumo outfits waddled in. I was only hoping that I was still out of the equation on this. Once we made our decision she was on to the next couple who I quickly realized was in an adjacent pit group in the same room. For some reason they agreed, and the two blobs wasted no time jumping on the couple. The sounds were not appreciated in our little corner of the room. It did not take long. I could only surmise that the male member of the other couple was emasculated beyond what he could have imagined before he agreed to it, and had to be very upset with himself. I could hear the satisfied sound of a female voice saying, "Thanks," to the blobs as they waddled off.

I could not let sleep fall over me as I lay on this pit group in this strange living room waiting for these amorous blobs to return, and have a go at me next. I was wondering how long this small fee that the other couple had paid was good for, and if it was involuntarily transferable to our corner of the room as I waited for daylight.

Were we supposed to get up and go now? I could sense someone was in the kitchen which was next to the living room. It must have been the Chinese lady. Someone was turning lights on and off in an obvious attempt to rouse us and get us out of there. Obviously she was going to have to try a lot harder to get us moving. That must have been another technique that was thought up during the strategic retreat. My misery at that moment made me black out.

***

PART II: I'M MILES AWAY[15] - SOUTH DAKOTA

LET'S GO OVER GROUND, TAKE YOUR HEAD OUT OF THE MUD BABY[51]

The next day we were on the road again, and there were constant calls coming into whatever had been inserted into my body during the various "limb reattachment" procedures. Now the alarms were accompanied by voices as if I had a speaker phone inside me.

"You need eye drops still," the voice said over the speaker. "We're sending the optometrist your way."

Oh, why wouldn't they give up? They just wouldn't. They just kept coming and coming. What was this eye-drop scam they kept trying to get us to fall for? No longer was it a transfusion, now it was the eye drops. Would this never end? Why did they want me so badly to return?

We did not respond, knowing to do so would give our location away or signal acquiescence to their request. It was obviously a trap. They wanted to get me, and beat me down, and keep me in their wicked hospital as I became one of those fat dudes running in place in that unholy liquid.

We kept going until we had made our way into what seemed like a National Park. The road was winding through a heavily wooded vista. We were once again driving up into the mountains. I could now see a visitor center in the distance and a parking lot. As we bypassed the parking lot we were aware of someone following us from the parking lot below. The driver had gotten out of the car and stood there holding up a bottle of eye drops.

The voice came through the speaker loud and clear, "The optometrist has you in visual contact, and needs to give you those eye drops. Please stop for him."

We did not respond; we just kept driving further up the road. The road kept curving back on itself so the man was visible to us the entire time. No matter how far we drove or what good time we were making there was someone right behind us. I couldn't believe how little progress we had made with my condition and getting away from these assholes.

The optometrist got into his car, and began to drive up the same road. We lost sight of him as we approached a tunnel and unfortunately the traffic began to slow. We came out of the tunnel looking out over a majestic canyon with the most breathtaking view. A bridge spanned over the canyon yet there was only one lane, and we were trapped as oncoming traffic made its way across. We could see the optometrist pulling up about five cars behind us. We removed ourselves from the car, and since I was obviously in no condition to run I was strapped to some sort of contraption on wheels. Becky pushed me to an ambulance right by the bridge and banged on the back door. The door opened, a blonde female EMT looked us up and down in amazement not really knowing what she was seeing.

"You have to help us," Becky said to the EMT breathlessly. "There's a man trying to get us back there."

Without any more hesitation she helped us into the ambulance. The doors of the ambulance closed, and I could hear the quack doctor's voice say over the speaker, "Our optometrist has found you, he's walking up to the ambulance you have just entered, please come out for your eye drops."

The EMT in the back of the ambulance then said, "Don't worry, you're safe now, you're safe."

Too much excitement. Once again, I blacked out.

PART II: I'M MILES AWAY[15] - SOUTH DAKOTA

***

HOME AGAIN TO YOU LOVE[52]

I could hear music wafting through the air as I had now come to floating in the attic of my house. God it was great to be home, finally. It was a dusty affair as I looked at all the items in it, however, these weren't items that were in there now. I didn't recognize these things, there appeared to be a lot of Beatles memorabilia up here just open to the attic air. I floated through the attic examining each item as I ducked and dodged the rafters. There were Beatle posters with the Union Jack, souvenir guitars, Beatle beach blankets, Beatle wigs, Beatle lunch boxes, a virtual treasure trove was up here. How did I not notice this before? Through the dusty humid air I could hear a scratchy recording:

As I write this letter,
Send my love to you,
Remember that I'll always,
Be in love with you.

Treasure these few words 'til we're together,
Keep all my love forever,
P.S., I love you.
You, you, you.

As I continued to float through the attic I found myself having trouble breathing, it felt like dust was filling my lungs, and I couldn't catch my breath.

I'll be coming home again to you, love,
And 'til the day I do, love,
P.S., I love you.
You, you, you.

As I write this letter,
Send my love to you,
Remember that I'll always,
Be in love with you.

    I continued to float around looking at all the things in the attic, why would someone put all these great Beatle souvenirs in here? There were some more items: Beatle stuffed dolls, a couple more lunchboxes, a Beatle throw, a Beatles tray showing the strange artist renditions of the four that made them look more like the Marx Brothers.

Treasure these few words 'til we're together,
Keep all my love forever,
P.S., I love you.
You, you, you.

As I write this letter, (Oh oh oh)
Send my love to you, (You know I want you to)
Remember that I'll always, (Yeah)
Be in love with you.

    As I continued around I began to realize that the attic was getting quite hot, and there was a great deal of light coming through the soffits. I would need to address this when we finally bought this place in forty years.

I'll be coming home again to you, love,
And 'til the day I do, love,
P.S., I love you.
You, you, you.
You, you, you.
I love you.

Finally, there was silence with the only sound being the needle running out the record. I thought I was home! I thought this was the end of my journey!

Part III – A Delicate Brand of Reality

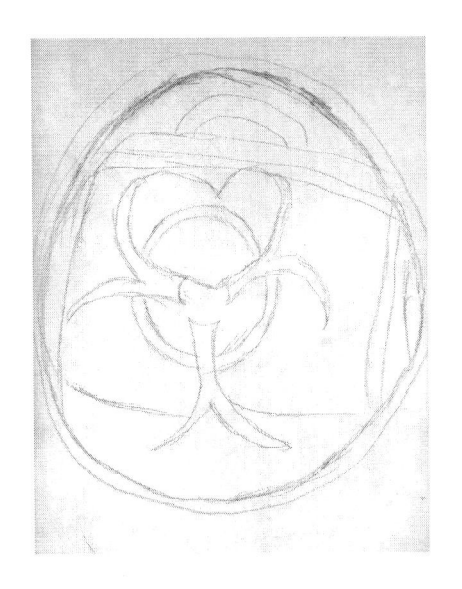

CHAPTER 12

Historic Site

The following risk factors have been associated with the development of severe GAS infections:

- *Minor trauma*
- *Injuries resulting in hematoma, bruising, or muscle strain*
- *Surgical procedures (eg suction lipectomy, hysterectomy, vaginal delivery, bunionectomy, bone pining, breast reconstruction, cesarian section*
- *Viral infections (eg varicella, influenza*
- *Use of non steroidal inflammatory drugs*[53]

JANUARY 27 - 31, 2009

WHEN I WAS ALL MESSED UP/AND I HEARD OPERA IN MY HEAD/YOUR LOVE WAS A LIGHT BULB/HANGING OVER MY BED[54]

The white ceiling, there was no mark on it, this was amazing, it was so pure, and I felt like I could look at it forever.

A male voice interrupted my peace, "Does he normally do this? "
A familiar voice said, "No, I have never seen this before."

Why were these voices disturbing me? I must impress them with my outstanding focus. I was going to keep at this until I bore a hole into that ceiling with my eyes. Nothing could keep me from this task. Something kept making me focus as if a major event was about to take place. I could not stop looking at this ceiling. Couldn't they see something was going to happen, and I must witness it?

She came into view, just off to the left of my field of vision. There she was. Becky. Becky! Sweet Beautiful Becky was here! I'm over here! Do you see me? I could not believe this. It was like looking at someone for the first time that you know so well. She looked beautiful, her face looked like it had the texture of a porcelain doll. She appeared to be lying on some scaffolding over me or floating, I couldn't tell. They were obviously preparing the building for the big event. There must be paint cans and cans of plaster and lathe all over the place. What in the world was she doing up there? She might get hurt. I thought we were in this together, and now she was distracting me.

I could only determine from this foolproof evidence that I was back in the old Confederate building giving it another shot. Or was this before I was hospitalized? The path of events was not clear, and I was having trouble coming to terms with the thought that I would need to rehash all that I had been through again. However I couldn't let those thoughts dissuade me from my purpose here, and that was to see something big happen. I didn't know what or when but it would happen. Now Becky was distracting me from it. The plan was that we would both lie side by side on the old wood flooring and stare at the ceiling. It was obvious that she had given up on this venture much to my disappointment. I could only figure that the male voice was some sort of doctor on staff in the Building. Once he saw that we were injuring ourselves he must have objected. This must have been a common problem for pilgrims such as us. I had never really been passionate about something that I could not fully understand. For some reason I was passionate about this.

Becky, without taking her gaze off me said, "Howard, the doctors say your lungs are in poor condition but you're going to be all right."

What the hell does that mean? I thought I was just a tourist lying here. How had they had the chance to check me over top to bottom, and tell that my lungs were in bad shape? I did not sign up for this!

I stopped this train of thought when I realized I was having trouble breathing and started to cough. The male voice said, "Maybe he'll respond to his parents. Where are they now?"

Becky replied, "They're at the other end of the building."

I thought this was perfect. My dad came with me and he was now at the other end of the building staring at the ceiling. He was also waiting for this wonderful event to take place. After a few minutes I heard footsteps coming toward the room. I heard he and my mom enter the room. Their entrance did nothing to deter me; I kept staring at the ceiling. That was all I saw, and that was all I continued to see. Becky turned her head to someone in the room. I could not tell what they were saying. It may have concerned what they were going to do with me. That seemed to be a big problem at this point.

My thoughts about all of this were interrupted by an incredible sound. Then I saw it! I could see it! It was happening! The ceiling was rising! It was rising! There was a beautiful chandelier floating over my head, and I started to cough more as I breathed in more dust. What was happening? The building was transforming itself into something else but what? The ceiling was rising, and the walls were becoming higher. Would it stop? When would it stop? It was as if a giant was stretching the building from top to bottom. I could not imagine how this would end. I didn't hear voices now. I felt alone, witnessing this event. My hard work at staring had finally paid off, and I was the one being rewarded because I didn't take my eyes off it. The wrenching of beams and wood finally ended. And there I was, and there it was, the finished product. The old Confederate building that I had come to see, and had used my body to defend had transformed itself into the White House. It was a spectacular sight.

It popped into my head, something that I had heard or knew. There was a legend that after the transformation of the Confederate building to the White House was completed the ghost or apparition of a Confederate barber/surgeon would soon appear. With the Confederate Building transformed he was now relieved and could go. After a few moments a figure appeared. It was hazy at first, just a silhouette against a window filled with light. He turned his head, and I could tell he noticed me. He walked over the creaky floorboards to where I was lying. The barber/surgeon walked up to me in his grey Confederate uniform, the dust from the old wool formed a cloud around him. He looked down at me and said, "Son, it appears you need a bit more taken off the sideburns." He touched the side of my face, and I could feel his calloused fingers run over my sideburns. As he turned to leave, his jacket left a trail of dust that I inhaled accidentally. It quickly filled my lungs, and I started coughing, and was no longer able to breathe normally. He didn't turn around. He left the building through a doorway, and I could see light shining all around him.

After a while I was letting what had just occurred sink in when I heard gunshots quickly followed by the sound of footsteps frantically making their way down the hall. The footsteps sounded like that of a lady's dress shoe. I somehow knew that it was the secretary that worked in the site of the Confederate building or the former Confederate building. She reached the room, and frantically informed us that the caretaker upon hearing that the transformation to the White House was complete had shot himself. He was so depressed that he no longer needed to care for the historic landmark. Somehow this had been foretold to me as I continued to stare at the ceiling.

***

SOME KIND OF NIGHT INTO YOUR DARKNESS COLORS YOUR EYES WITH WHAT'S NOT THERE[55]

Did you know that the new White House had a new section that was added on with the conversion? It's true. I was on hand to appreciate it, hung from the very wall of it. I was like a piece of art or something else just hanging there in this new stairwell that had just been built. Also, did you know that Martha White, the baked goods goddess, babysat for the First Family over many decades but when the Civil War came she was fired or nicely put, she was axed? Also true. Isn't it?

It appeared that someone had turned on a TV somewhere in the stairwell, and I could see a commercial for Martha White baked goods. The lines suddenly turned into the profile of Martha White at the conclusion. It was a comforting ad for baked goods. I like baked goods, and really don't get enough of them. Of course, I still seemed to have something in my mouth, and I had not eaten in what seemed like forever. That was OK. Martha was still around, and would be there when I was ready to have another go at a blueberry muffin.

So this new stairwell had just been built, brand new and quite unremarkable. I heard it joined the new addition with the old White House so for some reason I was stuck in the middle, not moving anywhere. Just hanging out seemingly forever was all I was to do. There was no natural light in here. It was just functional, built on the cheap. I could be in any office building anywhere. My belief was still that it was the White House.

Becky appeared to my left. She was quite stunning, and looked fresh as new fallen snow. She looked at me and asked, "Do you want to listen to some music?"

I nodded or somehow motioned that I would like to. She put some headphones on me and pressed some control in her hand. It didn't work and then it worked. I could hear the Beatles singing *I Want to Hold Your Hand*. The sound was so clear, it felt like I was inside the song. I had listened to it so many times but had never felt it like this before.

Over to my left I could see a lady in an old gingham dress like the kind worn in the nineteenth century with her hair done up in some sort of large hairstyle that I could not determine the configuration of. She was holding a broom sweeping up the stairwell. She looked familiar, like the nurse from the beauty salon except there was something else familiar. As she was sweeping she bumped into something. She looked up, and said sheepishly to no one in particular, "Excuse me."

Holy Toledo! I realized it was Martha White sweeping up next to us! Didn't anyone see?

Instead of having anyone notice I could only see Becky messing around with the music player and the headphones in her ears trying to get it to work by shaking it constantly. It was impossible. No one paid any mind to Martha White. It was time for me to go now, the webs I grew to loathe from the dirty Confederate hospital returned, engulfing the stairs, the webs were now in Martha's hair, and I was leaving again.

***

THE SONG IN YOUR HEAD IS NOW ON MY MIND[56]

Now we're getting somewhere, I was hanging once again from the wall except now I was in a doctor's office, and he would be able to get me back on the mend. How many doctors had this been? How many places had this been? Were hospitals and doctors lining up to have a crack at me? Was I still in the Confederate Hospital? Was this where I had been the entire time? It couldn't be. I had visual evidence of all those other places; I knew what I had seen. It was too brutal, too painful, too honest to be anything but real. At least I was not back in the old Firebird. There seemed to be some stability beginning to emerge in my situation. I was in the same place finally after the darkness came. That was some progress. I did miss being outside, this windowless environment, while stable, was a bit confining. The examining room was very clean with high ceilings and was quite narrow, perhaps ten feet wide. I was hanging from the wall and was again unable to speak.

Becky was once again on my left trying to get that blasted music player to work. *Throw it out! Throw it out! Get a new one please!* I yelled in my head.

But she wouldn't give up. She was being stubborn, and had to get it to work. As I saw her messing around with that infernal contraption I could see something or someone out of the corner of my eye. Someone had come into the room very boldly and not through a door on the ground level but up in the middle of the wall. They somehow had walked down the wall and onto the ground level where they examined some papers at a counter with their back to us. It must have been the doctor. He had on the white doctor's coat that lent credibility. I thought to myself that I should really get one of those to wear around the house. It would make me feel like I knew what I was doing at all times. He had a receding hair line, dark hair and wore glasses. He was probably in his forties. I hoped that there would be some answers given about my condition, and this mess could be explained in a clear, concise manner. He turned around to face me and Becky then without saying a word or even pretending to see us, walked across the floor right in front of us, walked up the wall behind us, and left through another door in the wall over our heads and was gone.

Oh, Goddammitt!! This is really getting to me, where the hell did he go? I thought ruefully.

The door continued to open, and close and the same doctor walked upside down on the ceiling, and then he disappeared into another opening somewhere, his footsteps making a racket on the tile floor. There he was again, examining something, never saying a word to either of us.

For all that's holy, please tell me something, anything! Will I live? Am I going to be nailed to the wall for the rest of my life? I thought pleadingly.

But he never said anything except flip through some charts, and walk right past us. He finally made his egress in a door behind us, and left the room. The room was now empty except for me and Becky. After a few interminable minutes, a door on the main level just below the door the doctor just departed opened. It was clearly not the doctor. It was some weird looking dude who walked in peering around like he shouldn't be in there. He had this crazy red hair, some weird tan and ridiculous looking teeth that were big and really white. He wouldn't stop smiling. I was beginning to think that this doctor's office didn't know what the hell was going on. Of course the lady at checkout would sure as hell know how much we owed.

Becky still hadn't looked up at anything as focused as she was with the music player. The weird-looking guy was wearing a white lab coat, and looked not unlike Yahoo Serious, the infamous 80s comic who I am thankfully still totally unfamiliar with. He saw me, and with a knowing look crept up closer and closer with that impish grin on his face. I couldn't move, I couldn't talk, I couldn't wiggle my body out of this cocoon in which I found myself.

Then as he was a foot away from me he held out his hand, and pressed something against my chest. "I'm giving you a sticker," he said with a tinny voice, and he slowly backed away apparently expecting some sort of thanks.

I looked over at Becky imploring her to look up, please, thinking, *are you seeing this?*

She finally looked up to see him as he slowly backed out of the room. I got a sticker but I was never quite sure if that was good or bad. Was I now marked for torture or to be treated to some horrendous comedy routine? Suddenly the doctor walked back in the door he had previously exited, and Becky said, "Some strange person put a sticker on my husband."

The doctor turned and looked at her with a look of one part frustration, one part fright and one part, where the hell did you come from? He said with great alarm, "Is that guy back again? I have told them to keep him out. He always wanders around this building."

This doctor's office definitely didn't know what was going on. I was not in good hands, that is until the bill came and said different.

CHAPTER 13

Slow Return

GAS infections usually occur sporadically. They are not generally associated with clusters of cases or minor epidemics.[57]

HUM ME A TUNE DOC!

A man came into the room. I was awakened by him messing with some tubes on me. I didn't know where the tubes were or why they were there. It was still as if I had just discovered my existence with no past and no future, no hope.

The man began to talk to an Asian guy nearby. The man was wearing a white lab coat so I guessed he was legitimate, it seemed that was the only badge that I needed for clearance. Then again I had instructors at the Merchant Marine Academy who wore white lab coats into class, and I sure as hell wouldn't let them get near me with a tube.

He asked the Asian guy a question and responded to his answer with a sort of mimic of the Asian guy's accent-laden voice. The man's mimic included a halting kind of speech. Perhaps my ears were playing tricks on me. I found this to be very rude but I supposed he knew the guy, and the mimicking was possibly only good natured ribbing.

The man then asked the Asian guy, "You have an interesting accent, where are you from."

I thought, *you mean the very accent you were just mimicking?*

The Asian guy told him that he was from a border region between India, and somewhere that was confused for being China yet was not actually China.

I found the questioning bizarre. I thought, *doesn't everyone that works in a hospital know everyone else? Well, I guess that mimic was rude after all.*

The man then turned his attention to my mouth. The man reminded me of my long time dentist in Tampa, Dr. Valentine, who I hadn't visited since 1995. Just to clarify, I have visited the dentist regularly since 1995. He wore glasses, was tall and had the same deep sort of voice with a slight Southern drawl. He was also very sure of himself, and knew what he was doing which to me more than made up for his rudeness. I needed confidence at this point. He did not acknowledge me in any way. He looked at my mouth, and began to pull off some sort of tape that was holding something inside.

"Good grief!" he exclaimed. "Why did they use this kind of tape downstairs? This is a bear to get off!"

He really expected no response to this inquiry, and began humming a tune as he slowly unwound the tape. It kept going and going like he was a magician pulling a hankie out of his pocket. Then he got to the part where the tape met the skin and the subsequent pain made me agree with the man's statement of why they used this type of tape downstairs, because it was really making my lips and the area around my mouth raw.

The word "downstairs" made me think of the who and the what that was downstairs. Did I have some history in this place that I was not aware of? Was I a piece of meat being moved from place to place?

I was getting really scared about how I was at the mercy of those I did not know in a place I did not know. I had no way of leaving or communicating. I just lay there as he hummed along, finished removing the tape, and began to reapply something else to my mouth to keep whatever it was inside. I had no idea what it was he had left in my mouth or why on earth this was necessary when I was just in perfect health, or at least I thought I had been. Perhaps I was always like this.

Worry filled me more and more as I thought, *had I dreamt my life?*

Then it dawned on me that I must be just a head or a monitor with no limbs or anything. Just some gizmo with dials that people would mess with, and there was nothing I could do about it. They didn't care if I was alive or not or even that I was a human. Perhaps I was just a head in a jar being kept alive for "Let's see what happens if we do this" purposes. I'm not stupid. I saw this very thing on *Futurama*.

***

GONNA KICK THE DARKNESS UNTIL IT BLEEDS DAYLIGHT[58]

I saw a tiny point of light. It was faint but I saw it. It moved from side to side and up and down. What a pretty light. There was nothing except darkness, and this little light. It was as if I was doing its bidding.

A voice in the darkness said, "Howard, follow this light for me, if you can hear me blink your eyes once."

I thought in a Ringo Starr, *Yellow Submarine* smart aleck voice, *Should I blink me eyes twice for no?*

I blinked me eyes, I mean, my eyes once. All of a sudden the room erupted in applause and excitement, and I realized that the tiny point of light was the extension of some human, perhaps the person that was holding me in this awful place. I was now wise to them yet excited that they were excited. I could begin to make out a few figures standing around me in the darkness.

First I thought, *how dare you wake me during nap time!* but I reconsidered and thought, *be cool Hoovie, play along.*

This was an easy crowd. Someone was acknowledging my existence. I demanded attention. I craved it! Let me up, and I will do any sort of damn trick you want. Do you hear me? Anything! Wait until I show you what I can do with a towel wrapped around a stick.

This initial response from following their simple command I thought was rather a bit of an overreaction. Didn't they know about me, and all of my awful adventures that I have had? I have been all over the damn country looking for a cure for whatever this awfulness is. Alas, it seemed I was for some reason a source of excitement for the throng crowded around me, and now everyone wanted to have their own personal affirmation of my responses and see for themselves the "Howard's eyes follow the light" moment. Perhaps they thought the doctor before them had not done it in a way that only they could or did not use the proper body English with the wrist in maneuvering the light. So I played along, and followed the next light, and blinked for the next one who requested, and followed obligingly. The excitement was at a fever pitch as if Willis Reed of the New York Basketball Knickerbockers had walked into the room as he had done during the '70 NBA Championship Series when everyone thought he was out for Game 7 and Madison Square Garden erupted. It was rather embarrassing but I would have done anything to leave this uncertainty. If only Mr. Reed had been there, he could have split this crazy throng down the middle and gotten me the hell out.

Excitement reigned each time I followed the instructions and did it a few more times. After a while I began to get a bit impatient with all of this and thought that I should be on my way by now. Certainly someone who can blink and follow a light can be independent and should be discharged. Please sir or madam, show me the way to the desk that says "Checkout" and I will be on my way. Now off with you and step lively.

Then someone with a roaring voice entered the darkness, and I sensed the throng part in front of me and I had a feeling it wasn't Mr. Reed. The boisterous voice introduced himself, "Mr. Hoover, this is Dr. Tale, your neurologist, I hear that there has been a breakthrough, and you're impressing people. Can you impress me?"

For some reason I was not impressed with his introduction, his position, his tone, the tenor of his voice. He sounded like the BMOC and I was having none of this cocksureness. I thought, *I am sorry, I have been performing for what seems like an eternity for this throng so sorry but you missed the show. Come back when I feel like it. No longer am I ready for my close-up. You be careful now and drive home safely.*

I just lay there in a non-responsive state. Dr. Tale shined the light at me and said, "Follow the light please."

I refused. No response from me.

He said, "Blink once if you understand."

Nothing, I was not doing it anymore. I wouldn't even blink me eyes twice for no. Sir or madam should have pointed me to the desk that says "Checkout" long ago. I should be waiting for a car, a Town Car would do, to take me somewhere. I knew not where.

"Why's he not responding, I heard that he was?" he said, not concealing his disappointment.

All of my bravado and defiance was then tossed out the window and I felt like a disobedient child when Becky piped up and said, "Howard, this is Dr. Tale your neurologist, if there is anyone in this room you need to impress it's this man."

This got my attention. Any man that may be a key to springing me would get the performance of a lifetime. I didn't want to end up like Jack Nicklaus at the end of *One Flew Over the Cuckoo's Nest* eating a pillow. So I did what he asked. By the way, I know it was Jack Nicholson, I just thought the golfer would have made for a more interesting scene.

"Follow the light, blink once if you understand," he requested.

I did it all. I impressed Dr. Tale to the four corners of the earth and the exam was over and I was saved from tasting pillow.

Wait, there was a final act, one of the figures said, "Now, give us a thumbs up."

I thought these parlor tricks were getting to be a bit of a nuisance. I thought, *of course, no problem*. I went to move my thumb like the Fonz had done on so many occasions. Holy Shit! It wouldn't move. Did someone nail the damn thing to me? Why couldn't I move it? This was terrible. What had happened to me? I worked and worked at getting it to move. I finally got the thumb to a somewhat upright position, and then had to let go. It felt like it would snap off with any more exertion.

"All right, great!" The voice said enthusiastically, and there was more applause. *If applause could sound patronizing, then this would be patronizing applause*, I thought. It was as if the voice could sense my cockiness from my ability to follow the light, and it wanted to put me in my place with the thumb request. I knew at this point that it wasn't going to be so easy, and my plan to get sprung would take a bit longer than I imagined. I did great following the light, the thumb? Not so good. Come to think of it, who needs thumbs anyway? The guy that was me in the green T-shirt and shorts getting up from the wheelchair whistling out of here seemed to be getting further out of reach.

***

TIME TO MEET THE SHIRT.

"Howard! Wake up Howard!"

The voice jolted me out of a daze. My eyes seemed to be already open like I had been staring but not really focused on anything in particular. The voice came from a man standing over my bed. Actually not my bed, a bed I found myself lying in. I couldn't feel anything at the moment and I was startled as my eyes absorbed his face which was two feet above my own. He was a balding man perhaps in his mid 40s, and I focused on his eyes for the longest time which seemed to be two different colors. The darkness wasn't getting me out of this one.

First I thought, *I thought I was awake. I have been through hell and I can't figure out what the hell's happening. Who the hell is this guy and why is he so pissed off at me?*

My thoughts took a turn toward concern as I saw the irritated look on his face, *this is serious, I gotta listen to him. He must be tired of me living on the dole just lying here doing nothing. I need to start earning my keep.*

He said, "Howard, I'm Dr. Rebefall, you're in very bad shape but you're slowly coming out of it. You have to work with us. You have got to wake up and get better. Nod your head to let me know if you understand."

I nodded which was the only part of my body that I could move at the moment. He continued to speak to me about various things concerning my condition; however, I really couldn't listen to him. All I heard was "Serious talk, Serious talk! SERIOUS TALK!" I hadn't been this frightened since the Dog People were gnashing at me. However, I realized I was distracted by something that I couldn't quite put my finger on. What was it? I should be listening though something was preventing me from giving my full attention. Was it fear? Was it confusion? No, those had been my constant companions. Then I realized what it was. Yes, that was it, it was his shirt! As it came into full focus I saw it for what it was, some sort of lime green monstrosity with a checkered pattern, and some other crazy ass colors that I hadn't realized had been invented.

I thought to myself, *keep listening, but Sweet Lassy Molassy! Where did he get that shirt?* It was crazy and was kind of freaking me out.

I realized as I tried to reverse engineer the shirt that a question had been asked. I thought, *Oh no, did he just ask me a question?* I didn't hear it so I nodded, hoping the affirmative response would not cause more trouble for me since I didn't need more trouble. I was in a prison for a reason I did not know, and I was going to agree with him to the ends of the earth. He saw my nod and took it as the proper response. Thank goodness. He then stood up straight, seeming satisfied with our exchange and looked up at something over my head, I had no idea what. He looked over at someone to the side of the bed, spoke to them briefly and left the room.

I was nervous and scared as hell over this encounter. I thought, *I screwed up and where's Becky? Where are they holding her?*

However, I kept thinking about that shirt, while I was scared shitless, that was the most amazing thing I had seen in this place, and I held on to that. At least I or the person that made that shirt hadn't lost our sense of humor, and it made me feel better that there was such a shirt in the world, wherever and whatever that world might be.

***

JUST NOD 'YES'.

"Do you need suction?" I was asked in a matter-of-fact fashion. I could not see her face. A nurse was standing over my bed. I could tell from her uniform, the ID badge, and the authoritative sound of her voice.

I was not sure what I had done to warrant this question yet I must have done something to get her attention. I could only think, *Suction?...I...*, and I stopped with that thought, and realized that this was beyond my understanding so I should just reply yes. Actually, I really didn't know how I was getting by in the general staying-alive department at the moment so I nodded in agreement and thought, *sure, what can it hurt?*

The nurse then picked up a tube lying on the right side of my bed and proceeded to pull out some sort of glistening fluid that kept coming and coming. It would not stop. Was it a tube inside a tube? How was it not spilling everywhere? I realized that that tube was in my mouth, and this glistening fluid was being pulled out of me. At first I reacted in horror then realized that the suction actually helped, and whatever discomfort I was feeling had now passed.

With a mix of horror and acceptance I thought, *Oh wonderful tube of suction how can I pay you back?*

It was such sweet relief, and I could feel the tube as it pulled the fluid out of me. It was an indescribable feeling. I felt sorry for the nurse

PART III – A DELICATE BRAND OF REALITY - SLOW RETURN

and staff. Who was going to clean up this glistening mess? I blacked out so I wouldn't have to.

***

I awakened in a dimly lit room, could it be the same room? This would be a first for me. Confusion still reigned in my head, not knowing who was in the room with me accompanied by a loud whirring noise that would not stop. It was just relentless. The room must have been on a plane, because certainly that awful sound had to be the plane's engines. Where were we flying to? I could detect a lot of commotion going on in the room. I didn't know how I felt about all of this however I did feel a bit restless.

I looked over and saw the nurse and Becky standing by the side of my bed. The nurse was doing something to me, and was standing really close to my left. I could make out an ID badge that she was wearing. It was a badge with the General Hospital logo on it. This was bizarre. Where did she get that badge? I recognize it as a place near where I live except I refused to believe that I was in General Hospital. I was not injured, what happened to me? Have I always been like this? My mind raced furiously to try and retrace my steps. However with the confusion, weakness, and drowsiness my mind was unable to get very far. Those things that happened to me before, were they real? What got me? The Confederate building or the body rebuild? I tried to ask questions but could not speak. All I knew was that it was horrible.

I looked to my left since that was the way my head seemed to be leaning except I couldn't turn it. On the bed rail were buttons that said "Radio" and "TV."

I must have been on a flight because only planes have such contraptions. I tried to lift my arm to point to the button. I wanted the Radio, I needed music. My soul felt empty.

Please! I pleaded so only I could hear me.

Becky said, "He looks like he wants something."

The nurse said, "Really, I can't tell what it is."

I kept pointing my head toward the buttons but there was confusion in the room as to what I wanted. I thought, *I paid for this ticket, therefore I deserve and demand all comforts and entertainment options herein. I'm sure the rest of the passengers are enjoying these options. I'm getting ripped off here!*

After a brief time of me unsuccessfully motioning to the buttons, the nurse finally said, "We just aren't communicating."

No shit! You think so? I can't talk or move so my options are limited here, I thought. The effort to try and resolve my dilemma subsided, and I slowly gave up. There would be no music for Howard, if that was my real name.

The nurse said, "I'm going on break." She left the area, and headed into what appeared to be a small room to my left.

I thought, *on break? How long is this flight? Where do you go for a break on a plane?* Somehow this small room provided the break space that she needed from me and my request.

***

ESCAPE YOURSELF, AND GRAVITY[59]

Whoops and cheers awakened me as I saw a lady in this haze at the foot of my bed. Extreme weakness and pain surrounded me along with great disappointment since I had never felt this low and helpless before. I felt like

I was floating and that I would fall at any moment. There was excitement in the air as the lady's face came more into focus. The curtains around the bed were drawn and she was smiling at me. She had on that putrid yellow smock, wore glasses, had blonde hair and appeared to be in her fifties. I could not explain her sudden appearance. She noticed that I was awake and others that were around the bed were excited to see my eyes open.

As for the floating, I soon realized that I had been raised by others into a seated position on the bed. The sudden feeling in my head was to faint immediately. My body felt like it would fall in on itself. Everything was shifting in me, and I could not stand the feeling. It was such exertion to sit there with even all of this assistance. Who the fuck would do this to me? I wasn't bothering anyone. They just looked so happy and excited. How much longer could I go on like this? Certainly they won't just hold me like this all night? There was no way I could get used to this but that lady's smiling face kept encouraging me.

There went my neck, whoever was holding my head up had let go. My head fell to the side like a doll's. It was soon apparent that the experiment could not last much longer. Perhaps it was performed for curiosity's sake. After all of this time on my back I was stunned and horrified to see how simply sitting up was putting me through the wringer. Slowly I was laid on my back again. The relief was immeasurable. I had a long way to go. Then darkness.

***

MR. MIKE

There was a true point of despair when I really wanted someone to be nice to me, to listen to me, or at least acknowledge me and then someone did. I looked up and saw coming around the curtain a balding white man with glasses who appeared to be in his mid to late forties. He had the friendliest face and voice and he was a welcome sight in all of this uncertainty. Come to think of it he might have been the therapist from the flight slinging those orange drink bottles around.

"My name's Mike," he said, "and I'm going to work with you in trying to get your body moving again."

I nodded or at least I thought I did. I was at everyone and everything's mercy at the moment. I wasn't sure what I did. He seemed to take whatever response I gave as an affirmative. He then removed the covers off my legs, and began to lift them.

I thought, *what in the world are those?*

I looked down and saw a pair of the skinniest and most discolored limbs I had ever seen. They were a purplish hue, and looked to belong to someone else but they didn't, they were attached to me.

Shit, this does settle it, I thought, *I did have my body rebuilt, and this is the horrific result.* I was hoping no one had really noticed, and that I could go along like nothing had happened. If they knew I was playing God with my body or not coming clean they might expel me since I was not fully committed to getting better, and worst of all I had held back information from them. It had happened before with all of the road trips and being tossed around like a hot potato. I don't want to get back in that car and fight the Dog People again!

Mike took my right drumstick, and lifted it gently. He then said, "We're going to try and get some movement in here so the muscles don't atrophy any further."

He was doing all the work at this point. I was just worried that those so called legs of mine would snap off at any moment. Who knew what kind of adhesive that doctor used in that freak hospital?

Not to mention the awful care I received at that hospital in the old Confederate building had to contribute to my sorry state. I thought I was in good hands now as Mike continued to work on my legs. There seemed to be a plan in place, something was getting done.

***

WHEN I'M FLAT ON MY BACK[60]

More evidence of my sorry condition was revealed as I lay on my back. My hands or what was purported to be my hands didn't really seem to be hands at all but some disgusting appendage. I was truly fearful at this point. All I could determine was that I was in a bed, and I was in a hospital. For the life of me I could not explain what was in place of my hands. What had I done to get here, and what had that quack doctor in NY done to me?

I studied the areas where my hands should be, and saw things that were huge and bloated and looked like feet actually. Had that been a little bonus? Transplanting feet onto where my hands used to be? Where were my hands? Why had I become so deformed? I tried to think of my past, and what could have led me here. Had I always been this ghastly, and this was what led me to the decision to have my body rebuilt? These things on the ends of my arms looked like a huge bunch of bananas, something that was not of this world. As I drifted off I began to think of what my children must look like, some sort of half human with long giraffe legs. Sure, they would excel at track and field but what about the rest of the time? What about the awkwardness in the hallways at school? They would be labeled weirdoes! I could see them running now with that giraffe-like gait.

As I dug back into my past to try and find some sort of connection between me and this hybrid species making I thought, *had I been some sort of quack myself playing God?*

The scene switched to me as a boy standing outside an older house with long steps leading up to a back porch. The house was in the middle of nowhere, and looked like a beach house on stilts except cheaply made, and in the middle of a swampland. I didn't recognize this place at all. As I peered under the stairs I could make out many jars with what appeared to be some sort of animal parts floating in a liquid. There were a bunch of these jars. In one jar there was an ear, another jar had a foot, and another jar had some wing, and then there was a beak in another jar. I slowly scanned each jar, which were all covered in spider webs.

As I gazed at the jars, I noticed the Beatles singing *The Hippy Hippy Shake* in the background. Had I dismantled animals in the swamp and stuffed them in these jars to make some sort of Frankenanimal at a later date with obscure Beatle songs as the soundtrack? We all knew what happened to Victor Frankenstein in the overrated *Frankenstein*, his creature ended up killing everyone he loved while he hid cowardly behind his embarrassment over having created such a monster. Sure, I might have gotten lambasted for referring to a classic as "overrated" however at the moment I didn't give a shit.

As I pondered Victorian literature someone grabbed my ear. I couldn't see who it was yet somehow I knew it was an older man. Then I realized it was my maternal grandfather, Pop. He died in 1981, and was the gentlest soul which really made me think that I had really screwed up as he picked me up by my ear and yelled, "I'll teach you a lesson for playing God!" I supposed my punishment was becoming the creature that I had set out to create.

Pop had died following open heart surgery in which hospital I was not sure. I figured the reason everyone was being nice to me and making sure I was going to live was because they owed my family. I kept saying to myself, *my God! This is the hospital that Pop died in, they know not to mess with me! The grandson of the one they killed cannot possibly go out like this too!*

My paranoia could not be assuaged by the fact that there was a Hippocratic Oath, and that even serial murderers would get the same level of care. To my way of thinking, it was risk of a courtroom tussle that kept this place on its toes. I felt there was no kindness here, just road blocks that had been set up to ensure that I was to never leave. Certainly some sort of key had been written that revealed how to extricate myself but I had no idea what it was or what the rules were. Someone out there was saying, "Now we play by my rules!" To which my reply was, "But I don't know what your rules are!"

I had to somehow be patient; however, I was very low on patience. I needed to know if my life was real or was a dream that had never happened. What's real now with the foot hands? What had become of me?

CHAPTER 14

London

Outbreaks of severe GAS infections have occurred in closed environments such as nursing homes and in hospitalized patients.[61]

PAPA'S IN THE INSTAFLATE WITH HIS HOSPITAL GOWN ON[62]

I was so freaking hot. I could not believe how hot I was and so impatient. I awoke to a bevy of activity in my room. There was a young guy in dark blue scrubs with this bizarre-looking collar that was transparent by my bed paying me no mind.

I may or may not be here but at least I can see what's going on, I thought in what defiance I could muster.

What was that I heard? Did someone mention London? Were we in London? I thought so. All of this activity could be explained by only one thing: I must have been backstage in the West End theater district. It was opening night, and we were backstage, and I would get an excellent seat to see whatever was performed. Did an entire hospital room often go overseas with a patient and become a dressing room? No time for explanations, everyone was too busy. I could feel the bustle, and the show was about to begin. People kept running in and out. Why would they fly me to London? Oh, I know, it was me they wanted to appear in the production. They wanted me, Howard Hoover, the first human to voluntarily have his entire body rebuilt. What I was mindful of was how I would appear onstage when I was in this bed. Certainly they wouldn't allow me on stage in just a bed. What kind of a show was that? There was much to do, besides learning my lines I first must get out of this bed.

As I began to move I felt a hand on my shoulder pressing me down. "Where do you think you're going?" It was Becky's voice.

I looked at her pleadingly as if this were my only shot. I somehow communicated that I needed to get out on stage since it was opening night, and they expected me to be out there. "No, you're staying right here," she said as if telling a child to stay put.

What? I thought with total exasperation. *You cannot be serious, even if it's a small part I should get out there. I have heard there's nothing like opening night at the theater.*

There was no arguing, especially since there was just a one-way dialogue taking place anyway. I was staying in my bed in the dressing room underneath the stage. I was damn mad. Even that guy in the dark blue scrubs that ignored me was going to get stage time! I could soft shoe circles around that guy.

"You have a visitor," I heard someone say trying to restrain their excitement.

I looked up and there stood a guy with a strong resemblance to Fabio though with a longer mane standing at the foot of my bed. "Hello," he said in some European accent. It was evident that he was a star in the production, and was awaiting his moment to make girls or guys swoon. Well, this guy doesn't swoon, Mister! And appearing on my stage too? Dammitt! What did he want? Did he want to push the knife in a little more into my theatrical dreams?

"I understand that you're in a bit of a pickle health wise. I would like to see what I can do," he said.

I just stared at him in silence. I didn't want to know what he meant by "pickle." I was really feeling hot, like I was sitting on a stove, it was just relentless. The discomfort was beginning to make me forget about the stage.

I now noticed the Fabio guy was wearing a ridiculous purple velvet tuxedo or whatever the hell it was with a cravat. He said, "I want to sing you a song to try and help brighten your spirits during this difficult time."

He walked over to the left side of the bed, pressed down on the blankets covering my legs, and began to sing some very derivative ballad song. It was the kind of song that I probably have had to listen to in my younger years on the radio while my mom was driving.

I was feeling really claustrophobic at this point and started yelling, "I'm so damn hot! I cannot take these covers anymore!!" I began to kick the blankets off of the bed, kicking Fabio's hands away in the process. The stunned look on his face said it all.

"Howard! What are you doing?" I heard someone say in surprise. This must have been a big star that I was refusing help from. Big or not we all know it was just a photo op for him anyway. Fuck him! I was not here to make him feel better!

I screamed, "I cannot take this anymore, these blankets are too fucking hot!" as I kept kicking and kicking away. I could hear my voice yet I wasn't sure if it was available to those around me.

The Fabio guy looked upset, and dejected, and shocked that someone would actually resist his charms. He left hurriedly without saying another word. Somehow without the Fabio guy there any longer I settled down and darkness came.

CHAPTER 15

Hazy Care

The most common initial symptom of GAS TSS is diffuse or localized pain, which is abrupt in onset, severe, and usually precedes tenderness or physical findings of soft tissue infection.[63]

ONE THING YOU CAN'T HIDE [64]

My socks kept getting pulled off. I would be staring at the foot of the bed minding my own business and someone would come in, lift the blanket up, and tear the socks off my feet. All I could see were hands and they were very interested in my feet for some reason. I was boiling hot, so I welcomed the sans-socks policy. The ripping away of the socks had no ceremony to it. The person would then pause as they examined my feet which I had noticed had become a ghastly purple.

Something happened. I'm in still in hell, I really fell into it this time, I would think mournfully. *This cannot be good.*

As I continued to lie there, the blankets were lifted further and my legs were exposed. They were skinny and still a dark purple.

What has happened? Was there an accident? I thought in a panic.

As I pondered my situation I saw an Asian man walking around the room hurriedly. I recognized him as the Asian guy the humming doctor had mocked when the tape was being ripped off my mouth. He wore a blue button-down sweater and was moving stuff to and fro. I wondered what country I was in. He resembled someone who should be escaping the clutches of Gamera. An alarm was going off. A noisy infernal racket, it came from this tall machine next to my bed. He would look at it and push a button to shut it off. The alarm had to be saying something but it was just being turned off and things proceeded as if nothing unusual had occurred. It must have been the "Everything's OK" alarm.

My eyes wandered around the room, it felt strange. It didn't feel like a room, it felt like I was still on a plane. Yes, a plane. Another damn plane! Where the hell am I headed now? The Asian guy was adding an international flavor to my journey. I must be on a plane, yes a 747 medical flight, they were wheeling me around the world looking for a cure or maybe not, maybe they just wanted to wheel me around the damn world like a hot potato. I must have had something so gruesome that I must now remain airborne forever.

There was someone standing meekly behind the Asian guy. The Asian guy noticed me looking at her and said, "This is So and Soichima, she's my nurse's assistant. She'll be helping me out during this shift."

She kept her distance and looked away as I looked at her.

I thought, *I don't know why she'd be scared of me, I don't bite... hard.*

After the brief introduction I continued my attempt to piece together events that had brought me to this point. I kept getting distracted by the Asian guy nurse who was running around like a chicken with his head cut off. He was constantly moving stuff hither and fro. It was exhausting to observe.

My gaze came upon a large sink across the room. It appeared to be a kitchen sink from the twenties or thirties with the wet porcelain counter surface that drains into the sink complete with ridges on it. On this surface I could see a turkey still in the wrapping, left there I assumed to defrost. Was this sanitary to have a turkey just sitting there in the hospital room? What's he defrosting a turkey for in my room anyway? Was it the holidays again? I couldn't take my eyes off of it, it was huge, must have been a thirty-pound bird. This must have been a holiday flight. It was just very bizarre to look at, and I swore for a minute there I thought I heard it gobble.

As I pondered this sound in my head I felt something let loose in my bottom. Something I had no control over had taken place, and made me embarrassed to think about.

I thought, *Oh no, Did I just shit myself?*

I heard something liquidesque hitting the floor like a pitcher of water had been dumped out. I felt terrible because: one, I was embarrassed, and two, I thought they were going to make me clean that mess up. Getting on my hands and knees and getting down and dirty with that mess was physically impossible at the moment since I couldn't move and I wasn't aware of the cleaning supplies that were available on the plane. Would this sponge work with that cleaner? Exhausting.

With horror, I saw So and Soichima walk over and look at the mess. She looked as if she had seen the second coming of Rodan. I felt bad that this was how she was starting her shift, a load of liquid shit on the floor. She disappeared and I guess was hoping someone else would see it soon and deal with it just like I would have done. All I could do was lie there and hope that my involvement in the incident was over.

A little later there was a commotion in and around my bed as I was cleaned up and the mess under the bed was somehow removed. I swore before I came in here I was potty trained. At least if I had lived the life I was led to believe I lived, then yes I was potty trained. The sheets were lifted off me revealing my ghastly purple legs. They were still there, and there was still no hope for me. It was useless to try and determine the course of events that brought me to this moment: a purple skinny legged deformed person with banana hands shitting himself on an international flight.

When I thought I could not feel any more embarrassed or down I heard Becky say all of a sudden, "It's Paul Boatealis!" and just like that someone entered the room on my right through some bizarre translucent glittery curtains like one would have seen on the *Merv Griffin Show*. Accompanied by wild applause and brass-driven talk-show music my boss entered with much aplomb. He didn't quite look himself. He was unusually tan with dark hair as if he had been to the George Hamilton School of Youth. It was very unusual except the wild entrance actually made me feel gloomier as I really wanted no witnesses to my current state. I felt weak and exposed. He walked over to Becky, who I now noticed was standing over to my left, to talk with her.

He was very jovial as he mentioned that he just realized he was on the same flight as us and his wife Nina was below. They were on their way to Bora Bora and they were looking forward to it. He then mentioned, "Incidentally my daughter's one of the nurses on the flight." He went on with what his plans were after the flight and did not really seem to notice my ghastly condition. It was as if we had just run across each other in a restaurant.

"First we're going to fly to Tampa so that a few of my friends and I can play my son Tommy's semi-pro team in baseball and I'm proudly the pitcher for our team," he continued.

Then the subject turned to me as he said, "We really regard Howard as a valued person, he has done so much for us and his new role has really worked for us."

I am never one to just take the damn compliment. In my head I was shooting holes in what he said as if I had been semi-fired and forced to work hourly because I suck at what I do. I was being very hard on myself, coupled with my stringy purple-ass legs, half a face, and my ill-controlled bowels, I didn't feel that there was much to work with.

Paul just kept standing over there by Becky and the conversation was beginning to die. Meanwhile, this international parade of nurses kept coming in and checking on me. There were the Asian nurses, then Indian nurses, a Hispanic nurse, a Middle Eastern nurse, and there was as my friend termed his sighting of an attractive waitress once, an Asian Sally Hudson, after a girl that we went to high school with. I kept thinking to myself over and over, *I need to tell him that one of my nurses was an Asian Sally Hudson*! If I could just hold on to pass on this important news.

Paul kept talking to Becky as I lay there helpless as the nurses moved my purple legs around. Somehow I just had to tell the doctors or nurses to please get him out of here. I didn't want him to see me like this anymore. I was tired of it all and wanted everyone to get the hell out of there. Feeling sorry for myself was becoming a specialty along with my paranoia and the questioning of everyone's competence. Paul finally came over to me and said "So, how do you think I'll do in the game? You know I'll be flying myself down there."

I don't know how I did it. I must have had a Stephen Hawking talking machine attached to me. However, I first somehow communicated to him that flying himself was dangerous as hell. He agreed and said, "Flying's the most dangerous thing you can do."

Then I communicated that he was going to get schooled in baseball and that his shoulder would get dislocated as if I was the Debbie Downer of soothsayers. He furrowed his brow at this comment. I suppose he thought he was pretty good and had great confidence in his conditioning being over sixty-years-old and schooling some twenty somethings. Finally, he said his good-byes and made a quick exit. I was relieved when that happened. Now me, my purply legs, banana hands, and stool-ridden bottom could once again relax and get to know one another.

***

KISS ME, I'M IRISH!

The plane must have been headed over the Atlantic again. This was really becoming 1984's *The Never Ending Story*. The origin story that is, for some reason I found the sequel, 1990's *The Never Ending Story II: The Next Chapter* too derivative. On this flight my parents were in attendance along with Becky. We were landing soon so it was only appropriate that I get my hair washed and my teeth brushed to do what, I don't know. Perhaps meet the press? I really believed that soon this would all be behind me, we would land and I would get off the plane and life could continue. The nurse, who introduced herself as Nora, was busy setting everything up. It felt like a casual loose atmosphere. I had a sense that I was going to be out of the woods of this whole ordeal soon.

There was no way to speak at all to Becky or to my parents but they were talking all around me. My parents could be very chatty so they of course asked Nora where she was from.

"I'm from Ireland, originally," she replied. It was a reply that was very much in keeping with the international flavor of the nurses on my flight. They continued to talk about Ireland which lent itself to my confusion as to where I really was at the moment.

I thought, *Are we flying to Ireland or are we flying from Ireland?* Even if I could speak I would never have the courage to ask lest the response be, "We're flying to/from Ireland you fucking nitwit!"

Nora washed my hair which I supposed needed it with the amount of bed head that must have seeped through. The water on my head just felt heavenly. I had been so hot lately that I could barely stand it. I just wished I could get some of that water in my mouth, I was so damn thirsty.

My hair was dried and the nurse started brushing my teeth. She said, "The toothbrushes in the hospital are not the best but they're better than nothing."

I didn't really care. At least the feeling of the grass in my mouth was subsiding. She pulled some attachment from out of the stand that was connected to the tube that was in my mouth that sucked the water. It was just like I was at the dentist. Well, not my dentist. My hygienist doesn't use air, she makes you sit up and spit, and with that I digress.

As she used the suction tube I began to wonder just how all of these tubes were connected. My last memory of these tubes was that they sucked something out of my chest and now they were being used to suction my mouth. Very impressive instruments they had on this medical flight. I just hoped some Clouseauesque nurse didn't hit the "Reverse" button by accident and put what had come out of me back while music from *The Benny Hill Show* played.

Nora put a new gown on me, which was a miracle given my limp-like status. It must have been like dressing a slab of meat in fabric. For a parting gift she laid those cursed blankets on me. As she tucked me in all around the corners she continued to utter "Shhhhhh!!!!" as if I was a troublesome child. Though I may have been acting like one with the shitting of myself and all, there was no need for that. The heat was relentless, I just kept trying to kick these fabric shackles off which was not possible since my legs didn't kick so it was more of a side to side shuffle. This movement caused her to tuck the blankets in tighter. I should have felt like a toasty cinnamon bun, but I didn't. I felt like a caged badger trying to gnaw off its paw to free itself. I was so uncomfortable with the inability to shift positions. The salon treatment with the hair and teeth had distracted me from that. Since it was over I realized that I was still stuck and the plane didn't seem to be landing.

Are we now flying past Ireland? Where are we off to now? Crap, I thought I was done with this, and the plane engines are so loud. It turned out my excitement of being done with this was unfounded. I was stuck and my discomfort was magnified by the disappointment. I would have asked but feared the response would be, "We were never going to Ireland you shit for brains!" The Answer Man wasn't very nice here.

***

MISSING YOU[65]

As the flight continued I just stared at the wall while the nurses kept coming and going. I kept wondering where the hell they went after they left me. It was a plane, was there some secret lounge I didn't know about with a platinum door called "The Platinum Club" that offered platinum level services?

My question was partly answered when I saw off to my left the same nurse that could not communicate with me open a door and disappear. Why was I so intrigued by this forbidden room of mystery? As I thought of all that I was missing in the fun zone my eyes just stared ahead. I was awakened from my empty wonderment when to my horror I realized the sofa that Becky had been lying on was empty. Oh shit, where was Becky? Did she not know that our flight was leaving and she missed it? I was unable to tell anyone. Had anyone else noticed this? Her book was open and I just knew she was in the terminal upset and fuming. I had already left her once on the runway in Pierre or Sault St. Marie, no, it was Sioux Falls. She was going to be pissed all the same and she would not be charmed by my ability to remember where I had dumped her last.

As if the pilots could read my mind I could feel the plane bank sharply and head in the opposite direction. I thought, *wonderful, they are heading back*. Somehow I knew I would get blamed for not telling them she wasn't on the plane in the first place! Shit! I could not explain myself out of this one. All the fuel and time wasted and with this being a polar route, there was no time for fooling. The other passengers were gonna go on an old style witch hunt looking for the responsible party.

Just as soon as my panic was reaching its climax Becky walked into the room as if nothing had happened. I was so relieved to see her. My relief turned to panic again. Now, the plane was headed back to the airport for no reason at all! Dammitt! I was going to be blamed for all the wasted time anyway. Come to think of it, why in the hell was I, the uncommunicative, paralyzed, bed-bound patient, responsible for headcount and the navigation of the aircraft?

I was still just relieved to see Becky, then again I was still rather upset over this whole Ralph thing and whether she was late because she was seeing him. I was going to ask her now. Right now. I was going to ask, "Are you dating Ralph?" I would do it. Now. Could I? Could I even speak? I was too afraid. I knew I had to put these thoughts to rest. I could not lose her. She was slipping away from me still.

I was still staring at her when she looked up and noticed me.

I thought, *she's so beautiful I can't even look at her. So certain and confident of herself, there are so many ways I love her. She's such a strong person and I admire the hell out of her, I just want her to know how much I love her.*

I felt terrible thinking she might be dating someone else. Would she be able to recover from my divulging to her my doubts over her entering the dating world? I didn't want to hurt her and I didn't want to see her reaction from such a question. Had she changed this much since I came down with this condition? Does she still hold what happened at the Plaza against me and this whole scheme which was my idea?

She slowly rose from the sofa and began to walk toward me. I couldn't stop staring at her and how she moved. She arrived at my bedside and had an expression of finality as if to say, "I know what you're going to ask so just don't go there, I'm here for you so let it be."

She then said to me, "Is there something you want to say to me?"

I shook my head and stared at the wall again.

CHAPTER 16

Theories

Invasive infections also include necrotizing fasciitis and spontaneous gangrenous myositis.[66]

FEBRUARY 1 - 3, 2009

The TV was on and I could see Steve Young and Rich Gannon and some other ex-jocks sitting around a desk next to a golf course talking about the upcoming Super Bowl but for the life of me I had no idea who was playing. Steve Young was relaying what was going through the players' minds at this moment. Then a story about Brett Favre's drunken depravity including wrecking golf carts and dressing up as a woman reporter had me confused to no end. To top it off I had heard that since some weather event had knocked off all communications to Tampa the outside word would not know the outcome of the game until it was well over. Toooo much stress, especially weather related, then darkness.

***

ARIZONA REALLY WAS A GAS/I WAS SCREWED UP IN A TOTAL MESS /MIND BLOWING ALL THE WAY, YOU KNOW[67]

No! This was not the same place! Where was I now? Did someone mention Arizona? Was I now in Arizona? Had I finally gotten off the plane and been unceremoniously dumped here? It was at least becoming apparent that all of this blacking out was saving me on boring travel time. Somehow we had gotten to Arizona. This condition I was in was really taking me all over the country. I felt rootless like I had no home. This was wearing my ass out trying to find someone who knew what to do with me. I guessed the doctors in Arizona knew what they were doing. I had no idea how Becky was finding all of this help for me and getting me to these places when I couldn't even move. She was just amazing.

I had heard from somewhere that the Steelers and Cardinals had faced off in the Super Bowl already. I was still smarting over witnessing the Panthers not even show up to play the Cardinals on January 10 in the playoff game that was so many flights and Dog People ago, so I was bitter about the Cardinals. Could you please figure out that they are going to throw to Larry Fitzgerald on a crossing route? The Panther defense prior to that game I was suspicious of especially when Derrick Ward of the Giants seemingly broke the 1,000-yard single-game mark in the final regular season game at Giants Stadium. However, in that playoff game they truly earned the nickname "The Escort Service." In the playoff game the only thing the Panthers didn't do was carry the ball to the end zone for them, truly gracious hosts. And besides what happened to the rest of the playoffs?

PART III – A DELICATE BRAND OF REALITY - THEORIES

Even though the terrible towels drive me crazy when the Steelers come to Charlotte in the pre-season this demise against the Cardinals was too recent and significant to overcome. I heard the Cardinals had won the Super Bowl and I was pissed off not only because of the recent events I had witnessed but for some reason I couldn't come to terms with the Lombardi trophy going west of the Mississippi. This was a strange stance to take especially since I had rooted for the 49ers during their Super Bowl victories. However, this time I had to make my opinion known.

An orderly came in to wash me, and when it came time to do my backside I informed him of my displeasure. It seemed that every time I was able to talk I got myself into hot water and this time was no exception. I said, "You don't deserve the Lombardi, it belongs east of the Mississippi!"

His already rough handling of my ass cavity was heightened at my invectives spewed his way. The pain was excruciating but I would not let it go. I went on, "Do your worst! You pussies can't handle what we got east of the Mississippi!"

He didn't say a word; he just continued to rub my labonza raw like he was on some mission of depravity. I didn't know exactly what my goal was here. I felt rebellious even though my ass was begging me to stop. What kind of hospital was this? Abusing patients for not liking the local NFL team? Don't get me started on the Arizona Wranglers of the now defunct United States Football League.

The orderly stopped the back porch rubbing long enough to ask, "You want some more? This pussy is raring to give it some more!"

I was defeated and said nothing. I and my gazonga had had enough for now. The Steelers would need to depend on another Arizona hater and his canetta to carry the banner. I slumped over and passed out.

***

CLOSE TALKER SALAD

I heard someone calling me "Handsome" and "Good Looking" through the haze. I hoped it wasn't that big orderly back in Arizona. This did something for my vain self. Certainly the voice was just being kind since half my face was missing. I thought I heard a story that it was a nurse that was a sorority sister of Becky's that was now working here. What a coincidence that she was my nurse and calling me such flattering names. Hopefully jealousy wasn't in the air.

As I saw her through the haze, I could tell she had dark hair, a big smile, and an enduring cheerfulness that just picked me up. I could not talk to her so I guess I was just supine, silent, and sympathetically handsome at this point to her. The haze was very deep so I could barely make her out. I could just feel her presence in the room. She liked to get really close when she talked to me and enjoyed getting a response from my multi-lingual eye blinking. I believe her name was Jenny. I could not be sure. She made it a point to talk to me all the time and treated me as an adult. I was always pleased when I heard her voice in the darkness.

***

BRAKE AND GAS

Mike had returned periodically to work my chicken legs out as well as my arms which by this point felt like the shoulders were glued in their sockets. He would slowly lift my arm and rotate it. It just hurt so damn much.

How long had I been lying like this, for everything to just stick in place?

I wanted to do a good job, all I knew was that I had the tube sticking in my mouth and it was not very comfortable and drove me crazy if I thought about it too much. So all I had to communicate with Mike were eager raised eyebrows and an occasional nod.

This day Mike began to work on my feet. I could barely stand the sight of those purple sticks and the feet with their red and purple highlights all over them. I didn't want to know anything about the why, I just wanted to do what they told me to do and hopefully everything would turn out all right. I felt like an animal, a hopeless caged animal that may have had a past though I certainly thought my future was up in the air. I didn't want to let Mike down. I had to finish this round of therapy no matter how exhausting it was. I had to keep occupied because it was either this or the Dog People would come back and get me. I was sure this place had something like that to threaten me in their back pockets.

Mike took the left foot. I have trouble saying "my" because it did not look like mine, it didn't look like anything I had ever seen before. He instructed me to do like I would do in a car and press the brake with the left and the gas with the right. I thought how ridiculous this was since I would never be driving again and thank God a clutch wasn't part of the session. For some reason I thought of John Lennon taking his driving test, I could see the picture of him with the other Beatles giving the thumbs up from the driver's seat. It was quite encouraging to me so I pressed on.

During this session I was overcome with something in my lungs that turned from a mild discomfort to a full blown coughing attack that would not stop. At this point in my condition it was by no means a boisterous cough. All I could offer was a cough that was as weak as a kitten's. Nevertheless, as I struggled to get up whatever was bothering me, I saw a nurse come in. She was faceless to me. She was wearing pink and she had that ID badge that always was so reassuring to me. It meant she was legit and she was going to help me. She offered me suction and I nodded since the horror of the first time had dissipated. Once again the tube was cleaned out as I could feel the liquid being pulled from inside me. It was akin to being forced to drive the bus from my lungs.

Mike stood back during this procedure and after the tube was re-inserted he asked if I would like to continue, I nodded and tried to continue however the coughing was again so prevalent we had to stop. My eagerness and bravado which was hanging by a thread suffered a setback as I had significant trouble breathing at this point. Mike once again stepped aside, and I felt so bad letting him down like that. I knew the session was over. Suddenly Mike's feelings took a back seat as I started to have a real urge to panic since now I could not breathe at all. I could see more nurses enter the room and again the darkness came.

***

GROSS ANATOMY VS. CRITICAL CONDITION

I heard that someone caring for me had the name of Dannette which was the name of a former co-worker of Becky's and with whom we still keep in contact. "Dannette's going to be checking your blood sugar," I would hear someone say in the room in my darkened state.

I thought through the darkness, *how bizarre that Danette has given up accounting and is now into medicine.*

I then heard the voice say to someone else, "Dannette checks Brian's [her husband's] blood sugar every night."

This was weird. First, would Brian consent to this? Second, was there a problem with Brian's health? Third, fourth, and fifth, was Dannette doing this because she was supposed to, because she hated Brian, or was Brian a willing practice pin cushion so that I might not feel so much pain? All these questions confused me so I welcomed the darkness instead of trying to figure it out.

Later, I would begin to see Becky except she was not in her regular clothes but this bizarre smock that was translucent yellow. A ghastly color that looked like this yellow cough syrup that tasted atrocious that I had to take when I was little. The memory of that made me feel ill but as I wondered what the deal was with Becky I noticed everyone was wearing this smock. Then it dawned on me. Of course, that was it! Becky must be in medical school. Everyone was in medical school now. It must be the in thing. How did they get accepted and how were they paying for it? Of course, money was no object in my world as I lay there in bed.

My thoughts on the subject were further verified when Dr. Rebefall would speak to Becky about my condition and would end each conversation with him saying, "Does that sound good to you?"

I thought, *Oh my, he's quizzing her. I sure hope she studied last night for this line of questioning and that my health or condition didn't spring any surprises for her.*

She would nod in agreement usually and after he would leave she would remain behind looking over me with a perplexed look on her face. All I could do was stare at her. How strange that she was in medical school and she got me for a patient in her rotation. Fate is a strange bitch. I had every ounce of faith in her that she would do a good job on me. I was just happy as hell that she was around to look after me. After a while, after his examinations, and his briefing of her, I wondered how long I had been in this place. How could she have applied and gotten accepted and now be in the middle of rotations in medical school? I don't even remember her taking the MCAT or even any premed classes. Man, I must have been in here for a long-ass time withering away.

So many more questions arose such as: Do we have children? Do we have a future together? Then the ultimate fear dawned on me: had I been in a vegetative state this entire time and created a life for myself based on just having met her? Did our story really ever happen at all? Was Ralph really her husband? The memories that were kind of floating back of our life, did I create them in whatever state I was in? I was too upset to think more on this topic. It was too painful. I was still just the monitor that everyone was looking at that could not interface with its surroundings.

***

Just when I thought that I had satisfied myself on the Becky in medical school question and still unsure if we really knew each other, I became more confused when I saw my mother, aunt, and uncle wearing the same garb. Did Becky even know them or had they just met?

I thought, *OK, I have the same relatives that I had when I came in here but why are they starting medical school at their age? You go guys! You're this many years young; don't let anything stop you from reaching your dreams! Shit Yeah!*

One night I awoke and looked over to my right. There sat my father, the self-nicknamed "Big Daddy," named so for the grandchildren since he did not want to be referred to as Grandpappy. He appeared to be kneeling next to my bedside in the same yellow garb reading this leather-bound tome of a book that appeared to be a Bible. I remembered when I was growing up my dad was not the one I would run to for medical advice. He was an attorney, and I would go to my mom. If I ever went to him either one of two things would happen: there would be no sympathy for the malady or there would be a medieval cure in store with lots of blankets, lying still, and leeches.

Big Daddy detected my gaze from the bed. He looked up and said, "Hey, it's me, Big Daddy."

I thought, *since when did Big Daddy start volunteering at the hospital?*

There was no consideration on my part that he was in medical school. At least there was one issue tied up in my head and I turned my eyes back up at the ceiling and let them close.

***

BABY ON BOARD, SOMETHING SOMETHING BURT WARD[68]

What I wanted to know is what the fuck did those assholes in that hospital in Manhattan do to me? I knew it was true, the highly contrived, I assumed, *Junior* movie coming home to roost with the baked-bean kid. All that happened in Manhattan must be true! Did they give me lady parts when I went in for my body re-build? Could a sex change actually yield a child because there was something weird going on at the moment. It's the middle of the night and I had been awakened out of a light restless sleep by someone that was now squirting gel on my chest. That can only mean one thing and I am wary of using highly technical medical jargon but this dude had a bun in the oven!

What the hell else could this be? She was a young lady in dark blue scrubs which was not what I had seen the nurses wearing. Does my nurse know the evil that was going on in here? Did the doctor know about this? Did that evil hospital send her to check up on me? I don't know if she saw that I was awake and I could not utter a sound. Perhaps she did know and wanted to just get her job done and get the hell out of there. This tube in my mouth was really beginning to piss me off right now. Not to mention I was so incredibly uncomfortable. My neck was cinched up and my feet and legs were hanging off the bed. Did anyone notice this? Plus my ass was killing me. My bony rusty dusty was taking the brunt of my weight and the discomfort kept reaching an all-time high. Why didn't she see my displeasure? Why didn't she tell me what she was doing?

She was wiping the gel off and applying it somewhere else. She put the cup on another part of my exposed chest and looked at the screen. An ultrasound, I was definitely pregnant. They were trying to check to see how badly I screwed up going to that hospital. Why did I do that? Why didn't someone stop me? I tried to retrace my steps through the insanity. What was the first step I took leaving the house? I must have gone to the airport and gotten on a flight. There had to have been moments interspersed in there where I could have reflected on what I was about to do. There must have been a beverage service, why can't I remember the beverage service!? What the fuck was wrong with me?! Now look where it got me, I am pregnant in South Dakota with no voice and very, very uncomfortable.

Howard Hoover, if that is your name, the life you knew is gone and you are here, wherever that is, a fucked-up shell of your former self. That vision of me getting up from the wheelchair and walking out of here kept getting farther and farther away.

***

I SAY A LITTLE PRAYER FOR YOU[69]

I woke with a start. I was flat on my back, it was night and the light over my bed was on as it burned my corneas. I pleaded in my head, *please turn that fucking thing off!*

I could hear voices in the room. It was my mom's voice and a female voice with a Jamaican accent. She was discussing my condition with my mom and suddenly the conversation turned to the power of prayer and how it can really turn the tide for someone in need. I just lay there and took it all in, they did not notice I was awake or perhaps I had my eyes half closed. I am good at having my eyes half closed yet having them look fully closed. The eye doctors have always had to hold my eyelids open so they can see into my eyes. Opening them too wide gives me a headache so in other words I have squinty eyes, not beady, squinty.

As I lay there the nurse said to my mom, "Come, your son needs to have a prayer said for him and I'll show you how we do that in my homeland. It's a powerful method when you stand over someone and join hands. The faith enters their soul and adds to the power of healing."

My mom just nodded. Usually she can get herself out of strange situations yet I think she felt anything would help combat whatever it was that was afflicting me. Plus, I didn't think that nurse was going to take "no" for an answer.

The nurse said, "Let us join hands over your son and pray for him."

I could feel my mom was opening the doors to all help and faith and she wanted to help me in any way that she could. I couldn't move as I thought about this. I just saw them come into my field of vision as they joined hands over me. I thought, *I must be in really bad shape right now.* To have a nurse see the hopelessness of it all and suggest prayer was a little too much to wrap my confused mind around. The prayer was over. There were no sparks, no crypt opening, and no melting Gestapo guy in black leather. Yet there was hope and that was all I could ask. I went back into the darkness.

CHAPTER 17

Questionable Companion

Group A streptococcal TSS is defined as any GAS infection associated with the acute onset of shock and organ failure.[70]

THE FOOT OF MY BED

I had the most interesting bed. I heard a lot about it as I lay there and no one thought I was listening. Staffers said that it was built for four-hundred pound wide bodies and not for tall people. There was one bed they knew of in the building that would have fit me comfortably but it was being used by someone who was around six feet eight. I was quite disappointed hearing all of this and wondered what in the world would happen if an NBA player was hospitalized. While my height was not abnormal it seemed to be for bed sizing. To make myself comfortable was akin to venturing into the unknown. It couldn't be done and was next to impossible. I couldn't move and it appeared all this time in the bed had made my caboose disappear because quite frankly my tailbone felt like it was stabbing my intestines. I had no padding back there and I was slowly and tortuously sliding down the bed where ultimately my feet hung off at a bizarre angle. I was convinced that if unchecked I would wind up in a crumpled heap on the floor since I had no ability to stop the slide on my own.

However uncomfortable the bed made me, it had an air mattress on it that made no small amount of racket. I heard that the surface of the air mattress prevented bed sores and was good for my skin. In addition to convincing me of the bed's overall comfort, action had been taken with repeated attempts to pull off the footboard but to no avail. I just kept slipping down the entire length of the mattress like a cartoon character. The footboard even had a little readout screen that I could see clearly which was strange since I am very, very near sighted and as far as I could tell I was not wearing my prescription spectacles or even a monocle.

The little blue letters flashed across the screen which measured about six inches long and two inches high. Names began popping up on the screen along with birth dates and dates of death. I recognized these names. They were my relatives. A name would pop up, remain five seconds along with a military rank if there was any and then disappear. Then the date of birth and death appeared for five seconds. This bed knew everything and it knew my family all the way back to before the Revolutionary War. Stuff that I didn't even know, it knew. A typical readout for my uncle and godfather who died the previous year read: "James Barantino, Airman US Air Force, DOB: Xx XX, 19XX DOD: Xx XX, 20XX." How did the bed know that? On and on it went listing his children, my cousins, Lisa and Clark. There was a Lt. Hoover CSN in the Civil War who died during a battle. There was a soldier from the Revolutionary War who survived and died in 1792. It kept going on and on, it didn't stop. Everyone eventually came up on the screen. My parents: "Herbert Clark Hoover, DOB: Xx XX, 19XX DOD: -------- Betty Bruce Hoover DOB: Xx XX, 19XX, DOD: -------"

Then it was my turn "Howard Webster Hoover DOB Xx XX, 19XX DOD: -------" Thank God, the bed said I was still alive, and I was so thankful. The bed was absolutely riveting. I couldn't stop watching it.

It had slowly become dawn as the soft light came through the window and I had spent who knows how long taking in the secrets of the bed. It would tell me what to do. I heard Becky stir by the window, she stood up. I had no idea that she had been there the entire time. She announced after some stretching and yawning, "I'm going to take the Babies to school."

She rubbed the sleep out of her eyes and yawned one more time and left the room. I was confused on how she was able to do that. Certainly we were in the mountains still and someone said it was icy and dangerous outside. After a few minutes the sound of car horns blaring outside my window broke the silence in the room. It sounded as if a truck was stuck getting up an icy hill grinding its gears in the process. The noise was awful. I prayed that Becky would be safe and be OK taking the babies in this weather. I stared back down at the screen to take my mind off the situation. The screen showed "Rebecca Lisa Hoover DOB Xx XX, 19XX DOD: ------- Iris Kate Hoover DOB: Xx XX, 20XX DOD ------ Phoebe Emily Hoover DOB Xx XX, 20XX DOD: -------, Henry Buchanan Hoover DOB Xx XX, 20XX DOD: -------.

To my horror I heard a sudden crash outside the window and a moment later a cacophony of emergency vehicle sirens ensued. I had a very bad feeling so I kept scanning the screen on the bed as it went back through its cycle listing all of my ancestors. I felt an uneasy sense of relief, nothing to report. Then suddenly an "Update" came up on the screen and it then changed to read "Rebecca Lisa Hoover DOB: Xx XX, 19XX DOD: February 2, 2009." I was beside myself with grief. I felt helpless and the notion that had I not been stuck in this hospital, she never would have been in that accident. I felt just absolutely worthless. Now my depression deepened because now I knew that when I got out, if that ever happened, I would be without her.

***

NIGHT OF THE RED-HEAD NURSES

It was dark outside and I had just awakened. Still devastated by the loss of Becky I took to staring at the wall once again. It all had to be a lie, except I had not seen her since the accident. The bed simply didn't lie. The depression, the discomfort, and the nausea on top of that was simply too much. Plus I kept slipping down the bed as usual and I simply could not push back up. My bed was still placed at a reclined angle. My feet were sticking out of it like Ned in *One Fish, Two Fish, Red Fish, Blue Fish* and my neck was getting cinched where the discomfort in my neck was unbearable. Plus I had this walking boot on my leg as if my transplanted chicken leg had fallen apart and this was holding it together. The fear of this and the heat it caused made me miserable. I just lay there not knowing how to do anything. I had nothing.

A nurse came in, she had red hair. *Becky?* I hopefully thought.

She came in and looked around but never made eye contact as her gaze around the room stopped just short of my bed as she quickly turned and left. A couple of minutes later a really short red-headed nurse came in, man she was short. That couldn't be Becky. I could tell she was short even from my height-disadvantaged locale which was compounded when a male nurse or orderly came in. He had short hair and a slight growth of beard and he just towered over her. They were whispering something. I couldn't make out what they were saying.

I just feared that they might start making out here in front of me. I knew they would detect my awkward stare, turn toward me and the guy would say, "Take a picture, it'll last longer", in a zinger that would be the ultimate embarrassment, as if I hadn't been humbled enough. That's how it must work in South Dakota.

They too abruptly turned around and left, their gaze never having come to my side of the room.

I thought, *What the hell is this? My room's not a lounge area to whisper in or a forbidden room of mystery, there's a person over here dammitt!!*

As I finished that thought a third red-head nurse came in.

Becky? I thought hopefully.

She entered the room, looked out the window and flipped her hair. This time I tried to wave at her. I was peering at her which seemed to do no good. She never looked my way and left. Did she feel the power of my gaze and just chose to ignore it? I knew if I was out in public and I stared at that very same person they would detect my gaze and rudely stare me down. Why wouldn't that expected social awkwardness work here?

I thought, *what the hell is out that window? What the hell is out that window?* Yes, I repeated the same question.

I knew I was just a monitor with some fake body; I just wished once that someone would come over and tell me that everything was going to be all right. I thought, *where's my family? What have they done with them? Where was Becky?*

Not only was she still pissed off at me for what I did at the Plaza, which seemed like a million years ago but she was gone forever. She died being pissed off with me. I saw it in blue letters. At least the bed was merciful and left out the "pissed off" part. How I wish I had her back. I would never do anything bad again. I just wanted to get out of here. Then the darkness came.

***

PARDON THE WAY THAT I STARE[71]

I must have dozed off, it was one of those times where you think you never will fall asleep again and then you wake up and there's daylight. I was still depressed as hell as I lay there, then all of a sudden a redhead came in, except this was a different one. She said as she brushed by my bed, "Hi Cutie!"

I was shocked and astounded. It looked like Becky though I was still unsure if I really knew her or just knew of her. She was wearing glasses, no doubt from her injuries at the hands of my seventeen-year old self and the accident. That was, if it was who I thought it was but how was that possible when the bed told me of her demise?

She took a seat over at the window. I just kept staring at her still uncertain if it was a ghost or my mind just playing a hopeful film. She had a slight smile on her face and she gave me a little wave. I wasn't sure if I knew her or not. I thought, *maybe she's one of the nurses trying to trick me.*

I looked away at the wall in front of me. I looked back at her. She was still looking and smiling at me. I looked away again and thought to myself in a hushed thinking-to-myself tone, *I think she likes you!*

I looked back again, she was still looking at me and smiling, I was feeling uncomfortable at such attention. I thought, *what does this siren think? Doesn't she know that I'm now a grieving widower?*

I didn't recognize her; however, she did look familiar. It was the strangest feeling in the world to have someone you haven't seen in so long and that you love so much all of a sudden appear to you when you are feeling at your lowest.

I was still playing it cool when she finally came over and said, "You're doing much better." After a slight pause she asked me, "Do you want to get married?" That question confused me. Had we just met and she had fallen for me? Boy, I still had it even with my rebuilt body of despair. Then it slowly dawned on me that it was Becky that was looking at me and I nodded in agreement since my voice was nowhere to be found. There was a dreamy sound to her voice that told me that everything was going to be OK and I relaxed and drifted away. She had forgiven me, she was still alive.

***

I'M DOING FINE, WATCHING SHADOWS ON THE WALL[72]

I was finally regaining a sense of my surroundings and what my room looked like as I slowly gained some contact with my inner self. I was in a hospital I knew, as for time and what city, that was another story. We must have been traveling by air and landed. Once again I was convinced that I had been bundled up and taken to London only this time I was in a hospital ward that was attached to Heathrow Airport. The hallway was filled with not only doctors, nurses, and orderlies but also travelers making their way to and fro. I recalled Becky telling me that Ralph, childhood tormentor and potential wife stealer, who had the superhero like combination of expertise in both legal and medical professions, would be getting off a plane soon in the next terminal. He wanted to stop by and be condescending toward me, I mean see me.

Good, I thought, *want to rub your superiority in my face? If I could hide under the bed I would.*

The good news was that he was married and his wife would be accompanying him, so my fears about him and Becky developing an emotional connection were unfounded or maybe he was a cheat and a wife stealer. As I re-found my new sense of security in my marriage I found myself actually looking forward to the arrival of Ralph. If I heard correctly he was going to talk to me about the dangers of smoking and why it was bad for my lungs and that my lungs would recover if I quit smoking because he has struggled with the same problem and had succeeded. While I was puzzled by the preachy reason for the visit, I was mostly confused because I had never smoked in my life so I didn't know what tower he thought he was preaching from. No matter what his thoughts were on my reason for being here I decided to listen politely to his sermonizing. At least I was going to get a visitor and I would do my best to stay awake to greet him and his wife.

The trusty foot of my bed was calling out all of the flights landing and departing from Heathrow and I could see the passengers rushing by my room to make their flights. What a great bed! It tells me what I need to know when I need to know it. Then I saw that Ralph's flight had come up on the foot of the bed as an arrival. How I knew the number of his flight I had no idea. I waited and waited and grew more and more disappointed as time passed. The foot board then announced that Ralph and his wife had boarded their connecting flight and had taken off.

Son of a bitch! I exclaimed in my head.

What a fool I had been. I had checked his progress and I waited and waited and they were off and gone back to the US. It might be true that I had nothing better to do, my ass was just lying here, but that didn't mean you don't send a note. I'm not going to be ignored, Ralph! As I realized that no one would be walking through the door for a friendly preachy visit, and what better kind is there, I started to feel really depressed and stared at where else? The wall, you're always there. You'll never leave me.

***

My staring at the wall was interrupted as a nurse came in looking hurried and haggard. It must have been the middle of the night. She appeared flustered and upset as did the rest of the hospital staff. I heard commotion in the hallway and I heard something about John Lennon. Then I knew where my time traveling had taken me. It's December 8, 1980 yet I am here in London and not looking through my closet as a thirteen-year-old overhearing Howard Cosell announce it to the world during *Monday Night Football*. I knew what had happened and not only that he was dead but I realized horrifyingly that I had 1980 medical technology keeping me alive. I could tell the nurses were trying to keep the news from the patients and were trying not to upset us. I saw one nurse come in and another nurse, a big country girl, get up off the floor where she had obviously been slumbering

"Are you working?" the nurse asked the slumbering one who I recognized as the one who could not understand my earlier request to listen to the radio.

"Yeah! I just needed a nap, I don't feel well," she replied with mock enthusiasm.

I didn't like this situation where my nurses were falling around me sick. How was that supposed to make me feel? I looked out in the hallway to see a doctor racing another nurse to the hallway bathroom screaming,

"Get outta my way! I gotta hurl!" Next, I heard the expected airing of the belly coming from the hallway. It seemed the staff was quite overcome by his death. While I was upset I didn't think it would have made me physically ill but we were in London and they must have had a special bond with the man. Also, I had over twenty-eight years for it to sink in.

Another nurse appeared in the room after the slumbering nurse had taken her leave for a brief respite in the "Platinum Lounge" to possibly get familiar with a platinum toilet. She turned on the TV hanging on the wall in front of me. She must have felt that I should know what the commotion was about. The TV appeared to be a model from the 1970s because that son of a bitch was taking its sweet-ass time warming up. It appeared to be a Wrangler brand TV with some sort of iron brand insignia at the bottom that lit up when it was being turned on. Since when did the jeans people start making TVs? The light was on yet there was nothing on the screen. I was really growing impatient over this. Was the damn TV working?

The nurse left and I was still staring at my wall waiting for this damn TV to warm up. There was nothing. I looked over to my left and saw Becky looking at another TV with an earpiece in her ear listening intently in a chair with her legs crossed. The warm glow of the TV was illuminating her face. I wanted a warm glow illuminating my face. Where the hell was that nurse? Could we get a TV guy in here to fix this? I wished I had the ability to get up and smack the hell out of that thing. Why wouldn't Becky tell me what was happening? She was probably watching a news report about the disaster. Oh well, I knew the story and what happened and there really was no sense in reliving it again or waiting for some piece of shit TV to warm up.

All I could do was keep waiting. So as I waited for the TV to turn on a nurse walked in and started to tend to something on my chest or somewhere. I was not really aware of where I was or if I really even existed since she didn't meet my gaze. She looked up at something over my bed.

Is it a TV? What the hell is this? You have the TV that I cannot see working above me and the one I can see is taking its time warming up. What kind of torture is this? I thought.

Her pocket started to glow; it appeared to be a cell phone. She pulled it out and answered, I started to laugh to myself. *Cell phones in 1980 were so ridiculous looking! They still don't know what one looks like or how small they'll become!* I thought in a superior way. What I found ordinary, they found amazing plus I had forgotten that cell phones were not at all small or portable or in existence in 1980.

The nurse left and I looked one more time at Becky staring at the screen and then returned my gaze to the Wrangler TV that was still in the never ending midst of warming up.

***

US AGAINST THE WORLD

Is that TV there just a prop or what? How could I get that thing turned on? What are they waiting for? Are they not bored by the silence? This was some new torture to have a TV on the wall and they wouldn't turn it on! I felt like I was back at my grandmother's house where it took an Act of Congress with various subcommittee meetings and UN Resolutions to turn the damn thing on! In fact, I saw three or four TVs up there, and a microwave! I hoped no one cooked anything smelly in that thing. If I smelled five-day-old tuna casserole being heated I was going to hurl. TV please!

Becky walked over to the side of my bed, thank goodness she was still here, and saw that I was awake. This must have been something after my impressive eye-blinking debut. I needed TV, if I could just somehow communicate to her what I needed.

"What is it?" she asked.

I had not the power of speech nor the power of movement, just my eyes. I started looking at the TV. She didn't know what I needed. I thought, *what torture! This was as bad as that flight I was on and they wouldn't turn the radio on for me. Are they joking with me? Can't they read my mind? I'm putting thoughts out there powerfully. TV!.....TV!........Please!....TV! I'll need to work my hand and start pointing.*

With all my concentration I could not get my hand to move. It simply would not. Slowly I recalled the hard earned thumbs up I performed for the doctors not too long ago. My hand began to move. Becky was looking down at my arm. She didn't understand my lack of entertainment travails. I didn't want to get her too concerned, I knew she had been through hell but I needed to move this hand. The hand was shakily moving, now I needed just one finger, one finger to move and point.

I thought, *what finger wants to do that? I need a finger to respond! Preferably the main finger.*

She was still looking at me, she must have felt powerless, I felt powerless, we were all powerless. This pressing need still made me think, *they're holding back on me. I have been committed to a room with a TV that's just a hollow box pinned to the wall. All of the TVs must be hollow boxes and they have one over my head so I can't see it to torture me, well played, but I'm going to call this bluff and get my TV. What is this? I have a finger pointing! Look at my finger! It's pointing at a certain place* on the wall, it's pointing over there at the TV! Please! TV! I cannot hold my finger up much longer! Please look!

Becky finally came to the realization, "TV! Do you want TV?"

I thought loudly, *Yes! TV! How are you going to get anyone to turn it on? They certainly won't allow it. They won't let me out of here! They must have it unplugged and the cable unplugged due to fear of electrical storms starting a fire and burning us all to a crisp!* I really did listen to my grandmother after all.

The nurse walked in and Becky asked, "He'd like to watch TV."

"Oh, certainly!" she replied. "Here's the remote, you turn it on with this button and change the channels right here."

This sudden offer of help made me think, *it's a trap!* It was too easy, but before I could second that thought the nurse grabbed the remote and turned it on for us. I watched as the magical glow came on. I thought, *I am alive! It is true, TV is still here!*

"Blink when you want me to stop," the nurse said.

And they're concerned with what I want to watch, glorious day! I thought.

She started a scan of the channels, then I saw ESPN and I blinked. "Fine, good choice we'll leave it on ESPN."

As the picture began to appear I suddenly became claustrophobic as if it was crowding in on me. Becky was standing by the bed touching my arm and I felt doubly claustrophobic and hot. The graphics for Sportscenter began to pop up and I started freaking out. The images were so fast I couldn't keep up with them. My brain felt fried just watching ten seconds of it. How long was this intro? Finally the anchors came on, they were smirky and self-important looking as usual and thought themselves funny however the news they began to provide was quite disturbing. I am quite the nationalist when it comes to sports and do not like it when the USA loses at anything. I was so upset when we laid an egg at the FIBA World Championships in 2002 even though that team thought the world was still the Harlem Globetrotter legendary foe, the Washington Generals. Now I was troubled as it appeared that all of these countries were challenging us to a duel in all sports.

I thought, *is there some sort of Sports Armageddon going on?*

First, there was a scene of a contest between the USA women's basketball team being mugged by a group of foreign thugs on the court. A US player injured her knee at the hands of some wicked foreign player who may have had a cricket bat hidden in her shorts and she was carried off the court. The dirty play continued when one of our men's players was raked in the eyes going for a basket in the opening seconds of a game. I could only assume we lost these contests. Even in tennis things weren't going well, as Andy Roddick was playing for his life in some monsoon somewhere and lost his match to some nameless foe. I hoped he hadn't wagered Brooklyn Decker.

I thought in a melodramatic fashion, *the horror of it all. The horror. The horror....*

Now as if things couldn't get worse our NHL teams were being beaten by some team called the "Canucks." What in the sweet name of Enola Gay was going on?

I could not take anymore. I realized as I was watching this USA beat down that I was crying. I was so filled with rage and disappointment at this whipping that I could not take it. The usual amusingly witty announcers also sounded a bit disappointed at the proceedings. I kept watching only because I worked so hard to get it nonetheless I thought, *TV? What have you done? Bringing bad news to me like this.*

I turned away. I could not watch anymore and I closed my eyes. The TV stayed on for longer than I would have liked. I somehow shook my head and got Becky's attention to turn it off but she didn't understand. Nothing seemed to work until I feigned that I was sleeping so someone would turn away this invited visitor who was now uninvited. It was like a vampire. Once you invite them into your house they proceed to go through the fridge, look through your mail, not flush the toilet, put their feet up on the furniture and you can't get them the hell out!

CHAPTER 18

Trust

Group A streptococcal TSS is mediated by toxins that act as superantigens. The exotoxins (superantigens) can activate the immune system by bypassing the usual antigen mediated immune response sequence resulting in the release of large quantities of inflammatory cytokines. The cytokines cause capillary leak and tissue damage, leading to shock and multi-organ failure.[73]

STARING AT THE WALL

I was staring at the wall one morning, had my eyes open just minding my own business, when my parents walked in the doorway. They were so shocked to see me, I wasn't really aware of why they looked shocked and pleased. My mom especially was so relieved. I supposed it was because I was awake.

"You look so good Howard," she said to me.

I suppose I did from whatever I had been through except I felt it was false flattery since half my face was still missing. At least I was breathing and somewhat alert.

I thought, *I'm just relieved to be in the same place each time I wake up and all that damn moving has stopped.*

They must have left the hospital when I was far from this good, and how I must look now must have been night and day for them.

Becky got up and walked to my side. Her voice sounded dreamy to me. She was talking to me like she was talking to one of our kids with a sweet soothing voice. I guessed for all intents and purposes I was a little baby at that moment, since I couldn't move or do anything but blink at them. No communication whatsoever, it was very frustrating. If there was a bright side I could at least make out faces and objects in the room. However, I still felt like I had done a terrible thing that I was trying to hide at all costs and I was looking for forgiveness without being able to ask for it.

As I sat there I had such discomfort in my ass that I could not lie there anymore. It felt like there was someone under the bed poking a spear straight into it or that Fabio guy with a hardened pickle. While that might be someone's fantasy it was my torment. If all my travels and all those hospitals I had been admitted and discharged from had taught me anything it was that I was not to say a word, that would only prolong my stay and put me back days if not weeks. That son of a bitch in the Confederate hospital did just that when I put in a request to get out of their dirty hands, and I was sure as hell not going to let it happen again. The pain was just pissing me off like a splinter under the skin that won't stop throbbing except this splinter was sticking in my parking place.

Dr. Rebefall came into the room and joined the impromptu party around my bed. I felt like a chimp in the zoo with all the eyes on me. "I hear someone's awake."

I just stared at him uncertain how to react. I remembered him and his shirt "greeting" me a while ago. I thought, *is he going to be mean to me again?*

He looked at me and could detect my discomfort since I was grimacing and squirming out of my skin. "Your butt hurts, doesn't it?"

That was a non-medical way of putting it. Shouldn't he have said my "posterior's nerve endings have reached a spear or pickle probing threshold" or at least say buttocks? I couldn't lie anymore, he had caught me. I could not deny it. The jig was up. The bill was due. The fiddler must be paid. If I had to lie here another second I was going to scream, but lie here I shall since my body was just a shell of its former self.

"We can give you something for that," he said.

I looked at him to detect a smirk, a guffaw, a chuckle, something to let me know that what was offered was a joke and not on the up and up. I was not a great reader of people at this moment be they of the human or dog variety. After this pregnant pause and seeing that his comment was all earnest, it was like the curtains had been opened and I thought, *these guys are trying to get me out of here.*

Like I had expected, he didn't say, "That will cost you another two weeks, Dickhead." "Dickhead," especially with the capital 'D' may have been a bit strong. I was not underestimating anyone at this moment.

I felt such a relief, a relief that I was finally safe from somebody trying to get me and take me somewhere to hurt me. That was the moment when I knew that they were helping, and I was out of harm's way from rogue doctors. It was certainly a huge step for me mentally but the physical and emotional toll was something else that I would have to deal with and would be slapping me around in the weeks to come like a poor job performance review.

***

WHO IS THAT?

As I lay there one day, maybe it was morning, maybe it was afternoon, at least the daylight was thankfully still there, I spied a group of people congregating at the foot of the bed. I noticed Becky was one of them and perhaps my sister was the other and maybe a nurse discussing something. Out of the corner of my eye I noticed someone slowly approaching the bed. She looked at me as if she knew me, knew me well. I had no idea who in the world she was. She looked like a woman in non-medical garb. She kept sneaking up to the bed and I was the only one that seemed to notice her at all. My initial confusion was turning to fear and was on its way to full-blown panic as her Chinese water torture approach appeared to have no end. What the hell was she up to?

Still, no one noticed her and I didn't know what she had in mind as she spied my feet which appeared to be poking out from under the sheet. Was she there to take my feet now? Her complexion began to turn from a black complexion to a heavily tanned look as she began to wiggle my toes as one would an infant's. Was I to giggle or scowl or curse up a storm? I didn't know, what I did know was that my brow was furrowed as I could in no way kick away this unwanted intruder as she continued to wiggle my toes. Perhaps she was joking with me before the foot removal began.

She then suddenly straightened herself up as she tried to join the group that was now beginning to notice her and her strange appearance. Someone in the group turned away to stifle a laugh as if they knew something hilarious had happened and were trying to ignore it.

Then it suddenly dawned on me, it was my mother! She was beginning to come into focus and this certainty grew as she began to speak. As she spoke she began to pull what appeared to be dark black band aids away from her eyebrows. Her complexion was still very dark as if she had some procedure in the hospital as well. What the hell was going on in my family and the elective surgery? Please stop! Learn from me! Save yourselves!

***

A NEW SENSATION[74]

I had a new sensation, and it was not good. First my purply feet were feeling awfully strange these days. Not only was there a general numbness to them, there was also this constant sensation as if I was walking in really dry grass not unlike a golf course with Bermuda grass that had gone dormant for the winter.

With my foot issue as puzzling as ever my attention was also drawn to this awful thirst I had. I mean this was worse than any thirst I had ever known, even worse than football two a days in August in Tampa or during Indoctrination at the Academy where all I could think of was liquid as we were cruelly marched by a Coke machine. This thirst permeated me down to the core. My throat was so parched, my mouth felt like dried up weeds; plus, I could not even open my mouth. There was an overwhelming sense of helplessness associated with it. I thought that my mouth in fact had grown over, the lips being permanently shut by some sort of grassy thread much like a scarecrow. Now I knew the hell of being Ray Bulger or an incompetent Batman villain. I could not swallow and there was something in my mouth that was preventing me from closing my lips just to recoup some moisture.

I could only think of water, sweet water which would be so nice. I could see three or four sinks against the wall. I was so hot and dry I wished I could pull that sink, yes that one there, and the one over here with its many faucets, I thought it had grown about two more since last time I looked, and drown myself in their wet goodness.

My only thoughts turned to immersing myself in water. *I want to go swimming so badly*, I kept thinking. The 2008 Olympics and the swimming competition, especially Aaron Piersol in the backstroke and the way they would jump in the pool before the race started. What a lucky guy, getting to compete in such an awesome environment. I would always cherish that if I were him, I don't think I would ever feel that type of invigorating experience again. Even though I am afraid of heights, the high divers even held my envy as they warmed themselves in the shower after they got out of the frigid deep end.

I thought, *man, I would live under that shower, I would never leave it. I am getting in a pool the first chance I get out of here.*

Since Becky was still in medical school under the tutelage of Dr. Rebefall I knew she had the means to help me with my dilemma and although she might get into trouble, I had to give it a shot. One night after she had brushed my teeth, well, it wasn't so much a brushing but a blotting, with the foam toothbrush to give my mouth a quick cleansing; I wouldn't release the toothbrush from my mouth. I just wanted to suck the sweet moisture off of it. The first couple of seconds was sweet liberty as the toothpasty liquid touched my parched throat. I felt liberated from my thirst yet I just wanted more and began to suck more. As this toothpasty liquid began to hit my stomach I became aware of a nauseous feeling that grew worse and worse. I suddenly began to gag on the toothpasty liquid and wanted no more of it.

I thought, *crap, that stuff is going to screw me up, I knew I never should have taken care of it myself!*

They had not let me drink anything for a reason and against their better judgment I had upset the apple cart by giving into temptation. I really hated power booting especially with something inserted in my mouth to God knows where. This incident taught me a lesson of not doing things before they were prescribed to me.

Although my experiment was briefly successful, I quickly re-entered the world of tremendous thirst. I was very depressed by the fact that my body could not take in any liquid no matter how small through normal means. I had to endure the thirst until such time that my stomach did not freak out. I hoped that Becky didn't get into trouble and that her grade would not suffer by trying to meet my needs. From then on I struggled with the pain but I always reminded myself to prefer the thirst to the nausea.

***

ALL BLURRED UP

Periodically, Becky would offer me my glasses to wear after I had awakened yet I kept refusing to wear them. My thoughts returned to how much of a dick I had been to her at the Plaza or how I left her on the runway or how I caused all of this mess with the body rebuild. Not to mention the three times she had died. I had been a real shit and I felt terrible about it. So in some grand gesture perhaps to make my case for martyrdom, I felt like I did not deserve corrected vision after all the horrible things that I had done. Now we're even.

My refusal was somehow a statement that I was sorry and that I didn't want to bother her with my trivial needs. So many people were already working on me, I was not worthy. For some reason it hadn't even dawned on me that I wasn't wearing them, for some reason I hadn't noticed that everything was blurry and fuzzy. I was really getting along perfectly fine without them. Perhaps I didn't want to show any additional signs of weakness that would be used as a reason to keep me here. Corrected vision might add at least a month to my stay.

***

THE NUMBERS FELL OFF THE CLOCK FACE[75]

The clock on the wall was very bizarre, I had never seen anything like it before. I guess in South Dakota they tell different time than where I am from, wherever that is, it must be an upper latitude thing. The clock was on the wall. I could see it clearly. It read 3:20 which I assumed must be in the a.m. since it was pitch black outside. However, the hours were skewed so the hours were shorter on the right side of the clock face and the numbers were closer together on the left side. How do people tell time here? It seemed to be some sort of bizarre local daylight savings time thing they had set up. Very asymmetrical.

Not only that but there was a penguin in the clock face and his tiny wings were the hour and minute hands. Instead of ticking, the clock made some sort of penguin yelp sound. This sound was driving me crazy. I wished they would take this damn thing away. It kept going, "Yip, Yip, Yip, Yip!" Do penguins really make that sound? It wouldn't stop. His wings were mesmerizing, they went around quickly then they slowed down. I was not getting used to South Dakota and its bizarre ways of measuring time. Like the Late Great Phil Hartman's character Unfrozen Caveman Lawyer might say, "Your ways of time measurement confuse and astound me."

So that was what I spent my entire night doing. Watching this little penguin yip and flap his wings around this horribly disfigured clock.

The next day, an old neighbor and friend was in to visit me as he had done on other occasions. He looked up and saw the clock and went to look at it. He must have been as confused in the daylight as I was in the wee hours by that confounded thing. I hoped he didn't get too messed up trying to figure the wings out. He was just going to get frustrated. As usual I could not speak to warn him of my similar experience.

Surprisingly, the clock had reverted to a normal form, and appeared as a clock should appear. I was flabbergasted when I saw the time. It was stuck on 3:20. Poor penguin must have gotten tired.

***

SOMEONE TO WATCH OVER ME[76]

"Tori was here," Becky said. I looked around, confused. Tori is Becky's oldest friend from high school and college and our family got along famously with hers. "Oh no, she was here when you were unconscious. She stayed for an entire week then she went to a conference in Columbia. She stayed up all night reading so I could get some sleep. She then slept during the day at our house. I didn't trust anyone but her to watch to make sure nothing went wrong. I just had this fear that you would be gone when I woke up."

I listened to her say all of this and tears were welling in my eyes. The thoughtfulness of someone to leave their family for a week to help out her friend was quite touching. Becky said, "People are just helping so much you wouldn't believe it. Clarice stopped by early on as well to see you. They all came from Greensboro and they had an American Girl tea party at our house and Hubert [her husband] played with Henry in the backyard."

I couldn't believe they were helping this much. My only lament at this point was, *why didn't you wake me up? We could have hung out.*

***

SILHOUETTES

I was lying there just alone late one night. I saw something in the corner of my eye just beyond my field of vision. I turned my head to the right, toward the door and standing there was a silhouette. Dr. Rebefall came to see me again. Had he been already in the room and I just woke up? Was he coming in to see me some more? He was just looking and I didn't know what to do. What could I do to get out of here? Should I look busy? Should I move? Should I lie still? Was he speaking to me? Should I respond? How? Was it just that I was here and I wouldn't get out and that was it?

I turned away to look at the wall, I could still sense him looking at me. I kept staring at the wall. Should I have looked back? Had I shown disrespect? Was there someone else in the room with me? Could I go now?

I could see out of the corner of my eye that he was departing, turning away. I guessed I wasn't impressive enough to get out. I then saw other people outside the room. There were my parents in the hall! Were they in on this too? Had I gone crazy? Was there anyone in this room now? What had I done? They looked serious and they were talking. What were they talking about? They looked back, turned and walked down the hall out of sight and I was alone. Perhaps they were discussing that evening's dinner party plans and had departed to act on them. I turned back to stare at the wall.

***

SILHOUETTES II

I was lying there one night looking at the wall, it moved, and it was entertaining and I could not take my eyes off of it. Dr. Rebefall walked in and stared at the TV above my head, something good must have been on and no one would even describe the action. It might have been an episode of *Sheriff Lobo* that really made you think about life as in, *what has happened in my life where I am now watching an episode of Sheriff Lobo?* Bastards. It appeared from the look on his face that it wasn't very good news. He looked down at me and looked back up at the screen. No, he should look at me! I was better now! You could really let me out, I would be good! You know I will be or maybe you don't! You have to trust this Half Face! My parents were having a Super Bowl party at their house, I think. I didn't know how I would get there but I would. They would be cooking ribs on their grill and I know that it would be delicious, even though the thought of ribs made me feel pretty nauseous at the moment. Please let me out, there isn't much time. Even though I can't move now, I will just lie on their floor in the basement and watch the game from there. Someone could roll me over. The floor would be so freeing from this damn bed that I am hanging off!

Of course this pleading was only heard in my head as he turned around. He was leaving and I was here again. The silhouette was at the door staring at me and I returned to staring at the wall. There were my parents once again talking to him, they looked serious, they kept looking back at me. I felt like a kid that had broken the neighbor's window with a baseball and was being taught many lessons, each more fiendish than the last.

I thought, *Good Lord would someone give me a timeframe here. I need to have some ribs that make me nauseous at the Super Bowl party! I have plans people, I need to leave!*

***

SILHOUETTES III

As usual, I was lying there late one night and I saw in the hallway a familiar silhouette and heard a familiar voice as it faded away down the hallway. "Charles Beardly came by to see you, Howard," Becky told me. An old neighbor, he and his wife are doctors; maybe he could get me out. "He talked to your doctors and checked on your condition."

I screamed in my head, *Charles! Get me out of here! True, we talk pretty irregularly and may only see each other at a mutual friend's place now and then but ya gotta help me! What better foundation for sticking your neck out for me is there?* I felt reassured that I had someone I knew with medical training on my case. He would get me out! I was wrongfully accused and shouldn't be in here. This was all just a big misunderstanding.

I waited and I waited and it appeared it was just a meet and greet, and I was no closer to getting released. The security here must be pretty serious if Charles had even been blocked from freeing me. I slowly put the pieces together that maybe I did have a life outside of here before all of this happened. Whatever it may be.

***

I'LL GO CRAZY IF I DON'T GO CRAZY TONIGHT[77]

I could not take it. I simply could not take it anymore. Lying on the bed, unable to move, it had gotten to me and I couldn't take it anymore. If I could only move something, only get up. The picture of me in my green shirt and tan shorts circa 1995 was slowly disappearing. I had no confidence if I would ever be the same again. I couldn't take it! I couldn't take it! I had to move. As someone who was bedridden for who knows how long and might be from this point forward I made a resolution to do something about it. What could I move? My hands wouldn't move, my arms certainly wouldn't move, my toes wiggled, sort of, well, not really. Ah! me head! Of course I could shake it. I thought that I would start swinging it and I could get some rhythm going because I was bored. There it went, some rhythm going. I may have had the tube still in my mouth but I would show them that I was still here and I could do things. I'm still a capable person. There it went, back and forth, faster! Faster! Damn you! Faster!

"What's wrong with him? What's he doing?" someone asked.

It was one of my nurses and I didn't know who. It was the middle of the night and I really needed to occupy myself with this swinging so their concern meant nothing to me. After checking me over the nurse could not figure out what it was that brought me to this Stevie Wonder like state. I was half expecting her to say, "This shit may be tolerated in North Dakota but this is South Dakota!"

"See if you can speak to him," she pleaded to Becky.

Becky rose from her chair and came over. I felt a little anxious, like a small child that had broken a lamp. So what! I could not stop. I would not stop. I was part of the Rhythm Nation. Would I be punished somehow? What more could they do to this rebuilt, impregnated joke of a body missing half a face?

"Howard, what are you doing?" Becky asked.

I couldn't speak, I couldn't reply, but I was doing this.

"Is something wrong?" she continued.

I continued.

"Howard, you have got to stop doing this," she implored me.

I just kept moving my head back and forth. My fear and anxiety continued. Stopping was not an option because I was moving and I was being a bad boy. I needed to prove to them that I was here, and I would get out. Even if I had to rock this fucking bed out the front door, I was going to continue.

The nurse then said, "I need to get the doctor."

Oh no, I felt like I was eight years old, I just hit my sister and my dad had been summoned. A few minutes later I saw it, the silhouette had returned.

I thought, *I am sorry you have to come and see this, Dr. Silhouette, for as you can see I cannot help it.*

Dr. Rebefall entered the room, "What's going on, Howard? Why are you doing this, you have us a bit concerned and you need to stop it."

I stopped for a second because I knew I was getting in trouble and I may not get out if I continued.

"Are you OK?" he asked.

I blinked or nodded or did what any mute, paralyzed person would to reply that I was OK, and then I continued moving back and forth. I did not like staying still. It was not me, not now.

"I don't know, I have never seen this before," he said.

The swinging he hadn't seen, but the rebuilt, half-faced, male impregnated body he had? The group continued looking at me for a while to see if this swaying was going to peak at some unpleasant point; it did not. I continued and that was all there was to it. I couldn't stop. I needed to break free from this bed! Concern still reigned as I continued through the night, I was driving them crazy. I just couldn't stop.

As I entered what seemed to be hours of doing this, long after the appeals to get me to stop had ceased since they figured I was doing no harm to myself, I noticed that someone new had come in and was standing by my bed. He was a tall young guy in scrubs. He stared at a monitor next to my bed as I continued my swaying. He looked at it, he looked at me, he adjusted something on me, and he continued looking at the monitor.

He finally said, "Man, if you're going to get better, you have got to stay still."

That comment resonated with me in a way that nothing else could. I stopped at that moment because it seemed that guy had the right answer to my dilemma, if I wanted to get better I did need to be still and I never swayed again.

CHAPTER 19

Interactions

Among patients who develop GAS TSS, a portal of entry cannot be identified in 45 percent of cases.[78]

YOU HAVE VISITORS

I was in and out that morning. It was tough staying up all night watching that hallway and all the activity that was going on and with the wall being its usual active self. The hall lights were on all night, the door was open and no one lowered their voice. All day and all night it was like that. So I was in and out of consciousness that morning, my body finally giving up, when I heard a voice say, "Howard, you have visitors."

I began to wonder who the rude SOB was that dare disturb me during nap time. It was hard work standing watch all night ensuring the Dog People didn't return to gnaw at my face. I opened my eyes very deliberately and quickly wondered what happened to my vision since of course I was not wearing glasses. I could make out the vague form of a man and a woman. They appeared to be my age. The man had a receding hairline.

The man said with a shit eating grin, "You're doing great, hang in there and take it slowly."

I suddenly was aware of the intense pain I was in. It enveloped me and would not let go. My sides hurt, every breath was a labor and I just felt lousy, virtually sinking into the bed. The nausea was unrelenting. I was unable to respond in my intubated state. I felt really low, I thought I would never get better, this might be the end. I could not do this, I couldn't, it was inescapable and it was hard, difficult, a pain in the ass. If death had wanted me then I didn't think I could have fought it. In fact, I wanted to give up right then if this is what life had in store for me.

But these depressing thoughts of surrender were not enough to suppress the thought, *fuck you, I'm in intense pain and I don't feel like being nice right now. You take it slow. This fucking sucks.*

The woman said nothing and stood in stunned silence. I treated them with disinterest and wished for the room to be clear. I closed my eyes to make them go away. I felt like an exhibit and was getting quite tired of it. I thought, *what the hell business do they have being here? You just let anyone in the door? I wish I could get out of this bed to kick some ass if it weren't for this whatever the hell it is that I have been bedridden for........ who knows the date? South Dakota gets cold this time of year.*

But the feeling dissipated as I answered my thought with a lazy, *can't someone else do it?* The darkness returned.

***

PUT YOUR MARK ON THE LINE

Problems outside my little world in this room were of no concern to me. I kept hearing talk of this refinancing of the house and what would need to be done in order to get me to sign. I thought, *poor Becky is having to deal with that outside-world stuff. I can't imagine how cruel it is out there. Please get me back to it!*

I would see a lady with a soothing voice come into the room periodically, she worked at the hospital in some capacity. I couldn't imagine working right now, I felt so low. I could hear snippets of things being discussed and I had no idea what was going on, only the words "house," "rate," and "sign." That was all I knew.

One afternoon I was awakened to Becky's voice. Becky said, "Howard, we have some papers we need to get signed to lock in our rate and refinance our house. This gives me the power of attorney to act on your behalf in order to do that."

I nodded, just happy to know what she was saying. I jokingly felt like a ninety-year-old man with no voice, getting a fast one pulled on him as he disintegrates into the bed and becomes part of the linen.

The hospital worker lady stood by. She held a piece of paper for me to sign. I could not raise my hand. I was still intubated at this time and it was dark in the room.

"Can he lift his hand?" asked the lady. "No? Then you can hold it for him while he signs. All you have to do is put your mark there."

Becky then gingerly lifted my hand as she placed the pen in my hand. I could barely grasp the pen as she slowly guided my hand to make a squiggly X on the paper. I thought how pitiful that X was and how hard it was to do even that. I fully trusted Becky with whatever needed to be done. With anyone else I would have thought I was in a Lifetime movie, however since I am not a chick then it would need to be a movie on the Spike channel.

***

BABY, BABY, BABY LIGHT MY WAY[79]

I didn't know how long I had been here, I didn't know how much of my life had been a lie, I didn't know if what I did before was real and now this was it. I didn't know how much more I could take. I was awake and something was in my mouth and I knew Becky was there. I could hear her voice, sweetly through the darkness. I could feel her sitting by the bed. Her voice was coming through to me from a great distance it seemed. She was talking to someone, responding to their questions concerning me. I could barely turn my head to see her but she was there. I knew she was there. I could barely keep my eyes open and the darkness.

I awakened with her standing by my bed. She wanted to tell me about what had been going on while I had been wherever I had been.

"Your office has been sending over meals, everyone has been helping out," she said.

I was extremely touched by this and the tears began to well up in me.

She continued, "The Babies are great, and they miss you so much. We miss you so much."

I was in disbelief, I thought, *you've seen them? Where are they? What are they doing?*

The frustration of not being able to say anything was really making it hard to take. I couldn't believe that they were still here. I wanted to ask so many questions, I felt so much relief. I did not imagine them after all. They had not disappeared like those poor kids in the Nic Cage flop *Family Man*. They were real, they existed.

I just looked at her, I felt myself just giving way because I finally realized that my children were still there, part of this world. They had been found and my eyes continued to well up. I knew where they were finally. I began sobbing uncontrollably.

Becky, shocked by my reaction, said, "I only tell you this because I wanted you to be happy and know that everyone has been coming out to take care of us. You wouldn't believe it. And the Babies are fine, don't worry about them."

I was happy, but you couldn't tell it. I was having trouble keeping my sobbing under control and I thought I was beginning to panic. My nurse came in and began to administer something to help me. As I went out, Becky said, "We'll buy you anything you want!"

The darkness came again.

***

ARE YOU READY TO LAUGH?

As the morning grew brighter I lay there intubated just staring at the wall, looking at the various shadows being created and destroyed by the advancing light. I had made it through the night and felt settled for the day. The tube in my mouth was a bit troubling, I had trouble getting used to it. There were so many things attached to me that I had to think to realize that it was still there.

It was one of those mornings when I had a pleasant equilibrium with my situation. The tube was working and I was staring away. Suddenly my dad walked into the room. Without a greeting or a hello he paused at the foot of my bed and started to go into a comedy routine. As anyone in my immediate family knows his greatest comedic achievement is to mock some of our neighbors when I was growing up by talking in an aggravating nasal voice with a heavy Yankee accent. Big Daddy immediately began talking in this voice.

"I would like to know how you're doing today. I have been hopping over the green stains from the dog in the living room. The coffee cake's beginning to spoil because of all the green stains. The A/C isn't on even though it's in the mid-90s outside and it's so rank in the house. You can hardly breathe in here." He then started to make a gagging sound, "My husband hasn't moved from his chair all day, I think he's dead from immobility."

He continued in this voice, performing for me. I was beginning to wonder where my mom was, where was everyone else? Where was the "Clear Room" button? However, the ridiculousness of the scene was beginning to get to me. If anyone walked by and saw this old guy talking this nonsense to a captive intubated person in this voice, there would either be confusion or a call for security. I began to laugh but my laughter made my sides hurt and I couldn't tell him to be quiet. I was stunned because he kept going on in that voice. Perhaps he wanted some sort of normalcy and didn't want to acknowledge my condition at the time and to make both of us feel better by talking about some common ground from the past. I think he was making himself feel better, as for me as I was getting kind of annoyed.

And with that he quieted down, sat in the chair by the window and began to read. Not a normal voice was used or a normal greeting. I thought I was going crazy at the moment. Where was everybody? I felt like Big Bird seeing Snuffleupagus on Sesame Street and no one else was around to witness it. I was much too exhausted to care and luckily my staring at the wall continued unabated.

***

IT SEEMED SO REAL TO ME[80]

I couldn't sleep, I was really uncomfortable. I had been lying here for how long? I didn't know what time it was, I couldn't see very well, yet well enough considering I was still in the midst of my glasses-refusal phase. The hall lights in all their glory were still on, it was night time, I was confident of that yet I still couldn't sleep.

I took stock of my room again. There was that microwave and my continued fear of it grew with the same thought, *if anyone heats up a hot pocket while I'm in here I am going to cast the gorge.*

There was that faucet that seemed to have grown a couple of more nozzles. How many sinks were there in here? One there on my right, one over on the wall facing me and maybe one to my left, I was not sure. There were what seemed to be a couple of TVs on the wall. There was one with that sort of spur symbol that was lit up that resembled the insignia of the old USFL Wranglers. That must be a very quality product. I still remembered that year they swapped cities with the Chicago Blitz which in hindsight really confused the hell out of me but no one else really seemed to care.

My eyes then settled on the medical waste box hanging on the wall where old needles are deposited. This really caught my attention, especially the label that was on the needle box. The symbol on it was morphing before my very eyes. I knew I had seen that symbol before but not like this. I studied it. How could I see it? I didn't have my glasses on. How was I seeing this? As I studied it further it became clear to me that it was a devilish man with a wicked smile and horns. I knew it was evil, one would think differently before sticking their hands in the box with that face on it. The evil devil face on it kept changing form and said wickedly, "Fuck yes, we have lots of needles for you! Ha! Ha! Stick your hand in here and see what you get!" Even placards were taunting me and they had dirty mouths as well.

The next stop for my eyes was the curtain that was sort of covering the doorway to my room. It was this putrid green color and the bags for the garbage can had a putrid pink color, the same color of the liquid those fat dudes were running in at that freak hospital in Manhattan that did all of this to me. I was feeling sick just thinking about it. The bag said something on it, what was that? Did that say *Beerfest* on it? I saw that movie not long before I came in here about those lovable lugs showing the Germans that Americans can drink, but I could not think of beer right now, especially drinking too much of it and barfing. That was what that must be for so I had two questions: First, why would a hospital agree to have a corporate sponsor? Second, why would a beer manufacturer choose a hospital, the least likely venue for partying that I could think of? Endora of *Bewitched* fame must have put a spell on the marketing decision makers at McMahon and Tate on that one.

I could not stop looking at that damn garbage bin with the awful color and the *Beerfest* logo, I was going to hurl with yours truly not being able to move out of the hurl's way. I didn't like to hurl, and I especially didn't like hurl in and of itself landing on my person. Then the window on the door to the room began to take on the same putrid tint of pink sick. I began to feel worse thinking of the things that can has held. I tried to take my mind off this color that was staring at me. The curtains that went around my bed also had that same type of color. I couldn't get away from it.

I thought, *please make this feeling go away,* to no one in particular.

I felt lousy, with the *Beerfest* symbols tormenting me and now the evil devilish man taunting me with a toast of, "Gentlemen, Here's to

Evil!." I wanted the night to be over. Please let the night be over. I tried to listen for anything in the hall to distract me. Unbelievable! It was pretty quiet out there. I thought Becky was asleep over by the window, but I couldn't be sure. I pressed my feet against the footboard; at least there was some sensation in my feet. I was so uncomfortable; at least it was taking my mind off the evil in the room.

***

COOPER

Darkness was abundant during this time. There were periods when my eyes actually opened and there would be light. During these times there was uncertainty as to what my eyes would find. Not that there were any expectations, this world was just one big surprise with nothing except uncertainty. However the level of the depths that I must have reached took a twisted turn when I saw him enter the room one day during one of these both literal and figurative eye opening periods. It was Cooper Lowry, Deacon of Local Episcopal Church. When I realized who it was I was not only shocked but a bit embarrassed. Shocked, that I must be in a low, low place for him to be there all in black complete with priest collar. Embarrassed, that there really hadn't been a personal relationship with him other than seeing him on Sunday mornings and hearing him announce the house for Habitat for Humanity and other outreach services that the church was sponsoring. I always meant to help. I always meant to volunteer. I just didn't. So in other words I knew of the Deacon Cooper Lowry, I just didn't know him. Here he was with me in a position of feeling really low not only because of my physical state but because he was at my side when I never came to be by his side.

Cooper brushed aside what was in my head because it was evident that it was not in his head. What was I expecting? Now that I was awake he would come in and say, "Finally awake I see? Maybe now you will come and do a little something more than sit down during a service." This harsh judgment that only my guilty mind could imagine was not forthcoming. It was obvious that he had already been there for some time and my conscious mind was joining the program rather late. There were no hijinks in my head trying to concoct a scheme that would have brought him there other than to see me.

It then dawned on me that this whole body rebuilding thing was something that he hopefully knew nothing about. It had really just put me in the deep end and here I was in such a serious state that our clergy had to visit. I knew this was bad, if he had found out that I had been playing God with my body who knows what the repercussions might be. I had a horrible secret to hide, I just didn't know who knew it yet, so I played dumb, a wonderful part for me.

***

ABOUT POLLY

Things were not progressing as smoothly as I thought they should be. Being in a bed twenty-four hours a day and not being able to move or shift at all had indeed gotten on my nerves. I figured that someone had to be watching me from above to see how I was doing. I could spy a small bubble on the ceiling across the room from me. Obviously I was being watched and not so much to see how I was doing but how I was being cared for. Since I was above reproach, it was the others who had to watch their behavior and what was better than working somewhere

where your performance was monitored on a minute-by-minute basis? Made one feel a little on edge yet my paranoid self didn't care as long as others were subjected to the rigid requirements that ensured my comfort. And my precious comfort had been suffering quite a bit.

It was obvious to me that Dr. Rebefall was in this control room somewhere in the hospital watching remotely, and I could communicate through the foot of my bed. The scrawling message wasn't just a tool for my genealogy or flight arrivals and departures to pass before my eyes but to do a little whistle blowin'. My nurse that day was Polly or as I liked to refer to her, Martha White. Yes, that Martha White from the White House, those were heady times. It was too bad that she had to befall my wicked foot.

I thought, *I haven't seen her for what seems like hours. Why was she not around? Of course, a quick message through the footboard should rectify this.*

I tapped out my message on the footboard and the scrawling message board came back, "Thanks for your message, we'll respond shortly."

I thought with a satisfied smile, *Ah, I am getting so much done without being able to move. Just lying here, tapping out inflammatory messages on my trusty footboard, the ultimate multi-tasker.*

A noise from the footboard awakened me from my self-congratulations when a printout of old dot matrix computer paper emerged from the top. It was obviously a receipt showing my complaint, an official document that I could keep for my records.

I panicked with a mixture of guilt and fear, *No! She'll know I'm a squealer if she sees it!* What in the world was the footboard doing? Besides, what does a receipt do for me? Do they think I can file or I have a filing cabinet in here?

As I rolled over the fear of getting caught in my head I was much relieved that I was under constant surveillance in case any monkey business or attempts at making me eat a pillow occurred.

Not much later I was typing out another delicious memo on the footboard when I saw a shadow in the doorway looking down at me. It was Becky and from her stance I could tell she was not happy. I had to keep typing or learn how useful my foot could be since my hands were obviously not going to do their part.

As I continued to have the footboard do my bidding, Becky finally spoke. "I hope you're happy with yourself," she said in a sarcastic tone.

Again I felt like a small child being reprimanded. I stopped typing and looked at the wall. I did not have the strength to look at her and thought, so that she may hear although I knew she couldn't possibly, *what do you mean, what could I have done? I have been in here the whole time not hurting anyone.*

"You got a good nurse fired today," Becky continued.

No, I thought. *I thought they'd have at least reprimanded her or put someone on me full time to fluff my pillows and such.*

I couldn't think anymore, the guilt strangled me. I felt terrible as I cursed the evil instrument that caused this. *Wondrous footboard, how could you have done this?* I didn't mean for this to happen, actually I did mean for it to happen. Come to think of it I hadn't seen Polly in a while. How terrible, what could I do? Perhaps I should tap out another message. Maybe Dr. Rebefall would listen to my appeals. However, I would do well to keep out of his way or I would be here forever and ever. I confided in him, and now I ruined a career.

I saw Polly come in the doorway, she looked out the window and then up at the TV. She looked cowed and was drinking something. It appeared to be a bottle of Orange Julius that the therapist told me I needed to use as both a weight and ice pack on that flight that Becky got kicked off of in Sioux Falls. Everyone seemed to be hooked on that stuff around here.

    I wanted to say I was sorry. I guessed they made you finish your shift in shame before you got canned or maybe she didn't know. How terrible for her. I knew I had better stay quiet and not make a fuss. Stay out of her way. I did wrong and I wished the floor had opened up and swallowed me right at that moment.

CHAPTER 20

Tough Love

Over 750,000 cases of sepsis occur in the United States each year, resulting in approximately 200,000 fatalities. Even with optimal treatment, mortality due to severe sepsis or septic shock is approximately 40 percent and can exceed 50 percent in the sickest patients.[81]

I'M READY TO SAY I'M GLAD TO BE ALIVE[82]

When the television went on the nurse would ask, "What would you like to watch." She flipped through. It was so awful. The action, the lights, the fast moving images were still freaking me out. I finally settled on CNN. The things going on in the world were really bothering me. There were stories of some woman using her uterus like a puppy mill. I couldn't get away from Octo Mom. She was being interviewed constantly. People were debating her right to exist. There was a house being built for her with twenty bedrooms. I had had enough of this, this fucking OctoMom! Now they were comparing her looks to Angelina Jolie. Ms. Jolie should sue for libel.

My viewing came down to one thought, *if I see any more of this fucking OctoMom I am going to tap on my trusty footboard!* I swore I wouldn't but this fucking Octomom business was pushing me! That was just manufacturing news. The news hounds knew that, been doing it since the first printing press. But this. Had anyone else realized this? In fact her name had been officially changed to "Fucking OctoMom." My venom however was not only limited to her as I directed invectives at the talking heads with their conversations about her. The damn fast talking know-it-alls! God, I sounded like an eighty-year-old shut-in.

The TV's strange relationship with me continued as I awoke another day to find it on and there was a group of people in the studio of some morning show talking about having survived something horrific a few weeks earlier. I didn't understand and was afraid to ask about something that appeared to be common knowledge. They even showed a picture of some Australian singer in a rubber life raft looking quite upset. The experience inspired her to write a song about it.

My first thought was that they had now manufactured some catastrophe since it was turning out to be a slow news day. It was beginning to dawn on me that this was obviously big news but I couldn't understand the breadth of the calamity or was it a joke?

My parents walked in as I was watching. My mom said, "You know Becky was on the same flight to Charlotte the Monday before this happened."

I totally misunderstood this comment and began to weep heavily thinking she had perished. With my intubated state I felt like a hopeless baby, she was gone and I didn't even know about it.

Seeing my alarm my mom quickly added, "No, no, she's OK, she has been here with you every day. She wasn't on that flight."

But I couldn't stop crying, just thinking about being in another world and not being able to help her or the Babies. What would have happened to the babies with this double whammy of losing both parents in the same week? It was hard to console me. My sensitivity was riding high.

***

A RUSE GONE WILD

My cousin, Sharon, and I are only ten days apart in age. A fact that I thought made me feel superior back in childhood when halves were thrown up as definitive mileage markers in age. A marker of maturity, if you will. These days and especially back on the eve of our fortieth birthdays I wished we were switched, I could have used an extra ten days of my thirties to do things that would be ridiculous in my forties. I still haven't thought of anything.

But we were forty-one by this point and I was hearing bizarre conversations between my mom and someone else about some sort of plan for Sharon to come to Charlotte to type her mother's, Aunt Grace's, poetry. The plotting went on and on concerning the vital point that someone could not be wise to her visit. It had to be divulged as being for another purpose and that poetry typing was a hot button issue that no one would question. Well, I had no idea that Aunt Grace had such a back log and that poetry needed to be typed right away lest it spoil. I wasn't going to argue with the voices even if they sounded crazy. The back and forth on this plan was astounding, so much so that I felt like I was in on it. Whomever this was intended to fool would be made to look the fool. I could not wait to see the looks on their faces when they saw that poetry was being typed or not typed. I was shaky on the specifics. I did get the feeling that it would be a humdinger.

Of course I had silence and darkness as my friend for a time when I was awakened by a voice that said, "Howard, Sharon's here."

As I opened my eyes I saw Sharon sitting at the foot of my bed but I felt like she was on my bed crowding me, the type of crowding that made me feel claustrophobic. It was kind of like when the underwear starts to cinch in a very bad spot. Plus, I was hot as hell and my bed did not need additional body heat thank you. After my flurry of internal bitching, invectives, and discomfort, I was pleased to see her smiling at me like everything was OK. I guessed that typing my aunt's poetry did not get the best of her. She was still in good spirits. I was pleased to see her for the five seconds that I was awake and my eyes slowly shut again and there was once again darkness and silence.

I heard voices talking about Sharon later and how she had to return to her home in Northern Virginia. That was a short visit. She must have really gotten fed up typing all of that poetry. I guess it was worth it because whomever they tried to fool I know must have felt quite the fool when the plan was revealed. Too bad I couldn't see it come to fruition with all that fool makin'.

***

THE TUNA FISH EXPERIMENT

"He was throwing up by the entrance!" I heard my mother exclaiming in the room through my haze. "All of these cars were backed up behind us and he just got out of the car and threw up in the bushes."

"There must be a big spot out there where nothing will grow now," I heard someone else exclaim.

My father once again ate something he shouldn't have and as a framed picture on the wall would do, I had to listen to this story over and over and over again with each new visitor. Actually, Big Daddy probably had a framed picture of himself on the wall in all the places that he had gotten sick. It really came as no surprise to me. When I was eleven years old, one morning during breakfast my sister and I told him the milk looked and smelled funny. With my mom and her voice of reason out of town my dad took it as a challenge and said boastfully, "Big Daddy will drink it!" Later that morning who should be lying in the bathroom a little sick? Big Daddy! Fast forward thirty years and I had to hear about the complaint lodged with the hospital. I had to hear it as an inside joke. I had to hear it referred to over and over. It was obvious that the Hoover men were in bad shape.

I could not speak, I just had to listen to it and I was getting a little annoyed with hearing about it over and over. One day I was sitting there minding my own business and in came Cooper. It was during daylight hours so the place was hustle and bustle. He greeted me and then my parents laid on him with the, "Don't eat the tuna fish story." It appeared my dad was in the cafeteria and my mom advised him not to eat the tuna fish since she thought it looked a little funny. Later that afternoon my dad had to be practically carried out of the hospital and back to their hotel. I heard how friends of ours that were visiting got to see him on all fours in the elevator as it whisked him away as he could only utter a faint greeting.

I also heard that he had to wait in a wheelchair by the entrance while my mom got the car and then the throwing up in the bushes occurred while traffic was stopped behind them at the main entrance to the hospital. Now, to someone with health issues of his own I could tell that the food-poisoning story was not getting it done for me, especially being told like it was for the umpteenth time. So Cooper was shocked to hear about this and how my dad was holed up in the hotel room for a couple of days just sick as a dog.

I thought, *sick as a dog? Really? You want to look over here and see this? Let me plug some of this shit into you.*

I tell you I had it up to here with that story especially since I was nauseous day and night. I did not want to hear about him being sick and certainly not about tuna fish. I was gagging already hearing about it and seeing the urp-colored can liner was not helping either.

As one might predict I had had enough. You could only push a guy that was intubated, bedridden, paralyzed, rebuilt with limbs of unknown origin, impregnated, half-faced, and multi-tubed so far. Some friends came in for a visit and once again my parents went in on the tuna fish again and they began to recount the whole entire fucking thing for me, the framed picture on the wall. I had had it. I somehow got the strength and anger to start pounding on the side of the bed with my foot and then my hand as I rocked my head back and forth in anger. I was trying to yell, I had enough of this shit. I wanted them out! My dad started laughing as he was escorted out of the room by my mom. I was left alone with my friends just pissed off. So I guess since I was not going to die at the moment it was fun time. I guessed everyone was glad to see some spirit in me. Anger was the best medicine that day.

***

THE TRICK IS TO KEEP BREATHING[83]

"You're doing great Howard!" I kept hearing my mom's voice say. "You're doing great!"

Great at what? I don't even know where I am. I'm in a dark place not doing anything. Am I alive or am I in eternity hearing that I'm doing great?

I had no answers at this point but it really felt hard for me to breathe right now. I just wanted to rest and not do anything, just let whatever it was pass over me. Please just let me rest. I kept getting awakened by, "You're doing great! Keep it up!"

Please leave me alone, please. I want to go away now. It was just too much work for me.

I heard Becky say, "Howard, you have got to breathe! Count with me: one, two, three, breathe!" in a commanding voice.

I knew she was getting me back for the whole Plaza incident by making me work when I was sooo motherfucking tired! *Why must I work at this, why can't I be left alone? I had my body rebuilt for God's sake. I want a refund!*

I actually had to work to meet her demands of breathing. I would take a breath and would just let go and relax and nothing more would happen. The demand would then come again, "Howard! You have got to breathe!"

I just couldn't do it. I was laboring, I had to be reminded. If she wasn't there I know I wouldn't have done it on my own. At this point I hated this. I hated what she was making me do. She was being a hard ass and I couldn't cope with this anymore. I didn't understand because I remembered being wide awake. Things were OK then, well, relatively OK. Why did I have to work so hard now? Wasn't I out of the woods yet?

My mind started to wander to things I would rather be doing like wanting to get to my parents' house for the Super Bowl party. I didn't know why this weighed on my mind; they had never hosted a Super Bowl party before. I just kept reminding myself that the Super Bowl was about to happen, I had to get out of the hospital.

I was called back from my daydreaming by Becky's voice again, "Howard, you're not breathing, you have got to breathe!"

Dammitt!! She was making me focus, focus on breathing. This was hard, had she ever tried breathing on her own?

Her voice continued, "Breathe!!! You have to breathe!!!"

Then out of the blue I heard my mom's voice, "You're doing great Howard, but you have to breathe!"

Oh, teaming up on me are you? I could take it, or maybe not. If I was having trouble breathing I didn't see how I could possibly take on the both of them.

Becky took my hand and put it on her stomach and began counting out a rhythm for me to follow. I was so tired and lazy, please no mas! I wanted to stop then. She wouldn't let me stop, this went on for a while, it seemed like an eternity. Was this my life now, someone reminding me to breathe? I could not do this. I slowly slipped into unconsciousness.

***

BRIGHT LIGHTS, BIG OPERATING ROOM

I awoke to the sounds of voices. I opened my eyes to a bright room. I could hear two men talking, one young, and the other older. I could see the young one had on a mask and a cover over his head. I was someplace different. I heard the young one say to the older one, "I did quite well on that procedure, don't you think?"

You conceited asshole, I thought. *You're complimenting yourself when I'm in my vulnerable weakened state.* I gave him the glaring of a lifetime.

The young doctor stopped talking as if he suddenly realized that he was being watched. He slowly looked down at me with a look of surprise in his eyes.

I thought, *that's right, I'm on to you.* I then shut my eyes.

When I woke up, Becky was cheerful when she walked in the room. She was no longer exhorting me to breathe but was very affable. She told me about her co-worker who had been through a similar ordeal of breathing. The same ordeal? She was kicked by a horse that nearly detached her head! What do you mean the same ordeal?

She didn't seem to remember that I had cursed her before with the breathing demands so my day was already looking up. Day, yes, it was morning, not night when the MICU ghosts came around to haunt me. I felt much better, more comfortable. I questioned these good times and why they were here after the awfulness of getting me to breathe on my own. Why was she leaving me alone now? Was there a magic wand they used for me? Was there something they pushed on my monitor that solved my dilemma of having to work to breathe? I had no idea, I played along acting as if nothing had happened but something did. I did notice that no longer did I have some appendage hanging out of my mouth, the feeling was very liberating. *Please don't let on that you know!* I kept pleading with myself, *or they'll put whatever it is back in!*

***

GARDENING AT NIGHT[84]

I awoke and found I was looking up at some machine hovering over me and could feel something hard and smooth under my torso. I heard a few clicks and the hard and smooth object was removed from my underside. A male voice said, "Thank you." The machine was rolled away and he was gone.

For some reason I was pissed off. *How dare they treat me like a slab of meat! Did they think I was that easy? That would never happen again! Resist! Resist!*

I was aggravated with myself for having let my guard down when my thoughts were interrupted by the sight of a young girl slowly rolling this machine around in the hallway. I dubbed her "Cherry Soda Girl." I didn't know why, she just reminded me of the fizzy drink. She had not stopped in my room yet, I guess she was meant for the more serious cases but maybe I was too serious for her to see. She just seemed like a breath of fresh air to the horrible nights in the MICU as she snapped her gum going from room to room. Speaking of cherry soda I could have really gone for some then, my mouth felt like dry straw.

There was a bevy of activity in the MICU that night for some reason. My eyes were always drawn to the door to see what was coming next. My eyes could wander along the wall where I could see into the room next door. There was a window in the wall and for the life of me I could not figure out how I could see next door. It was as if I had X-ray vision. This place was laid out very strangely. Through the window I could see a gathering of people looking down at the person in that room. There seemed to be a lot of instructions being given. I wondered if I have had that much attention paid to me. I really hoped I had righted my ship and could get out of here and that I wouldn't have to see that group looking over me so seriously.

One person in the gathering was particularly physically imposing. He was a big guy who looked like he was built out of stone. I called him Mike Singletary, one of the Bears' great linebackers now ex-head coach of the San Francisco 49ers. He didn't exactly look like Mike Singletary yet that was the only name I could come up with. Now that was the guy that would be able to pull my ass up into bed and stop me from sliding. On second thought, he might have pulled so hard I would have ended up standing on the headboard and of course falling on my face with my ass wrapped around my head.

At that moment I was slipping down and I wondered if he could come over and pull me up without the heave ho to the headboard, of course. He would need no help at all. There would be no call for the army of ant nurses. The discomfort began to embrace me in its evil clutches. It was like having a nasty itch that I could not reach.

I could see Mike Singletary leaving the room next door, and to my surprise he paid a visit to my room as if he could sense my brain waves. He took about five steps inside and looked around. He was bigger than I previously thought, his arms the size of tree trunks. He was wearing the dark blue scrubs that according to Becky identified him as a respiratory therapist. Becky said that the guys in the dark blue were nearly impossible to get help from. Their scope of duties seemed to be so narrow.

He paused a moment and said to me with surprising care in his voice, "Are you comfortable?"

I felt so flattered that Mike Singletary would care about my comfort but at the same time I thought it was a trick. If I shook my head with a "No," he might respond with a "Tough Shit!" So with that little tidbit of negativity in the back of my mind all I could do was nod my head stupidly. I didn't really need to bother him with my obviously awful uncomfortable position. He returned my nod and left.

Realizing my opportunity was gone I yelled in my head, *do I look fucking comfortable?*

***

WE HAVE A REMEDY, YOU'LL APPRECIATE[85]

This pain I had been feeling periodically, well, I had figured out finally what it was. I had been pinned with shots in my stomach and I was getting quite pissed off about it. One nurse would come in and lift my gown up and dammitt to hell it hurt.

Becky asked, "What's that?"

The nurse replied and what I heard was, "It's a specially developed medicine worked up and patented here in our hospital."

So they had some witch's medicine they were sticking me with so I could just stay the hell here and not ever move? I thought, *they just want to torment me, don't they? The pharmacist here must be the hospital owner's cousin and he begged the hospital owner to let him use this crazy shit he worked up and to put it of all places in the stomach.*

"Ha! Ha! We will say it's for good but it's really for evil with discomfort the only goal!" They would have both responded. Conspiracies seemed to follow me around like a bad rash.

"How often does he have to have that?" Becky asked.

"Every eight hours," came the reply.

There was something else I could look forward to while I was here. This was going to be great. Now, that's sarcasm.

"But why in the stomach?" Becky asked. Thank God she was here to read my mind and ask my questions.

"It's the only place with enough fat on his body for the needle to enter," came the reply.

I had no arms or shoulders and I thought with the way my ass had been hurting that that had disappeared as well. I was very depressed by this, that my body had in reality gone away. I had really found no good way to take this shot, my strategy was to tense up. That didn't seem to work and actually made it worse so I tried to relax as much as possible. Perhaps this would become old hat in time but it sure as hell was not right now.

As I looked at the needle being brought into the room once again I thought, *let's just get it over with*.

***

COOPER II

When I began to see things in the real world Cooper would talk to me about what I was going through and all the things that had been done to me. After which I thought that only an abduction and release by aliens would have been less intrusive.

He talked of his own past health woes, and that his doctor, who I confused with Dr. Rebefall, would not let him go on a mission trip to the Caribbean because he was so sick. I felt like a comrade in arms with him and was irritated that Dr. Rebefall would not allow him to travel. He assured me that the folks at the hospital knew what they were doing. I might have known that, though I still felt trapped and I unreasonably thought that I should be on my way by now. He assured me that I was in good hands; however, I still could not understand how he was able to fly back between South Dakota or wherever we were and Charlotte like he was doing. It must have been costing the church a fortune.

I learned over time that Cooper was a true Godsend during the early days when no one thought I would make it. He comforted my Dad when my Dad was beside himself with grief. He sat with Becky in the ER when I was laid out on that first day. And he paid the ultimate price by having to hear the tuna-fish story.

***

SHE'S A MAN BABY! [86]

"Mr. Hoover, it's time for your medication," I heard an effeminately male voice say.

Who in the hell are you? I thought.

He looked like a version of a guy I knew from my childhood but this time effeminate sounding and with a weird haircut and darker hair. The haircut was in some salad bowl style on the front and the hair looked like it was waxed on. A hair hat, if you will. Even though I was no longer intubated, it was still my timely good fortune not to be able to speak, so at least I had a thin layer of protection. So I just nodded.

I saw on his ID badge that his name was Curtis. I could feel some doubt creep in about Effeminate Curtis, as I began to refer to him. There was some tension in the room as I could tell Becky was not a big fan of his caregiving methods. He left the room and walked in a style that I found had been cultivated more for shock value. I realized that walking style was no accident when he returned walking the same way with the damn shot. Yes, that goddamned shot they stuck in my gut that I later learned was a blood builder but to me seemed like a quack's idea of a good time. I had my eyes open but whenever I would lie there and finally get my body to a still enough place to fall asleep, there would come Effeminate Curtis right in my face once again with his questionable breath.

I studied Effeminate Curtis and his movements and even in my altered state I found him one part annoying and one part entertaining. He had a gait that I found especially interesting. It was more of a prancing shuffle actually. He walked like an effeminate Frankenstein with his arms extended forward and his hands hanging listlessly.

I thought, *hell, why oh why?*

I had this fear that some old friends would pop in for a visit and instead of talking to me would ask, "What's with the nurse? That's the nurse you chose? Where are the hot nurses? What is wrong with you?" Not to mention what the Dog People might have said. Their snarling faces would have a fucking field day with this.

To which I would reply, "I swear there were hot nurses here a little while ago. I don't know what happened."

"Sure there were," would come the disbelieving reply, "and you probably sent them away."

"It's not like there is some nurse menu where I immediately went to the "Strikingly Effeminate Male" list," I would reply in a desperate defense of what was mistakenly seen as my choice of caregivers. In my mind they would have none of it; and the visit would go on with Effeminate Curtis prancing around the room getting in the way of our now awkward bullshitting.

Dammitt! Not only were my fantasy friends annoying, there seemed to be no way I could send this Effeminate Curtis on his way. He told me to get some sleep and truthfully I wondered how I was supposed to do that with him slinking around here.

I couldn't sleep, my discomfort was great. It appeared that they had given me something they kept referring to as Milk of Amnesia to put me out. Effeminate Curtis appeared ready to have me fall asleep yet like a small infant in the crib with his hours mixed up I simply found it impossible. After having been on all my whirlwind travels, I had to absorb all of the stability that I could even if it had Effeminate Curtis front and center.

Once sweet darkness had overtaken me Effeminate Curtis stuck his fat face in my half-gone face once again to wake me. Why was it that my falling asleep schedule fell only five minutes before my wakey time? When I was awake he would have the nerve to poke his head back in the door and exclaim with some sort of girlish shriek when he would see my eyes darting back and forth. I was once again being suspiciously troublesome. This was my activity, Effeminate Curtis. I stare at the wall at night so get used to it.

It was time for the shot to the gut once again. As I braced for what was to be another painful moment I glimpsed a female standing behind Effeminate Curtis. She was wearing a white coat. She must have been a doctor. Still, it wasn't at all evident why she was there. She seemed to be admiring Effeminate Curtis's big fat caboose. I was waiting in sweet anticipation to finally have the shot over and done with for the next eight hours. As he was bending over me she slapped him on his big fat ass and said, "I just love looking at that tushy!" He immediately stood up straight and let out a shriek that would have embarrassed a school girl. Howling with laughter he came over to her with his arms out and his hands hanging limply. This guffawing went on for what seemed like an eternity as I kept slipping down in the bed, getting exceedingly uncomfortable while they laughed their asses off.

Eventually, this huge ass joke that I had to witness died down and he was able to finally focus on me. He turned around and finally gave me the damn shot and he was the worst at it. The absolute fucking worst, I shit you not.

On those occasions that I would slip further and further down into the bed, Effeminate Curtis would be summoned to take care of the situation. As he entered the room there would be a pregnant pause and a long sigh as if my ass was keeping him from something. He then would leave the room in a huff and return with another nurse. They would each take a side of the bed and he would utter matter of factly, "one, two, three," and lift. It was no surprise when my rectum felt like it was going to remain in the same spot. My ass nearly came out of my body a few times during the lift with different nurses but these lifts were the worst that I could remember with the exception of what Mike Singletary might have done.

And with that he would turn around and leave the room. However, the motion of turning around for him required clearance because the arms were always extended, always in front. No pillow fluffing, no adjustment from the burly move. It seemed that Becky was becoming more flustered with him. She couldn't find him when I would have a problem, and there was a sense that we were bothering him. I was very hopeful that the daylight would turn him to vapor, bring something better and not him and his high voice.

CHAPTER 21

Speech

Approximately 80 percent of patients have clinical signs of soft tissue infection such as localized swelling and erythema, followed by ecchymoses and sloughing of skin which progresses to necrotizing fascitis or myositis in 70 percent of cases.[87]

FEBRUARY 4 - 9, 2009

NOW IS THE BEST TIME OF YOUR LIFE[88]

Time was growing short for me, I could feel it. It was the weekend and with the free and easy feeling a weekend will bring there was obviously stuff going on. A positive energy was in the air. I finally slept some that night, and I had a new nurse, Teresa, who was my day nurse. Things were a little more jovial and she was full of good news with regard to my condition. They were small steps but there had been talk from Dr. Rebefall that I would be able to speak one of these days.

Of course, the weekdays and weekends held no meaning for me, however this seemed like a Saturday somehow which was a relief since the days had not had any feeling until now. My parents had come into the room and were milling about that morning. Soon after Teresa came in, my dad somehow had found out she was from Germany and he had visited her hometown when he was stationed over there with the army in the 1950s. It had to be Danzig or something like that, a place that got bombed badly. So they talked about that for a while. Whenever I heard these conversations I always felt like an outsider, like I would never get to see any of that again. It was so removed from where I was at the time. It might as well have been a different galaxy. However, if the conversation had turned to South Dakota, I would have ruled the roost.

After things settled down and Teresa had done all that she had come into the room to do, she went back into the nurse's office where I could see her through the glass. I didn't know if she could sense me looking at her but she would look back at me periodically as if something was going on or she had good news for me. I had no idea what the day would bring. I could feel a buzz. My trach was still in and I was still unable to speak. The feeling that things were moving for me kicked off when Dr. Rebefall came in and said that I would be talking soon.

I couldn't remember the last time I had the power of voice. What would I sound like? Effeminate Curtis? If that were the case I would just stay mute, thank you. What was I to say? What I said had to be meaningful and thought provoking. Something that would really get those on hand thinking and never forget. Simple, yet stylish and of course that meant no, "Get your hands off me you damn filthy dirty ape!" That would be the opposite of a good impression. I knew I had to think on this one. Perhaps something from a carpe diem derivative movie that Hollywood pops out every year. I just couldn't think of one. Wasn't some obscure character from *The Office* in one recently? "Suck the marrow from life!" the obscure character would say from some building ledge as some romantic interest looked on admiringly. Such a profound message usually stuck with me for an average of twelve minutes after I left the theater.

Thoughts of profound movies were interrupted when a new doctor came in by the name of Dr. Fine. My mind kept drifting to the Three Stooges and a short that they appeared in that was set in a hospital. They were constantly being called over the intercom, "Dr. Howard, Dr. Fine, Dr. Howard." Thankfully this doctor had not the sadistic humor of a Stooge, in fact he was all business as he looked at my trach tube and matter of factly said that I could go down to a smaller gauge and be able to speak. I supposed this meant that my lungs were getting stronger and I would be able to begin breathing on my own. As for the hole in my neck my common sense wouldn't allow me to figure out how something smaller could stay in a larger hole. I didn't really want to know, I only hoped this guy knew what he was doing. I found myself in that very paranoid state where I didn't trust what was going on around me. I had no idea why I was this way, this was the best hospital that I had been in so far, and it certainly beat the hell out of that Confederate hospital.

As I pondered this I realized that the fitting of the smaller gauge into the larger hole would be occurring at this very moment. There would be no special room to take me. No appointment to make. Right here in this bed, this would be done.

Dr. Fine was a young-looking guy, maybe even younger than me. I couldn't believe a guy this young that I had never seen before was about to take something out of my neck and put something else in. I had to trust him, what else could I do? I let all of my fear go and trusted that he did not miss the one class where they taught this procedure.

Certainly he hadn't fooled the entire hospital, and certainly he didn't come off the street like that weirdo that had pressed a sticker on me.

Dr. Fine wore round glasses, looked very smart, in a delicate genius sort of way, had short brown hair, and he was going to do something that I was glad I had never seen or felt before. He began to fiddle with my neck; I couldn't look, yet unfortunately I could feel it. The feeling was strange, obviously with something sticking inside my throat. It didn't hurt but the thought of it did. I tried to relax as he re-inserted something else in my throat. Then to top it off, he installed the infamous cap so I could speak. I had no idea how this thing worked, I supposed it allowed air to pass over my vocal cords. In order for it to work I had to press on it.

I repeated horrifyingly the instructions in my head as I heard them, "Press on the hole in my neck." This was weird. I didn't know if I could do it. And with that, Dr. Fine was gone; yet I had a feeling I would hear the words, "Dr. Howard, Dr. Fine, Dr. Howard" again.

Teresa took the cap and showed me how it worked. If I wanted to speak all I had to do was press down on it. What would I sound like? Would I sound like Rudolph when he first spoke? Would I have the vocal range of Julie Andrews? Would I be practicing scales with Mariah Carey? One could only imagine. I felt terrible because Becky was not there. My parents had left the room possibly to return something to Marshall's as they seemed to buy the entire store when they visited. After nights of thinking of what I would say the only thought left to me was, *I do not know what to say.*

Dr. Rebefall had spoken about this for weeks but all I could think of was, "Hello Cleveland," a salute to Spinal Tap. That was too obscure or, "Good night Springton, there will be no encore," even more obscure and what did that mean in relation to this event? "The dirty ape" comment was off the table since it was deemed by me and any other right-minded person to be too rude. These people did bring me back from the brink. So I had nothing. All of those years of profound movie watching and this was all I had.

Teresa was too impatient, she had to hear me speak, and I could not hold back. I was just surprised Dr. Fine had not hung around to hear. Suddenly a young girl came in the room to ask about something. I had seen her before. Why, it was the one and only Cherry Soda Girl

She was finally going to speak when Teresa whispered in my ear, "Tell her 'Go Away.'"

That's it, that's my moment of verbal brilliance? "Go Away?" This couldn't be. Becky still was not back and the young lady was waiting for a reply and I said to myself, *sorry Cherry Soda Girl*, then I blurted out a weak, "Go away."

Teresa laughed. Cherry Soda Girl was shocked. I was sorry. Then Cherry Soda Girl stammered, "Oh, that's OK I can come back later."

Teresa said, "He was only joking."

Yes I was, sorry my first words were rude but I guessed we had to have a laugh around here. My first words, "Go Away," still made me feel terrible. I sat and sulked thinking my new power was used for rudeness.

How the scene was supposed to play out was that I would say, "Profound thought for you to think about always."

With that comment cameras would click and flash bulbs would go off as those in attendance reached for paper towels to either scribble on or dab at their tear-filled eyes. As they frantically searched for primitive writing implements they would say in awe, "Slow down bedridden guy, this stuff is gold!"

Becky came in soon after and Teresa was quickly at my bedside telling me to tell her to, "Go Away." No, actually she didn't. She said to me, "Tell her 'I love you.'"

I was the one feeling like the ape at this point. I said it, "I love you."

I could really only make out Becky's figure in the doorway but I could tell that she was taken aback by my sudden vocal fame. I was so happy that she got to hear me say it. All those days of wanting to say I was sorry, all of those days of not being able to tell anyone how I felt, or thank for thinking of me, or to ask what happened, I could finally do it, talk. They would not have to teach me sign language after all or have me use some dry-erase board like Bubbles the chimp, and in turn I would not be flinging my stool at them. I was slowly coming back.

***

TO THAT SAME OLD PLACE THAT WE LAUGHED ABOUT[89]

My voice was back! I could not believe that after all this time of not being able to communicate it was here. As if on cue my parents came in and I said "Hello" very nonchalantly. Their reaction was of surprise, gratitude, shock, and yes even some awe. My only concern was the button on my throat that I had to press in order for any sound to come out. This was no easy task and I am squeamish about pressing on things connected to my body. So naturally I wasn't pressing hard enough. My voice was not coming through, not even with the assistance of Dolby.

It seemed when word got around that I could talk the world began to gather around my bed. Lorraine came in and appointed herself the button presser. I don't know what her skills were in this area but her confidence seemed to be overwhelming and something I could not argue with. It was just wonderful to catch up with everyone on the goings on in their lives. No matter how much we talked it seemed the confusion in my own mind seemed to stay the same. I still had my own theories of what happened, of where I was, and I had a road block in my head on the cause of my current circumstances. Reason and confusion were butting heads inside of me, and it was going to take a while for the two to come to some understanding.

CHAPTER 22

New Normal

Invasive infections associated with GAS TSS have been reported with increasing frequency, predominantly from North America and Europe. There an estimated 3.5 cases per 100,000 persons with a case fatality rate of 36 percent for streptococcal toxic shock syndrome. Up to one-third of these cases developed GAS TSS in reported case series. A higher rate of TSS of about 50 percent has been described in patients with necrotizing fasciitis.[90]

I WOULD LIKE A FROZEN TREAT

What was that strange machine sitting next to my bed? It had something swirling inside it and there was a man that sat next to it who paid me no mind. One morning, before I had regained the power of speech, he came in and without saying a word fiddled with something on my chest, snapping things into place like I was some sort of doll. He never said a word to me. I thought, *Dammitt! At least ask for permission to touch!!*

Becky appeared by my side and said, "Dr. Strester has been with you since your first night here, she's your nephrologist and she's very smart."

Yeah, I muttered to myself, *if she's so smart then why am I still in here?* When I really should have thought, *hey dickhead, if it wasn't for her you would have found out what was above that tree.*

Dr. Strester walked into the room as if on cue and introduced herself. She was very tall and seemed very determined. She announced that she had cold hands and would be examining me.

I was so hypercritical. I thought this whole Dr. Strester thing was some New Age/John Tesh music/incense/touchy feely dead end since I had no concept of what kind of doctor she was when what I should have been thinking was how lucky I was to be here. I should have been thinking and remembering this as a blessing.

My ignorance knew no bounds as I lay there impatiently and heard the banter between Dr. Strester and the man by the machine who I dubbed the Delicate Genius. He may have dubbed himself that too, who the hell knows? This hospital from my perspective was full of them. I was still getting a little agitated that I was being ignored as he described his trip to the Galapagos Islands with his wife recently.

Are we near there? I wondered. All I could think of about the place was George Costanza's made-up trip as a marine biologist there to study sea turtles. Obviously, I kept silent on the matter.

As I continued to stare at the sweet treat machine and received no offer, I simply gave up. However, the sweet treat machine wouldn't give up on me, with its alarms and constant high pitched whirring that kept waking me up. Every nurse I had seemed to have had to come in and turn it off. Did this alarm mean anything? Should I be concerned? If the alarm kept going off did it lose its meaning?

What it must have been was an Icee machine and from personal experience what I did know about these Icee machines was that they were infamous for being out of order. I remember growing up in the

1970s being so excited to get an Icee at the local neighborhood Sears and the out-of-order light was always on. It seemed to be doing the same thing here in whatever year this must be. When the Asian nurse was on duty he just kept turning it off. Did he break it? Did I break it? Even if I did break it, I and Gamera would have pointed the finger at him, if I could have pointed.

I was awakened again to see another male nurse looking at the sweet treat machine as the alarm went off. He looked like some Vincent Price character from some black and white horror movie. I could actually see him in black and white. He kept coming in to turn off the alarm.

Would someone please switch this sweet treat machine for another, it obviously didn't work especially if no one was going to offer me one. It must have been the same one that was always out of order at the very same local neighborhood Sears all those years ago. I would have taken a cherry red one since I could see that was the only flavor that was swirling in there. Although I did prefer a good Coke Icee, cherry would have to do. Now off with you lad or lass and look lively.

Once, before I had regained the power of speech, the Vincent Price nurse came in to respond to another alarm. I spied on him examining the gauges or buttons or whatever was there. Perhaps he was pretending to understand what it meant like most people do when they open the hood of their car. I really hoped that wasn't true.

Someone spoke up in the room, "Someone's watching you."

Vincent Price looked startled and looked down at me, "Holy cow, I didn't know he was awake, I have never seen him awake."

I truly didn't know if I was awake or not, but I would take any interaction I could get. I felt like an infant that had seen a shiny object that I couldn't take my eyes off of.

Thank goodness by this time I had regained my power of speech because I finally was able to clear things up once and for all concerning this machine that was both friend and foe. One day Becky was sitting by my bed and I thought this was as good a time as any to relay to her my wants, no dammitt, they were needs, as the machine taunted me with its deliciousness. My thirst was still prevalent and I couldn't stay silent any longer. I got up my nerve and asked her, "Do you think they'd give me a sweet treat?"

"What do you mean?" she asked.

Confused by her answer since there was this huge-ass Icee machine not five feet away I said, "Over there, the cherry red stuff swirling around."

She said, "No, you can't have that. You wouldn't want it."

I thought for a moment at this stonewalling and said, "But I do."

"No, Howard. That's your blood swirling in there," she said.

"What?" I asked not really knowing what she said.

"Your blood, that's a dialysis machine. It's cleaning your blood since your kidneys shut down," she said carefully, knowing I should know the truth.

I was speechless. Dialysis? Me? That's for old and sick people or people with diabetes. Not me. Not an impregnated, rebuilt guy with half his face missing and all manner of tubing sticking out of him. Can't be. I didn't want to let on how totally in the dark I was on the topic so all I said was, "Oh." I didn't know which to be more disappointed with, that I was on dialysis or that I wasn't going to be getting a sweet treat.

As I lay there with my disappointment I was still weighed down with regret over my elective surgery. I had to finally confront this monster burden by unloading it on Becky. How? She might freak out that I had broached the subject at all. I then mustered my courage and said very tentatively, "Do many people undergo the body rebuild process?"

Becky looked at me quizzically and said, "Only if you're the Six-Million-Dollar Man."

Shocked by her answer, I thought, *shit, if we can't have a serious conversation then forget it.*

***

THE NAME THAT SAVED ME

I kept hearing a name over and over again while I was in and out of consciousness: "Jeremy Sherwood." As in, "Jeremy Sherwood's the one who saved him."

"It was like a nuclear bomb going off in his body, it just doesn't happen."

"Million to one that he could have gotten this."

What the hell was this all about? When I finally awoke, my parents and Becky were raving about the doctor named Jeremy Sherwood. "He absolutely made the changes that saved your life when you needed it most."

"He was here when you were at your worst."

"He said you were minute to minute, then ten minutes to ten minutes."

"You should have seen him hit that homer over the wall for you." Wait, that was Babe Ruth.

"He's a young guy, looks a little like Doogie Howser."

"He was the one that took the reins in the ER and was the primary doctor looking over you."

"What almost got you was *Something Something Comegys* [Streptococcus Pyogenes]."

To all of this confusing chatter all I could utter weakly was, "Is he around?" as I thought at the same time, *why would former basketball great Dallas Comegys want to try and kill me?*

"No, his rotation on you ended and Dr. Rebefall took over," said Becky.

I felt like I had missed so much. Not being appreciative to someone for saving my life was really bothering me.

"I would like to meet him," I said and I didn't mean Dallas Comegys.

"We'll see what we can do," said Becky.

She asked the nurse whether Dr. Sherwood was around. "I don't think he's in the hospital today," she replied.

"If you could tell him that Howard would like to meet him that would be great."

"Okeley Dokeley Arteley Chokeley," the nurse replied. She must have been working a triple shift.

Not only was I thinking about what to say to someone that had saved my life but what was it like to come and go from the hospital as one pleased? I couldn't understand the concept of such freedom which I had taken for granted for so long. At least the word had been passed and he would come and see me. I wanted to show off my newly opened eyes and my non-Bubbles-the-Chimp mannerisms.

***

WHILE YOU WERE OUT

"David was here," my mom told me. I immediately took on a feigned expression of fear as half joke/half serious.

"When?" I asked.

"He was here that first weekend. Drove through the night to be here on Friday and stayed until Sunday," she replied.

My brother was the king of all-night driving. I don't know how he was able to stand it. No matter the time of night he would pile him, his wife, and his teenage daughter in that car and drive. I could never do that. I feared the Leatherfaces and their faux detour signs too much on the highway in the middle of the night.

As I mulled this over and the time commitment involved I had forgotten that my mom loves to dial a number and give you the phone without warning. Before I knew it she had done that to me. Without the ability to move I was caught. She said, "Leave David a message, he'd want to hear how you are."

I gathered my thoughts as I felt I was on a stage in some backwater production of *Les Miserables*. *What to do? What to say? Shall I leave a message for my brother today?*

Once the instructions to leave a message ended and the offer to leave a call back number was not answered, I spoke shakily, "Thank you so much for coming up to see me. I really appreciate it." As I continued this uncomfortable monologue I felt like I was being graded on grammar, enunciation, and might as well throw diction in there. Finally, I broke down completely and said, "I love you."

My mom took the phone away when she saw this. I continued sobbing as she said something else and hung up. I had trouble calming down after that, there were no more calls from that point on.

I felt vulnerable and emotional. I had gone through hell, and I was so happy to be around and having those around me who loved me.

***

POLLY RETURNS

There she was! Martha White…I mean Polly, back again. I heard someone exclaim upon her return, "You're back!" She was one of the best nurses and I was so thankful that everything got worked out, no thanks to me.

"I had three days off," she said to the welcoming voice.

I took this to mean that she was suspended for three days and she had to really offer a good explanation to Dr. Rebefall on why she was so derelict in her duties in not serving my ridiculous pillow fluffing demands. Such absolute power had corrupted me absolutely.

Maybe she carried a grudge. I figured it would be best not to bring it up. By this time I could talk. I had the tube removed from my mouth and so I should have said hello but I thought it would be best that she just not remember. She had to remember. Best not to remind her.

She came in a bit troubled by some problem next door. It seemed that another nurse or some lady next door required a great deal of help or was incompetent. On the other hand, it could have been a demanding relative not too keen on having Polly out of the room for too long or another troublesome footboard had introduced itself to an all too willing patient's foot. Polly didn't say anything directly to me as she adjusted and worked on something that was on my chest. I had no idea what it was; it seemed to be the central part of everyone's concern. Everyone had to snap something on it and I had no idea what "it" was. I was getting used to the myriad of colors and such coming out from under my gown so much that I could have bet that I had an amplifier plugged into my ass.

In any event, I could see the darkened figure of this old lady ambling into the room. My immediate impression was that she was too damn old to be caring for anyone. Thank goodness I didn't get her as a nurse.

I kept praising myself as being no trouble, the perfect patient except for the getting nurses fired part. However I kept wondering if Polly had noticed that it was me yet.

As the old lady was sent away with an, "I'll be there in a minute" response, Polly began to let off a little steam about the hospital or perhaps some unfair treatment that I could only assume was caused by me. I couldn't stop thinking about why she had to remind herself about all of this trouble and her changed attitude all due to me. I was already beating myself up over this, couldn't we just move on? To my relief she never brought up the suspension and I never touched that footboard again.

My parents arrived later that morning and Becky had to leave to go to work. I couldn't believe she was still holding on to that job with the incomprehensible duty of attending medical school. It was obvious that this had to be true with the amount of time she had been spending here.

As I felt simultaneously comforted and puzzled by this scenario, someone asked me if I wanted to listen to some music. My parents were as oblivious as I with this modern new marvel that was on my tray table that could actually charge your Ipod while it played so it wouldn't die after thirty minutes. I had never seen anything like that in my life. Polly looked at it for a second and said, "This is new."

I laughed or I thought I did. I didn't want to send her into a rage after our history. *Be Cool Hoovie*, I thought to myself.

"My husband's better at this stuff than me," she said.

"What does he do?" my mom asked.

"He works in sports for a local media outlet," she said.

That raised the question in my own mind, *what do I do?* Perhaps her husband was a sports blogger or something. Who was to say? She didn't really add much to her statement to make my foggy mind think of anything else, except that I could have blogged a few things about the Panthers' latest playoff disaster against Larry Fitzgerald.

Polly tried a few buttons and was getting frustrated. She then tried the remote. Nothing seemed to respond, it was just like that damn Walkman that Becky had in the stairwell of the White House. Polly must have known the problems this thing caused. She had been there sweeping up as her other persona, Martha White, in her gingham dress.

As none of this background information seemed to pierce the scene, Polly held the clock radio/Ipod player in both hands out in front of her in a pleading fashion and said, "I can save your life, but I cannot work this thing."

I had to laugh and said, "Becky's the keeper of that thing, I have never seen it in my life."

She pushed a button on the Ipod and said, "Oh, it's working. What would you like to listen to? One of your playlists?"

"Okely Dokely Artichokely," I said. What the hell was wrong with me? I hadn't worked a third shift.

She began at the top of the list and said in an unsure voice, *Aunt Ellen's Favorites*?

At this I started really laughing. I was embarrassed yet humored. *Aunt Ellen's Favorites* was something I had set up before all this happened. There was some sort of connection to my past and *Aunt Ellen's Favorites* was it! There was reality here. *Aunt Ellen's Favorites* certainly wouldn't come to me in an alternate universe. Once this realization drifted over me I was so relieved I couldn't stop laughing but was rather embarrassed that my "humor" had seeped through the fog. Aunt Ellen was my dad's sister and she always had this persona of having a good time. Somehow I had collected all of these crooner/big band CDs over time so I had figured her formative years were when this music was popular; ergo, I had all of this music on one playlist, Aunt Ellen's Favorites. I had to say, "No," though to playing it, I didn't want to be put in the geriatric ward. However, maybe I should have because whenever I think back or do an impression of Aunt Ellen I cannot help but be in a good mood.

Not waiting for this internal monologue of mine to resolve itself, Polly instead pushed "Most Played" which was a bit dirgy yet not so embarrassing. "Aunt Ellen's Favorites" would have been better. At least it did break my perceived icy relations with Polly and all seemed to be coming together in the world.

***

SIT UP STRAIGHT

During one of my physical therapy sessions Mike attempted to do the impossible and had a surprise for me at the end of the session. With all the on-the-back time I had been through this was easier said than done. After the usual leg and shoulder exercises he said, "Now let's get you to a seated position."

Before I had a chance to object to this cruel advance in my treatment I was pulled up in the bed. I was being held nonetheless; I just was not in love with this position. As expected, my neck was not on board and my head kind of just hung there with my chin attempting to find a comfortable resting spot on my chest.

Mike lifted my chin with his hand. My head didn't want to follow and I was losing energy fast. He said, "Now lift that head up to get some air into those lungs, now doesn't that feel better?"

I nodded weakly hoping this would end soon. It did not feel better though. I felt like a whale out of the water. The forces of gravity were too much for my body which was accustomed to being flat. I could see his point, but I would have preferred hiring this task out.

After a few seconds of this attempt I was laid down gingerly in the bed.

***

WHEN ARE WE LANDING?

That incessant humming was beginning to get to me. There was no way that wasn't from the plane. I could see only sky out the window so that was enough proof for me that we were flying and landing periodically but I was in a hospital so how could a hospital be in the air?

Maybe it was. My question would of course be treated with disdain so I best just keep silent. Perhaps it lifted itself all on its own during the night and landed in the same place day after day. This seemed like a lot of effort and for what gain?

I was confused as I tried to pry apart the puzzle of the floating hospital. The whole thing made no sense. I concluded that I might as well accept that I was somewhere in the mountains in a hospital that flies at night and get on with being inside it.

One morning around dawn I was getting very antsy and was wondering when we would be landing finally. We were in the air for what seemed like hours. Of course, I had nowhere to be or to do and I certainly would not be leaving after it landed. However, I was a bit alarmed that Becky had to leave sometime that day to look after our supposed children who I was still not at all certain existed. I didn't know if they were just telling me what I wanted to hear.

I finally drummed up my courage and asked, "When do we land?" I had the fear that I was really stepping out on a limb here asking questions and being bothersome.

Becky replied, "What? We aren't flying."

I was shocked, absolutely shocked. All this time I thought we were flying. I was relieved but frustrated at the same time because I had worked the entire thing out in my head. I was just certain that we were flying. What else would explain that incessant noise and all of our travels? I was still skeptical yet my expression was one of acceptance. I was in an ordinary hospital that did not fly at all. Just a building? That just sits there? What's the point of that? I could not accept this so I asked again only this time in my head, *got it, but really, when do we land? We have been floating around for hours.*

***

THE DOG PEOPLE SLEEP TONIGHT[91]

I was down, just depressed, lying there. My adventures had been coming back and were colliding inside of me. As I rolled everything I had been through over in my head, my thoughts landed on the Dog People and what they must be doing now. Were they after me? Were they plotting to find me? Certainly they were still pissed at me for whatever I did. I couldn't leave it. I couldn't get out of that horrible place I had been in.

After a while Becky noticed my troubled look and said, "Howard, what's the matter? It looks like something's bothering you."

I didn't know how to come out and say it gingerly since she was in danger too, but I just had to say it, "I'm thinking about the Dog People."

There was a long silence from her and then she asked, "What Dog People?"

Oh, poor thing is suppressing the memory. Certainly she must know. She fought them off with me. It was so clear or perhaps she had her own name for them such as "Canis Humanoidis." However, I was taken aback that the self-titled description that should have said it all only added to the confusion in the air. I replied, "The Dog People that attacked us in the cave."

"Nothing like that happened," she said puzzlingly. I didn't remember her being so talented at forcing horrible moments from her memory. I sat there in silence and stared at the wall.

Later in the day a therapist came in the room to see how I was doing.

"How's everything going?" she asked.

"Good, getting back to normal," I replied.

Becky added, "He has had some concerns about Dog People coming to get him."

Without missing a beat the therapist said, "It's the hospital's policy not to allow Dog People past the lobby."

I was so relieved by this and she answered so quickly that she must have had to deal with them before. The Dog People, if they ever found me, would be stopped by some surly security guard in the lobby in a blue blazer holding a radio very authoritatively. I felt my body relax at this news, but I was still concerned about them milling about down there perhaps looking for knick knacks in the gift shop just waiting for my release. That was for another day. As long as I could be assured that the next being I saw round the corner was not going to be emitting a squealish chatter and ready to scratch me the hell up, I knew I could relax.

Now, it was time to worry about those Native American boys with the broken glass. *C'mon you little fuckers, show me what ya got!* Bravado getting me in trouble again.

***

LOOK INTO THIS FOOTBOARD NOW, TELL ME WHAT YOU SEE[92]

"Hey come over here, you need to see something," I said to Becky.

Although my airplane theory and my Dog People theory were untrue, and the jury was still out on the body rebuild and male impregnation theory all of which I still had a difficult time coming to terms with, I knew my ace in the hole, the footboard, would prove my sanity. It was there in black and blue, a screen of incredible information and power. Flight information, ancestral records, and the ability to fire people just with the tap of a foot. It had it all. I was now in a position to relay this information to Becky. Perhaps she could help me unlock its secrets. Since we were alone in the room I could confide in her lest they take away my secret weapon. She certainly wouldn't tell on me. My earth shattering discovery taken away? No way.

I motioned my head over to the footboard. It was ready to give information. I could sense it. She simply had to see this. She got up from her chair and walked over to the side of my bed.

I said with great anticipation in seeing her reaction to this wonderful marvel, "You have to see this."

"What?" she said.

I tapped my foot on the footboard, it was my magic wand. "Down there. Don't you see? The screen tells all about our family."

She looked at the tiny screen on the footboard and announced, "It says 'Instaflate Activated.'"

I looked from her to the screen, I couldn't believe it. I thought, *Instaflate Activated? What does that mean?* "What does that mean?" I repeated out loud.

"It means the bed's inflating, you're on an air mattress. That just means its working," she replied. She looked back at me hoping I was kidding, and if I wasn't that my disappointment didn't take too much of an ugly turn.

I kept looking at the screen. It did say it. "Instaflate Activated." I was crushed and could only mutter an, "Oh." I couldn't believe that the bed would hide its secrets from others when I needed it the most. There was nothing special about any of this. The wool was literally pulled from my eyes. The bed never offered up any secret tidbits after that, it was pissed off with me since I betrayed its confidence. I was hurt because the magic of the bed was gone and I felt I had lost a friend.

***

GIVE IT TO ME STRAIGHT

Dr. Rebefall was back again one morning to check me over during his rounds. Once again the socks were pulled off as he examined my feet. Everything was still a purplish hue, and I was beginning to realize that the longer they stayed that color the worse things looked.

Becky came to the bedside as the exam continued.

After looking them over closely he finally spoke, "It's a shame, looks like you're going to lose that toe….."

I couldn't believe it, *why? WHY!? WHY!?*

While I assumed his sentence was finished he continued, "…… nail."

***

MY FUNNY VALENTINE I[93]

The activity in the room was a funny thing, it ebbed and flowed like the tides. At times I felt like no one knew that I was there and at others it was like you had to take a number to see me. Usually it was the physical therapists that would come in when the bevy of activity was at its peak and they would need to return. Mike came in one such day and had to leave when he saw that I was being poked and prodded. I wanted to progress and get out of here and the only way that was going to happen was the passage of time and tolerating the things that they had to do to me. However, it was difficult to see the doctor come in and the TV go off, because that meant there was business to be had. I would really grow alarmed when the curtain would be pulled around the bed. That sound of those curtain rings sliding on the curtain rod sent shivers through me. It still does when I take a shower. *Psycho* has nothing on it. If someone needs privacy in the MICU, a place that sees everything, then something serious is going to happen.

Mike finally got his turn with me and began working me over. Things were harder than ever especially since I was now awake more and more and I could sense my own mortality and weak body. It was quite discouraging. He would expect me to push on this or that or bend my leg this way or that. My legs looked like spaghetti, my arms looked like spaghetti. Whatever had happened to me, it appeared like my body was rejecting my new limbs from the rebuilding and his job was to clean up the mess, which I thought was impossible. For the thousandth time I thought, *again, why did I do that body rebuild?*

On this day he had me sit up on the side of the bed for a moment. This seemed as large a task as raising the Titanic in that movie, *Raise the Titanic!* Thankfully that was all I was expected to do was sit there, and it hurt like hell. I was fully awake for this moment and I did not like it. As my head flopped forward uselessly on my atrophied neck, Mike encouraged me to raise my chin as he put his finger under it to raise it.

He said, "Now see if you can raise your head and straighten your torso to really get that air into your lungs."

I did it, but I didn't like it. It was terrible.

"There, now doesn't that feel better?" he asked confidently.

Hell no! I thought.

On this visit he looked like he was deep in thought after our session. I had no idea what day it was, or month, the date, or even the year. Was he discouraged or encouraged by the day's performance?

He said, "Valentine's Day's coming up, have you thought about getting anything for your wife?"

No! I thought, *it's Valentine's Day already! It was just Christmas! Where has the time gone?*

As Becky will attest I am not good with holidays with Valentine's being the worst. I am still recovering from Christmas and thinking of stuff to get her and the Babies and everyone else if that memory was really true when this holiday comes up from nowhere and my gift idea queue is exhausted. I know it's there and I know it's coming up but maybe if I ignore it, it will go away. I like doing the giving once it's done, it's just that thinking of new creative things makes my head hurt. That's why romantic comedies make me nervous when outlandish creativity grows horns and a tail and makes all of us shlubs look like brain dead bodies. And now when I am at my absolute weakest in a location that still has yet to be determined, I still cannot get away from this holiday.

Mike continued, "I think you're making progress so I have been thinking that a wonderful Valentine's gift to your wife will be to walk across the room to her and hand her a flower."

There were so many things wrong with this picture. *First of all look at me, so unless it's February 15 and you are talking about next year then fine but there is no way that I'm going to be able to do what you are saying. Second, I am going to look like some weirdo and freak her out like that large insect that was trying to become a human at the end of Mimic II, and by the way that ending is testament to why there* was no *Mimic III*. [Unfortunately, I found out later that there is indeed a *Mimic III*.]

He continued unabated, "I'm going to talk it over with my team and see if we can make that happen."

As he finished up he looked up at the TV over my bed and then looked around for something to write on. He took some brown paper towels from the dispenser and wrote on those.

That didn't look too official. I guessed this hospital didn't provide notebooks; maybe there was an embossing station on the floor. I just hoped he wasn't writing down a reminder about Valentine's Day and to see *Mimic II*.

CHAPTER 23

Field Trip

Chest radiographs and arterial blood analysis should be obtained following initial stabilization. These studies are used in combination with other clinical parameters to diagnose acute lung injury (ALI) or acute respiratory distress syndrome (ARDS), which frequently complicate sepsis.[94]

THANK YOU FOR THAT SMILE UPON YOUR FACE[95]

Becky popped in one morning like a ray of sunshine after having seen the Babies off to school and said, "I heard a new song on the radio that made me think of you, I have it here and thought you might like to hear it."

For some reason my musical tastes run 15 years behind the times with any group that I have never heard of. They have to age like a fine wine or a foul smelling cheese for me to begin to appreciate them. I know it's crazy, but it's true. God, I just quoted Christopher Cross. So with that attitude I have resisted Becky trying to get me to listen to anything post 1994 except U2 and those Smashing Pumpkins, they're going places. In my weakened state I agreed.

What she played was the Jason Mraz song *Lucky* featuring Colbie Callet.

The song's opening lines, "Do you hear me, talking to you?" immediately struck me as my time being in a nowhere state.

And Colbie's reply, "Boy I hear you in my dreams" (except I'm the boy not the girl) followed by "Lucky to be coming home again," sent tears to my eyes.

It was all true and hit home. Like David St. Hubbins said in *This is Spinal Tap* as they stood around Elvis's grave: "It's a little too much fucking perspective." I still love hearing that song and it takes me back to that time and that place that I physically never want to be again.

***

HOW DO YOU SLEEP?[96]

I would really feel left out when the announcement would come from whoever was visiting that now was the time for them to get something to eat. *I love that, go off and eat in some fancy restaurant with champagne flowing and socialize*, I would think bitterly.

There would be a large oak-paneled banquet hall where they would sit as they swilled their wine and ate their at one time cover-laden dishes before the floor show began, "Wish you could be here now Howard!"

The pattern was usually this: they, whoever it was, would go off to eat at 7:00 p.m. maybe it was 7:00 a.m. I don't know because time had no meaning in here and the penguin with the swinging wings on the clock wasn't yipping the time anymore either. Lazy bastard. So if it was 7:00 p.m., they were going to take their sweet-ass time with all of the ribaldry and saunter back into the room at 9:00 p.m. This was the part that got interesting with the question, "Then what?" Did I need to receive them again? By this time I wished they would just stay away. It seemed when I needed them they weren't there, and then when they were there I could not get rid of them. As one could imagine, this was a rather confusing situation and I was very pissed off about this conflicted state.

My mood took a turn for the better as I could make out Becky over there, sitting, taking it all in. She was there, I knew it, watching. That made me feel better, more secure. When the moment of departure would come and they had gone on to dinner, I would just continue to stare at the wall.

When they would return, and it would feel like they were gone for hours, they would usually say, "You're still not asleep, you must sleep."

The possibility was just not there; it hadn't been there for quite some time.

I said, "Enjoy your meal?" and added in my thoughts, *great I enjoyed lying here doing nothing. God, I cannot wait to get the hell out of here.*

***

I PROMISE YOU ANYTHING, GET ME OUT OF THIS HELL[97]

There was a general ruckus going on. I couldn't tell if there was anyone in the room with me or not, be it family, friend, or Dog Person. I had a feeling that I might be headed somewhere on a field trip. It was late afternoon and it seemed I had to get somewhere before the end of the business day. It all seemed so exciting. There was Polly going around talking on her cell phone frantically trying to arrange something for me. I was to be taken somewhere and I didn't know where.

Could I be getting discharged now? My, the wonder of it all! I might be home tonight lying somewhere. I didn't give a damn if I was unable to do anything but lie there, it would be better than here. I wanted to go home! Hooray!

Polly still talked on her cell phone, which I by now realized, was not from 1980. It was from today and possessed 2009's latest technology offering. I always liked the way the nurses' pockets would glow when someone would be trying to call them.

As Polly spoke it sounded like I was needed somewhere and I would be taken there very soon. She got off the phone and began to pack stuff onto my bed. I guessed I would be staying on my old reclining friend for this trip since gravity seemed to be a bit too much for me to overcome at the moment, but my spirits did rise a little if nothing else. It felt like a knife had been cut through the boredom that had surrounded me. I had never been out of this room, at least not that I knew of; it was going to be wonderful to see the scenery that went on backstage. However, it seemed my bed would be a bit of a challenge as it had been the scourge of all that had tried to move me. Some sort of braking system had been installed on this bed that proved unfamiliar to all that touched it. Polly messed with it for a while after unhooking and re-hooking my various tubes and such so that I would be completely mobile. There was so much work involved to ready me and so much she had to take care of that I felt awful that I couldn't help out or at least point at different areas. I'm a skilled pointer.

Although my ability to speak had returned by this time, I had no idea what to say. I realized that none of my family was there, nor

Becky. I had no idea where anyone was and what they would think when I wasn't here. Worry filled my thoughts about their reaction and where I was going, but I had complete faith in Polly and she made those thoughts vanish.

Polly pushed my bed toward the hallway and there it was, the outside of my room. Backstage! Wonderful! I hoped I was allowed out here and that the doctors knew that I was going somewhere official.

Polly placed a small monitor on my bed which was the first time I got a glimpse of the screen that everyone had been looking at all this time. It was a multicolored wonderland of sights and sounds and I had no idea what it was reading. She then put a binder that seemed to dwarf the biggest encyclopedia I had ever seen on the bed by my feet. That was mine? What the hell was that? Was I in that much trouble and pain? I knew it was serious but good Lord what had I done to myself to cause such a treatise to be written about me? This having my body rebuilt business certainly caused a lot of paperwork for everyone. Not to mention the file from the evil Manhattan hospital which must look like some cracked leather-bound *Necronomicon*.

Other questions filled my head such as, *who put the chart together? Where does the stationery come from?* I had a lot of other uninteresting questions to ask as one could see; I was just happy my foot wasn't crushed by it.

We started making our way down the hallway. This was fun for me but I didn't think Polly was having a good time with the cursed braking system. I didn't care. Well, I did, because it was Polly. However, whatever empathy I had for Polly at this time was brushed away by the sense of freedom this trip offered. I felt like a prisoner on yard time. I would take any of this at any moment even though I had no idea where we were going. I wished everyone could see me out of the room. Where was everyone?

Suddenly Polly had a tough time going up an incline in the hallway when who should suddenly appear but MIKE! He was there looking like he was about to head home with a bag over his shoulder. He got behind the bed and helped push me over the incline and we were rolling. I hadn't seen Mike in a while; I hoped he was not disappointed that I was not walking yet and my Valentine trip across the floor would probably be a bust. *I swear Mike, I have been working. I'm just not doing it now because I have to get someplace hopefully that's tons of fun as you can see*, I thought.

We headed toward the elevator and I continued to see familiar faces. There was life going on beyond my door. I felt better about this already and my spirits were really lifting. There was that doctor I had seen with the *Cold Case* hair talking to someone; everyone looked at me in amazement. They were all calling my name like I was Bud Fox heading into the office in *Wall Street* except I didn't have any funny quips for them like, "Great Carolyn, doing any better would be a sin...", "Takes one to know one," or "Shut up!"

We headed down the elevator with a couple of other doctors and nurses. Small talk was had. With the small talk, I felt like I was part of the group. You folks here in Winston-Salem are indeed the best. I didn't know why I thought I was in Winston-Salem and when that changed from South Dakota. Charlotte still was outside the realm of possibilities as my location. I guessed I needed to get better wherever that may be so, I resolved myself to just being quiet and letting it happen.

The elevator stopped somewhere and with a shove we were out in a hallway with no natural light. We must have been in the basement hopefully and not the mortuary. Polly, my bed, and I headed to a door that opened in two opposite directions and entered this room with this loud continuous humming noise.

I am usually pretty good at tracking segues when the topic changes in a conversation, but I have no idea how this subject came up or what prompted it. Polly began to relay a story to someone about what happened at her house recently. It was obvious that she really had it on her mind since she was finally at a point to wait and recover from the tasks that had to be completed to get me down here. She relayed to those of us present that recently, while she was inside reading to one of her daughters, an eight-year-old boy was playing out in the back yard with her youngest daughter who is five. Polly said she looked up and the boy had pulled down her daughter's pants and she was flabbergasted as to what to do. She knew the parents and a get-together was coming up in the neighborhood and she had no idea how to handle the situation.

I was just looking back and forth at the conversation that was occurring over me from my familiar spot face up on the bed like I was at a tennis match. The story was stopped at that point when whatever it was we were waiting for was finally available for me. I was rolled into this room with these enormous machines with digital readouts all over them.

I found the digital artwork on the screen to look a bit dated from my judgmental place and with a totally unqualified opinion of medical equipment. I was still convinced that we were in Winston-Salem. We had come out of the mountains and I was slowly getting back to Charlotte but I wasn't quite there yet. So I dismissed the equipment as being too dated and was certain that Charlotte had better and more up to date facilities. I went so far as to compare it to the tool shed size machine into which Dr. Bruce Banner inserts himself at the opening of *The Incredible Hulk* TV series. Perhaps I might have had the privilege of turning into the Hulk after this if I was only in Charlotte. However, I realized I was getting angry enough over my short bed and my feet hanging off of it that I didn't need whatever poison that machine had up its sleeve. I kept thinking that I must not show my disapproval or discomfort since any scowls on my part would set me back two weeks. This must be true, or I might end up be being held here as a permanent mascot.

There were two men in white scrubs that greeted Polly inside the room. My bed and I were treated the same: indifference. Strangely though, after this greeting I suddenly felt very protective of Polly and did not trust these guys since she was the only woman in the room. I hoped they treated her with the full respect she deserved. I don't know why I was sensitive about that or protective of her, but she was my nurse and I didn't want anyone mistreating her. As one could see, if anything did happen I was in no way, shape, or form to do anything about it, unless that machine's dial was turned to "Hulk" or even "Moderately Fit Male" and please not "Effeminate Curtis."

The two men in scrubs lifted/rolled me off my bed and stuck me on a smaller gurney. "Have you been busy today?" Polly asked them.

"Yeah, it's been a very long day," one of the men answered. "You're the last one," he said to her but was really meaning me.

It felt very basementy in there like I was at the center of the earth. I had no clue where I was and there was no one there except Polly that I knew so it felt very much like a road game for me. I was rolled to the center of the room and the constant humming of the machines continued.

I had no idea what was going on or what was happening. This certainly did not look like the exit to the hospital but a glorious internal field trip. I was feeling a little anxious and had no idea what I was there for. All I could do was look at the ceiling and hope that this wasn't the end of my time here on earth. Maybe it had been explained to me dozens of times, I could not be sure. There was some reason why I was there, and I had to believe that it was for my benefit. Polly wouldn't trick me.

I was placed on my side since I was unable to do so under my own power. My shoulder was in immense pain due to all muscle having disappeared since this all began.

One of the two men examined my side after my gown had been pulled up and all dignity had flown out of the room. Who was I kidding, that had happened long before this. There was something of interest going on there.

"This may hurt a bit," the man said.

I became very aware of an immense pain in my side that continued until I felt the sensation of something inside me being moved around.

Polly came over to my side and said to me reassuringly, "He's good at doing this, it'll be over in a second."

I was then rolled to my other side and the same procedure was done with the same level of pain. *This isn't a fun field trip at all*, I thought half in jest but I wasn't really feeling the jest.

After the pain had diminished they raised my arms and put them over my head. I was very aware at how stiff I had become and how the muscles go on vacation without any movement. It had been weeks since I had done anything like this and it was a very depressing feeling. My arms wouldn't even go over my head without some encouragement from one of the men. I thought my arms were going to be ripped out as I grimaced and gritted my teeth as they resisted all movement. I couldn't allow myself to yell since I was still paranoid about being locked up in the hospital for the foreseeable future if I protested.

The gurney along with me, its unwilling passenger, was then shoved into the tube with the Dr. Bruce Banner digital readings on it. Some may feel claustrophobic in those tubes, but I felt safe since I knew they couldn't jab me with anything while I was in there unless it was a special jabbing machine.

Whatever they needed at the time was registered after several minutes in the machine and I was removed and rolled out of it. It takes so long in those machines that sometimes I wonder if I am part of some prank where the theme is "Let's see how long this guy will stay in this thing before he says something."

One of the men in the white scrubs then began to talk to Polly about what had been done and how successful it was. All of this talk was beyond me. I felt no responsibility toward it even though it was my body. There was just a blank space inside me as if they were talking about someone's car that was in the shop and it had blown a gasket. I had no strength and I continued to stare at the man in the white scrubs since there was no other place my eyes could comfortably gaze without looking like I was deranged. I began to study his face, and as if the power of my stare made him notice me he stopped talking and looked down at me briefly. Why would my stare work here and not with the parade of red-head nurses? He looked quite shocked and uncomfortable that there was a human lying there awake as if I had just popped into the room. He pulled away from my gaze and continued talking to Polly. I suddenly noticed that I had been rudely staring and looked away. Getting caught in a stare is embarrassing, so it was good to see that I was still aware of some social graces.

With the threat of the poking and prodding over, I was taken to a side room where Polly continued the story of her daughter to a young male that was fiddling with my gurney absentmindedly as he heard the tale. I just looked on as the two of them discussed this and I could not help but feel like I should have some input and pushed my brain to the limits should I be called upon. With two young daughters of my own or at least I thought I had two daughters, this act would have concerned me as well. With the recent prodding of my sides I was doubly annoyed and could only think of scare tactics as the solution. One of my favorites was finding a big kid in the neighborhood with a big dog, and to instruct the two of them to scare the hell out of this kid. Sort of an evil Shaggy and unreasonably insane Scooby Doo.

The young guy began to put his two cents in, and he was greatly annoyed as well. He insisted that Polly should not tolerate that and go straight to the parents in so many words. I was prepared with my answer when Polly finally looked down at me, and asked, "What should I do?"

I was struck dumb with being included in the conversation, and all of my piss and vinegar was taken away. I choked out a lame, "It's a tough situation, I don't really know." As only a woefully ineffective diplomat could. She then nodded, and looked disappointed that I had no solution to her problem. The evil Shaggy and unreasonably insane Scooby never got a shot. It was a solution that would have worked in the 70s and no one would have been the wiser, but in these times I guess it might be the lead story in the local news.

Finally, Polly rolled me back up to my room; it was around 6:00 p.m. and almost the end of her shift. Dinner time for normal people but no such thing for me I guessed, since I had the feeding tube. I hadn't eaten anything in weeks, and I still had no appetite. She rolled me back and I was in a hallway waiting for something to happen. I was just hoping that the field trip was over. This rabbit wanted to get back to his cage.

She looked down at me and leaned over the gurney to reassure me with a caring look. At that moment I thought my friends and family were all around. I don't know why, but when she asked, "How are you doing? Are you OK?" I did this face that I used to do when I was a kid with my brother David, sort of a Joker "let's kill Batman" Face. So I wasn't comfortable with offering a solution to her problem, but I was comfortable making this face? What the fuck was wrong with me? I thought it would get a big laugh since everyone was there and the appropriate audience would certainly appreciate it. Polly's reaction was one of dismay and shock as she quickly stood upright. Not the reaction she was expecting, and I was flabbergasted that I made the face. I guess I was feeling psychotically loose and needed some levity at that moment. Then again, all she had done for me and I had to make a shocking face. I don't even know if I had my glasses on but I could see her reaction clearly. Realizing what I had done, I tried to salvage the situation with an, "I'm doing OK." She nodded and said, "Good." And I was wheeled back to the room.

I don't think Polly was my nurse again after that and I was very disappointed that she wasn't. She was a great nurse and I had full confidence in her. She was a true advocate of mine. That was a wonderful field trip and it seemed she had gotten things moving with that adventure. Too bad our time together ended with my Evil Clown face.

***

DOCTOR, DOCTOR, GIVE ME THE NEWS[98]

Someone please answer this pressing question I have of why someone needs an infectious disease doctor to undo the shoddy body rebuild and male impregnation he had done by a shoddy doctor? The news of this need came to me in the form of an older doctor, whose name

I didn't quite get and had forgotten in no time, but he said he was the infectious disease doctor. I thought this was perhaps some connection my parents had to get me out sooner and needless to say a gross overreaction. At least they were trying to do something for me.

The doctor mentioned basketball in North Carolina. My mom is from North Carolina and my parents met at Wake Forest University so there must have been a connection between them and the doctor I supposed. Where was he from? The CDC? Was the CDC that interested in my case? I had so many doctors in here I could not keep them straight, but infectious disease? I didn't know how each one knew what the other was doing. They seemed to like to examine me. I thought they were quite the reactionaries. It was similar to Alice or Carol Brady's reaction when one of the Brady kids sneezed, their asses were bedridden for a week. Hopelessly depressing. All I could say was let them have their fun; my rebuilt impregnated body knew the real answer.

Two infectious disease doctors traded shifts on me. One was older as I mentioned, I saw him only once. He was very boisterous and the other was younger, he looked like a resident from Scrubs with a receding hairline. He was more low key and I saw a lot of him. He would come in and see my Ipod docking station and comment, "You seem to be set in the way of electronics."

I replied with a weak, "Yes," but really wasn't sure how all that stuff had found its way in here.

The younger one usually came in in the morning and would take his time washing his hands in the sink, turning his head to look at me while he did. I guessed it was just to get a sense of what condition I was in and not to see if I was going to attack him with a sock full of pennies.

I wondered as I returned his look what it must feel like to have water running over one's hands? Why did I take that for granted at one time? If I did ever get out of here I would always revel in the feeling of being able to wash my hands.

The older doctor examined me and talked to me about my likes and dislikes. I had no idea what I liked but I knew what I didn't like and that was being in there.

"Do you follow basketball?" he asked me.

"Not really, some pro," I replied feeling like I had been living under a rock.

He sounded like a big Duke fan, because he said that once he went to a Duke game he was smitten and he always followed Duke from then on. He was passionate about it; however what I really wanted to know was when I was going to get the hell out of there. No one really seemed to have an answer but would come in and look and would leave me hanging. I was afraid to ask and feared the answer to the point where I was content to remain ignorant. I still had no idea why an infectious disease doctor was around me during my stay there. You could explain it and explain it; I just was not going to get it.

Of course I must say during this time the amount of doctors that saw me was quite astonishing. I had neurologists, nephrologists, pulmonologists, cardiologists, the infectious disease doctors, and the doctor that coordinated my physical therapy. I don't recall a vibeologist or alchemist. All that brain power was working on me. Before this happened I had only been in the hospital to get my appendix out, and now I was here with these fine minds in sort of an open-ended situation. I stumped them and I stumped myself, but at least I was alive to see the show.

LIKE A HOOK

Even though the power of voice had been returned to me, I was still unable to relay my displeasure later that day. My head was full of opinions; however, my voice didn't seem to find the words to relay the message. The displeasure stemmed from these tubes that were still in my sides. Lord knows why they were there. It must have been some method in keeping my legs attached. I guess that evil hospital didn't just use adhesive.

Dr. Rebefall came into the room and said, "We're slowly unplugging and that continues today."

Forgetting I had a voice I just stared. I was now finding out that sometimes it's better to have an excuse not to speak like, *because I have this tube sticking in my fucking mouth!* or something just as poignant.

My Ipod docking thingie was playing the Eagles in my room in a continuous cycle ala *Speed* all morning. It seemed to be stuck on this playlist and I just was unable to move from my familiar position of perpetual stillness to change it, and even had I been able to my hands felt like a big bunch of bananas and would not have been up to the task. Who put it on the Eagles in perpetuity? It must have been that Yahoo Serious guy skulking around here again with his stickers. It depressed me and made me think of the times when I was able to accomplish simple tasks. However, the excitement to have my voice back and the notion that I would not be going through a Coco the sign language gorilla/white board/eye blinking communication phase lifted me out of those thoughts.

Dr. Rebefall had me lie on my side, a motion that was still akin to moving heaven and earth and which was quite excruciating. My shoulders were no more, I was just lying on bone and to stay upright like that was just killing me.

He examined my sides, looked them over and finally said, "It's about time these came out, we had better see about it."

With that he left the room and I thought nothing much of it. Since it was daylight and I was keeping the hours of a vampire, I somehow was able to fall asleep. I was awakened shortly thereafter by Dr. Rebefall. He was with another doctor and Teresa was standing by his side looking on. I was asked to roll onto my side again where the shoulder pain began immediately like before.

"Take a look at this," Dr. Rebefall said to the other doctor. "How would you go about getting this out?"

I was in pain on my side hoping they could resolve this soon, balancing like this was a feat of physics.

The other doctor was I assumed a surgeon and was young. He was tall, well, everyone was tall to me, had a goatee and glasses and was a little overweight. He said, "You have to grab it, it's like taking a hook out of a fish. Be careful. If you don't get it just right, then it'll slide back in and you'll have a real problem."

Dr. Rebefall looked on with his serious gaze taking it all in. He seemed like he was stern but that was only a reaction to the seriousness of my situation, and I knew he was kicking ass to get me out of there. He said, "Very well, thanks," and added to no one in particular, "We might as well do it now."

The other doctor left and it suddenly dawned on me that Dr. Rebefall was going to be handling this by himself. I thought to myself and I am glad that I didn't say, "Wait, why can't that guy do it?"

I was nervous and I was hoping that Dr. Rebefall did not have my attention span because I know me, and one time hearing something and then doing it two seconds later, well, I didn't like to think what the consequences would be, especially adding anxiety into the mix. At this point I was projecting my ability and confidence on everyone else, which really amounted to nothing. At least my mind was getting a steady nervous workout. Waking up and having a voice was a good start. It still didn't mean I was out of the woods; there was much left to be done. Apprehension, my old friend, enveloped me more and more with each passing day since I was awake to see this stuff happen and not in South Dakota where the Dog People were pricks, but at least predictable.

Dr. Rebefall turned to Teresa and told her to get various instruments that had very specific names and were in a different language: a scooper, a gouger, a doodle, and a Doogie Howser. Teresa procured these items and came back to the room. I kept reassuring myself that at least this wasn't the dentist's office.

As Dr. Rebefall examined my sides he noticed the music that had been playing non-stop by this point and remarked, "The Eagles? You're really dating yourself here, Howard."

It was playing *Desperado* from 1972. Too bad *The Long Run* wasn't on, at least that's from 1979 and is relatively recent?

I was irked by this comment. My wit gauge was running on empty and I just said a lame, "Yeah." When I should have said, "Yeah, but I remember when I was in high school in the mid-80s I proclaimed, 'No more albums by ex-Eagles please!' Too bad I didn't realize it was such a golden age with the *Smugglers Blues, Building the Perfect Beast* and *The Confessor* becoming the soundtrack of my senior year." Match

Point, Howard. Come to think of it, had I said all that they may have gotten the restraints out.

As I lay there staring at this dried phlegm on the side of the bed that the last patient must have left and that I had just now noticed, the thought finally dawned on me that this was going to be done here. Right now. In the room. Why couldn't Dr. Goatee be doing this?

I tried to keep my brave face on as I heard those cursed curtain rings rubbing against the curtain rod as it was drawn. I guess pain was the name of the game at this point. I was still not used to it. Teresa tried to comfort me, "He's good, this won't take long at all."

After a local anesthetic was applied to the spot he did something that caused the same amount of pain that I had experienced prior to my Bruce Banner experiment in the basement. I was just hoping that the guy that had adjusted the tube had done it correctly. That seemed like years ago. Funny how I thought I was being released then, I was so far from that.

The good thing about the pain in my sides was that it took my mind off the pain in my shoulders. Like a fish hook indeed, now I knew what a fish felt like. I was still shocked that these tubes were inside me. I was worried. What good was worry, especially now, when everything was beyond my control. After a little while, the first tube came out so I was happy that Dr. Rebefall had neither my attention span nor nerves. Now it was time for the other side. I feared lying on my other side and snapping that shoulder. Hopefully Dr. Rebefall was getting better at this and I hoped I was easier than a carp. The pain was immense in my sides as if someone was placing a drill into it as I grimaced and ground my teeth. This side may have been quicker but it didn't feel like it.

It was over and I was laid on my back once again, another step was behind me. I never saw the tubes or knew how big they were and there was no disturbing collection that I wanted them to be a part of. I later learned they served a vital function in getting my fever to go down by draining the fluid that had collected between my lungs and my sides or so I was told and not to keep my legs attached. Where this fluid went I had no idea. As always I chose ignorance over unpleasant knowledge, never to be denied my ignorance.

CHAPTER 24

Questionable Freedom

The complications of TSS are severe. They include bacteremia, acute respiratory distress syndrome (ARDS), disseminated intravascular coagulation, and renal failure.[99]

HIGHLY RECOMMEND IT TO PEOPLE YOU DON'T LIKE

Why won't someone protect me from myself? It was getting late in the MICU. Night had come a few hours earlier and lo and behold outside it was dead winter dark. As usual, the night brought fear and the unknown to the MICU. It felt like anything could get me and anything could happen. I would will myself to stay awake so nobody or nothing would catch me off guard. Once I had gotten the new-found freedom of flipping channels, I was able to keep the night at bay for a while. Nothing could keep me from flipping now that I knew that I would not get into trouble for doing so. As I flipped past the talking heads, smug ESPN broad necks, and whatever the hell Fucking Octomom was up to, I finally came upon a black-and-white movie that looked intriguing. Gregory Peck was in a bedroom with a woman that appeared to be Audrey Hepburn, who was asleep and she would not wake up. Perhaps she had had her body rebuilt too. I did not understand the set up but I stayed on the channel only because some commercial hadn't popped up and my, this looked rather saucy for black and white and appeared to be taking place in Rome.

Around ten o'clock my parents came in to see me and my dad sat down in the chair to take in my discovery. "What are you watching?" he asked.

"Something that looks intriguing. I can't seem to turn away from it," I replied.

We continued to watch it and it dawned on me how weird it was that we were watching TV under these circumstances. I was feeling much more relaxed at this point, and I thought I was out of the woods which comparatively speaking I was, but when you are still in the MICU I guess you aren't really in the clear yet. We were just watching and it reminded me of the times I would join him in his room to watch whatever trash Showtime was showing as we would laugh at the unintended humor of *Body Chemistry II* or the always dependable knee-slapping situations of *Red Shoe Diaries*.

The clock was going on eleven o'clock. I was wondering why no one had told me to turn off the TV yet. Until that someone did I was going to make it my personal mission to see this movie through to the end.

My parents had decided to call it a night. I didn't know why they were visiting so late. They usually cleared out right after dinner and a brief final visit. Where was Becky? I was a little confused but my mind had to focus on other matters like why I was watching this. It was good to have goals no matter how preposterous.

My good friend, thirst, then decided to visit which was worsened by one scene in the movie where Mr. Peck approaches a group of adolescent girls in a public fountain. This scene struck me as strange. This fountain was huge and the girls are lounging in it like it's a swimming pool. Who knew what kind of bacteria was lurking in that petri dish? This and the likelihood that they could be cut on some of that sharp granite really concerned me. I breathed a sigh of relief when the school marm suspected Mr. Peck of being a pervert, got in his face, and chased him away. Atticus Finch was never treated that way. Atticus Finch wouldn't have taken that shit.

While this movie's intent was not to be a horror movie, its scenes seemed to have that effect on me, especially the one where Mr. Peck and Ms. Hepburn visit the infamous stone face with the beard. Mr. Peck declares some legend coming true if one puts their hands in the statue's mouth. There was water running from the face's mouth and it seemed to be moving. I had no clue what was going to happen when he steps in and sticks his hand in and screams, alarming all those around. So scenes that accentuated water were not helping me and my thirst. It was a small price to pay to ensure that his and Ms. Hepburn's character bonded.

Then the unintended horror of the movie was summed up with my thought, *will this damn movie please end?* Even the wise cracking expat friend of his couldn't save this abomination. Why didn't I just turn it off? What had been denied to me for so long I felt like I had to do, even if I didn't enjoy it. I was *carpe dieming* the best way I could and it sucked.

Ms. Hepburn finally returned to being a queen or whatever royal title she had and I was annoyed that it was almost midnight and nobody had the good sense to make me turn the TV off. I wished there was a Code Blue for patients watching insufferable cinema.

Mercifully this horror had come to its awful end so I turned off the TV, finally. Needless to say I was quite spent trying to pay attention to a black-and-white movie. Maybe two colors and a lack of explosions was what I needed. I finally found out the name of the movie was *Roman Holiday*. I had never heard of *Roman Holiday* before and have never heard of it since. So, I realized that it wasn't the commercials that necessarily made a movie bad.

Once the TV was off I was hoping that Mr. Sandman would find me. As usual he couldn't. Was he really trying or just being lazy? I couldn't sleep, I just couldn't sleep. I kept staring out in the hall. I could feel the activity around me. I couldn't move. I didn't know what to do as the hours slipped away. No one would pay attention to me, and even if they did I wouldn't know what to say. The nights were the scariest.

I then eyed the remote and thought, *maybe they're showing that movie again.*

***

WE DECIDED TO HAVE A SODA/WHATCHA FAVORITE FLAVOR? [100]

"I'm excited about your nurse today," Becky said. "He took care of you when you were out. He's a great guy with two teenage daughters. He is divorced but he gets to spend time with them as much as he can. He's really a cool guy. You're going to like him."

PART III - A DELICATE BRAND OF REALITY - QUESTIONABLE FREEDOM   291

If Becky was excited then I was excited. She had seen the good, the bad, the ugly, and the Effeminate Curtis so I imagined that any endorsement from her was something I could count on.

I could see him through the window to the room next door as he was preparing to take over the shift. It was the Vincent Price guy who I saw earlier in black and white. Damn, he was in such good spirits with having to start twelve hours dealing with me. I felt bad for him. Thankfully he had a brighter outlook than I did. He didn't look like any Effeminate Curtis so I was not worried with what the shift would bring.

Finally he stuck his head in the door and introduced himself. It was so far so good, he seemed down to earth. He began to look me and my tubes over and Becky asked him how his daughters were doing.

"They're doing great but their rooms, the house, there's always a mess it seems. I often have to say 'Can't you just pick up some of this mess?'" he said humorously. Well said.

I knew what he was talking about with his views on messes in the house or so I had imagined what that must be like. I could see my house, my daughters' rooms, and messes but what I didn't know for sure was if they were real or imagined.

It still looked like it was going to be a good shift. There had been talk from Teresa the day before of me drinking something once I got my trach removed. Now with Mr. Price here today the rumors proved to be true.

"What'll it be?" Mr. Price asked me leaning into the room from the doorway.

I was shocked, positively shocked; I had been thirsty for so long. My mouth felt like it had dried grass in it, my throat felt like concrete and I was being asked what I would like to drink. Things seemed to be moving fast this weekend. It was a fine Sunday and Mr. Price was asking me what I would like to drink.

My mind was abuzz as I kept anticipating that the next words would be, "Only joking! Of course you can't drink anything, it would come out of your trach hole in a cartoonish way. Silly fool."

I managed to put these fears aside as I thought hard. I didn't want to screw this up. What should I choose?

All I could muster was an, "Uhmmmmm."

Becky chimed in, "How about a Welch's grape soda?" Articulating it just as my old roommate from Kings Point, James Strain did way back in '87.

Seeing no other option I could just utter a, "Yes. One of those."

Mr. Price replied jokingly, "Going high octane I see."

I didn't really understand the comment as he left. Should I change my order? This is what it must feel like to get handed a million dollars and to be told that you can spend it on only one thing. My mind was racing with not only doubt about the Welch's grape soda but about what was transpiring in general. So many questions that I had such as: "Am I to be released with my Welch's Grape Soda?" or "Will they give me a to-go cup?"

Mr. Price returned with not Welch's Grape Soda but Nehi Grape Soda. That would do since I was not really a connoisseur of grape soda, how could it be any different?

Becky poured the bubbly purplish liquid into the cup; it fizzed wildly. I was given a straw and I was nearly blown back into the wall from the strong carbonation. Ladies and Gentlemen, People of Earth, I implore you to never kick off drinking liquids again after a long lay-off with grape soda, the carbonation will indeed send you back to the Stone Age.

I drank half the cup appreciating the liquid except after a while the carbonation was burning my throat and overwhelmed me. I could not go on and I regretted my decision. I would have made the wrong decision anyway without the suggestion. The regret would become magnified with what the night would bring.

The night began well enough; however, as it went on things began to go awry. With the foolproof flexi-seal somehow firmly attached to my anal canal the Nehi began to test the limits of the adhesive used to keep it there. The buildup of gas in my intestines came in waves and the need to expel this horror was crucial to my insides. I tried to fight it as long as I could as there were people in the room and I had a strict "No Release" policy in mixed company. This however was a pain that I never experienced before and there was no way around it. This evening was going to hurt. The word "Help" was unfortunately not in my vocabulary by this time.

I kept gritting my teeth yet that only hurt my teeth as the awful gas kept me up all night. Sleep was something I was finally trying to attain and I actually may have attained it on this night were it not for this deadly purple juice. I finally gave in and rescinded my "No Release" policy. However my common sense had taken a vacation since the flexi-seal I soon realized was acting as a de facto cork and severely limited a means to release the stress. The bubbles in the flexi-seal and attached bag would make it appear that I was smoking a hookah pipe through my ass.

After what seemed like hours of enduring this pain, I had finally had enough. My tentativeness to ask for help slowly faded away with my butt hurting and the nausea it wrought.

I finally said to Becky, "Can you get a nurse please?" as I thought, *I gotta the badda gassa!* (in a politically incorrect pseudo Italian voice).

The nurse came in, and I don't know how she did it but lo and behold the horror of the Nehi Grape Soda was calmed and I have not had a Grape Soda since. My shield of paranoia was slowly being drawn away.

***

A CHAIR, A CHAIR, MY KINGDOM FOR A CHAIR

As the Nehi incident indicated, things were going pretty quickly as my wakefulness had returned. Mr. Price had said that they would put me in a chair before he went to get me that ever powerful Nehi. I was very anxious over this development. Did the doctors know about this? Had he just gone off half-cocked and thought I was being a lazy slob and needed to get my ass out of bed? Was I actually going to be that guy I had imagined in my nightmares that would get up out of the wheelchair and walk off? I was in a state of alert as Mr. Price was getting my Nehi. He left the room to locate the chair that would welcome my bony posterior.

It was a Sunday so Mike was off. I hadn't seen Mike in a while. He was sending in his associates to watch over me. He mentioned one female associate as if I should know her, "You know, she's the one who's about to get married."

I would nod and think *I do not know who that is*. I didn't wish to argue. Maybe this was a hot button issue for Mike that I knew who he was speaking of. Whoever they were, they always seemed to turn up when I was at my lowest just to pick me up emotionally.

Mr. Price finally returned with a chair, and it looked totally out of place in the hospital setting. It had a strong resemblance to a chair one might find on the showroom floor of an Ethan Allen with a high back, covered in light brown leather cushioning with a dark wood finish on the legs and back. For all I knew it could have been snagged from some unsuspecting doctor's office who would soon hunt it down passionately and give me a long, stern lecture on the wrongs of stealing once he found it. What a dick. Mr. Price was not bothered by this daydream of mine as he brought the chair in and set it down. My first thought was how in the hell was the transition from this bed to that chair going to happen? I had not been out of the bed in weeks, and I was a bit nervous over leaving my hated yet safe home base.

Mr. Price called in one of his friends who was on the floor at the moment. He was a tall, well, everyone was tall to me at that moment, guy that was quite athletic looking. All of my tubes and my catheter had to be moved with me. There was so much to think about. I hoped they were allowed to do this as I didn't want to get them in trouble. To my thinking there was always some higher power that was not in the room at the time.

They lifted my prostrate body from the bed very gently. I was surprised that they thought I was heavy; I felt like a shell of my former self. Perhaps there was something left of me after all. Without their help I would have had gravity taking me for an unwanted journey to the floor. They got me into a sitting position on the bed, carried me to the chair, and lowered me gently. My socked feet were touching the floor, the hardness of which felt foreign to me. The sensation was so different, it was as if I had never sat in a chair, never been upright, never done anything. I felt like a baby that needed constant attention and reminding. As my ass hit that cushion, I felt every bone in my rear twinge with pain. I simply had no ass and the pain was excruciating as my tailbone drilled down into that cushion and found whatever hard piece of framing was awaiting it. It was hard to sit up straight. Mr. Price and the respiratory therapist, I believe his name was Chadwick, left me once they saw that I hadn't spilled out of the chair after the first ten seconds, but I couldn't guarantee how the following ten seconds would go.

Mr. Price asked, "Do you need a pillow to sit on?"

"Yes!" I said. Someone still had to offer, I couldn't seem to think of what would solve my discomfort yet.

As Mr. Price left the room he said, "We'll try it for twenty minutes." I didn't think I could stand the first twenty seconds.

As the sensation of sitting up overcame me I could not believe I ever took sitting in a chair for granted. I always thought pushing my bed everywhere was quite dramatic and a little over the top but thank goodness they did. Just sitting here was awakening every weakness in my body where the ability of the trunk of my body to remain upright was severely lacking since I had no ass to ground me. My legs felt like pieces of spaghetti just brushing the floor. I was at the start of a long road, yet I kept reminding myself to thank God that I was here and able to experience it.

Becky sat by my side as we watched television. I tried to concentrate on the screen but it was hard. I was trying to settle myself the entire time by keeping my focus on an object on the wall to maintain my balance. The faintness, the weakness was overwhelming. I tried to push through shifting my weight from one ass cheek to another however the pillow amazingly did not cushion enough of my bony behind. Certainly I had been there for at least ten minutes.

Finally giving up on ignoring the clock I asked Becky, "How long have I been sitting here?"

She replied, "Five minutes."

I was having a hard time digesting that answer and said, "You gotta be kidding. How am I supposed to get to twenty minutes?"

"If you can't, then you can't, don't worry about it."

I feared that my inability to accomplish the twenty minutes would prolong my stay in the hospital, wherever it was. Twenty minutes is out but I could make it to ten minutes, certainly. As I tried to reach my goal leaning on an arm I could only think of the flexi-seal in my ass, the catheter up my wang, the remnants of the trach tube, and the lines that were all the colors of the rainbow in my arm and chest as reminders of what should not be.

I once again concentrated on the screen. What was this I was watching? I didn't know, wait I do know. There were two commercials that drove me up the wall much more so than *Roman Holiday* if that was possible. One was the Verizon network commercial showing a map of the United States and its networks crossing it; that one really made me dizzy. There was also this ad about a man that has lost his way from his wife's cooking and so she sets lights out along the road and sidewalk that leads back to their house. I found this ad to be very unsettling, the man had lost his way and needed to get back home all because of baked goods? Get your ass back home!

"How much time now?" I asked hopefully.

"Ten minutes," came her reply.

"That's it, I cannot go on."

I continued to wonder how people could sit, it was so uncomfortable. I analyzed it and just didn't see how it could work even at my healthiest. I felt guilty about needing to lie down again, to give up, the shame of it all. It would look like I wasn't even trying. Even after all of that dubious motivation I said, "I can't do it. Get me back into bed."

As soon as I had released this admission it was as if my effort had gone, my spirit had departed and the lightheadedness became stronger.

"OK," Becky said, "I'll call Mr. Price."

As expected in the MICU there were cases more taxing than my bony ass in the chair dilemma but Mr. Price was great in responding to my hardship. He poked his head in at that moment and asked, "How are we doing?"

"He needs to get back in the bed," Becky replied.

"OK, let me get my help. Chadwick!" and Mr. Price was off to look for Chadwick.

Mr. Price then came back in to check on me. Good thing I gave up when I did, I began to realize that by the time they got me back in the bed it would be twenty minutes.

"Chadwick! Where ya at man?!" Mr. Price half humorously called out down the hall. I thought what a great combo they made. I would really like to go out drinking with them sometime but all of these tubes in me would certainly raise a few eyebrows in whatever bar we went to, especially the ones hanging out of my ass and pistol. Hey, at least I wouldn't have to wait in line to use the can like a sucker.

It was strange having two men my age caring for me at the time when I was at such a critical transitioning phase. All of those small female nurses would be called in like an army of ants just to raise me up in bed and here only two guys were needed but they still struggled.

After a few more minutes Chadwick showed up which was quite fortunate because I couldn't take much more of the sitting. My warped perspective of time was still telling me that a few minutes in the MICU seemed like two hours; in the end I would be saved from my first attempt at sitting.

Chadwick was apologetic about his tardiness, "Sorry but I had to help this really heavy dude down the hall. Guy must weigh about 240 lbs."

I wondered how heavy that guy was when he got in here.

Since my neck muscles were still nowhere to be found, my head flopped around as they somehow lifted me up into the bed. It was a trying journey. Looking down, my eyes focused on Chadwick's shoes. They were some sort of croc hybrid shoe that was dark blue. I had never seen anything like it before. I looked up and caught Chadwick's gaze; he was grinning at me once I got into bed. I could not figure out if it was an encouraging grin or really a grimace with all the exertion that came with trying to get an ill-balanced piece of dead weight from Point A to Point B. Perhaps it was a grin of encouragement but a lot of sympathy as well. I felt two foot small as I thought that I really would have liked to have gotten in the bed on my own. I really was not lazy. I would get there.

Once my weight became fully supported by the mattress I felt extreme relaxation. I didn't care if Instaflate was saying, "I knew you would be back, you bum, giving me a hard time. Well, you can waste away in that chair, you and your bony ass."

After this imaginary harangue I knew that I must have really offended Instaflate.

As I lay down I felt tired, deflated, defeated. Mr. Price asked what I wanted to watch and I really didn't know. I didn't care.

"You might like this one, it's a thriller with Denzel Washington," he said as he stopped flipping the channels.

I couldn't make out what it really was so I said, "Sure."

What I got for my "Sure" was a movie about a kid dying in a hospital, a hostage situation, a police sniper no one knew about hiding in the ceiling, Denzel going crazy, and of all things that short turd from *Entourage*. No, not the one with the beard, the one who is always arching his eyebrows and thinks he is the shit. If I had seen the bearded guy then my ability to walk would have come back in an instant as I left the room. I got all of this from the one episode of *Entourage* I have seen. I really don't watch it baby.

So I endured the movie and I really was depressed about seeing such hardship in a hospital, but I didn't have the heart to tell Mr. Price to change the channel, he had talked it up so much so I laid there and endured it. So there I was. Things were progressing. I got some Nehi, I sat in a chair, Denzel was depressing the hell out of me, and I had an evening of gut-wrenching gas to look forward to.

CHAPTER 25

Relief and Fear

Renal failure is present in all patients by 48 to 72 hours and many patients require dialysis for 10 to 20 days. In patients who survive, the serum creatinine concentration returns to baseline within four to six weeks.[101]

THE GLASS IS OVERFLOWING

Becky came in one day with some surprises from the Babies. She held in her hands some drawings they had made for me. They were all so wonderful and they touched me. I wanted to see them all at once and take them in. I couldn't believe I was touching something that they had made, they were actually real. There was an actual connection to them. Now I knew and the doubt was gone, I do have children.

Becky said, "Also, I have another surprise." Before I knew it she had pulled out a pint beer glass with the Budweiser emblem on it. As it tapered up from the bottom, it curved outward and curved inward toward the rim. I had not seen a glass like that before and it looked rather fragile; I feared for it.

"Who's that from?" I replied as I continued looking at the glass.

"Kate won it when she went out with the Indian Princess tribe."

"What was that?"

"Your tribe went on an outing to Jillian's this week and we arranged for one of the dads to pick up Kate and take her along," she said. "She won this playing skee ball."

I was so touched. Kate had taken a shine to skee ball and the system of earning tickets for prizes when we had visited my parents the previous summer. She was putting her new-found talents to good use and cashing in her winnings to get me a prize.

"She thought you would like it, since you like beer," Becky said thoughtfully.

I laughed and began to cry at the thoughtfulness of my seven-year-old daughter not getting herself something and thinking of me. I couldn't believe I had a little girl that would be so thoughtful to her daddy. I used that glass with great relish from then on, but the fear of its fragility never left me. I would get antsy when somebody else touched it, even looked at it, since it was so significant to me. I stared at that glass all day. After a few close calls of it almost falling off the tray, I sent it home with Becky. The thought of it falling and breaking was too much for me to bear. It would have crushed me. I needed for it to be safe and home was the best place for it.

***

I CAN BREATHE AGAIN[102]

Becky announced one day, "The Babies don't believe me when I tell them you have been asleep. They're having trouble believing you're still around, and I really have to provide them proof that you're still here and I'm telling them the truth. It's getting harder and harder to go home with the questioning."

I was upset, upset that the Babies could not count on me to be there and that I was away from them. I was as lost as I thought they were, and not seeing them had really started to get to me. I had been in here forever. I had just disappeared one day and they needed to know I was OK.

She continued, "I want to bring the video camera in to film you saying hello to them so they know you're still here, that I'm telling the truth, and that you're working to get better."

I was on board but a little anxious about this. What would they think of me just sitting here with my half-missing face? Wouldn't that upset them? I felt like I was in a hole looking up to the surface and they were still far away in another time and dimension. I had so many questions: How had they been doing? What had they been thinking about all this? I was there for them all the time and I just disappear? This must have been a living hell for them.

In any event I agreed that proof was required for Becky to get back into the house. Even Henry I heard was not buying the "Sleeping" bit. Proof had to be provided.

"That would be fine," I uttered. Usually I have to mull things over in my head but to give them something from me was what I had to do and it was a wonderful idea.

The following day she brought in the camera. She laid the get well cards they had made for me on and around the bed. My half-melted face must have looked terrible to them with the intact half having been visited repeatedly by the Butter Man. The Butter Man was an imaginary figure I thought up growing up in Tampa, Florida. With the high humidity it felt like someone had coated my face with butter at all times. Thus who would be responsible for such a dilemma? Why, the one and only Butter Man! Whether he was a villain or superhero I could not tell, he just did a job that I detested. In any event the amount of butter was getting out of hand even during the winter months, and I had a strong desire to remove this unwelcome sheen. It would be disturbing for them to see me this way but it needed to be done. The half-missing face? That would be fine. The shiny sheen of butter? Too horrifying.

I had been thinking of what I would say, it was hard to know what sounded good in my head and what sounded terrible out loud. See my "dirty ape" conundrum. Becky started up the camera. I hadn't felt this put on the spot since my interview on our wedding video right before the ceremony. That time I was hoping the camera man would offer me a smile or some form of encouragement yet there was nothing so I must not have been as funny as I thought. I was facing this same dilemma at this very moment.

Becky began filming. She started talking to me, "Hello Babies, we have a surprise for you, Daddy Hoover!"

I said, "Hello to you Babies from me, your very own Daddy Hoover! I'm coming to you live from the zero gravity chamber where I have been kept for I don't know how long."

That was all the levity I could muster, I was at a loss as to what to say next.

"How are you feeling?" Becky prompted.

I felt a little puzzled since I did not want to tell the truth, instead I said, "I'm feeling better and will be home soon."

Becky filmed the cards on me and went up and down my torso and legs. I must have looked a fright. I didn't know if I wanted them to see me like that but they had to know I was alive and not part of some Newberry Award winning *Wrinkle in Time* plot.

"Daddy's drinking some grape soda over here," Becky said as she panned my tray with the cup and the straw sticking out of it.

"Yes," I replied.

"Is it strong?" she asked.

"Yes, very spicy," I said.

I then sort of wandered off. I didn't know what to say and I was getting confused and also upset. Thinking of my condition and my state was really beginning to depress me, and I was more silent as my uncertainty grew. Becky continued to make small talk and my answers grew shorter and shorter.

"Anything else you want to say to the Babies," she asked.

"I love you and will see you soon," I said and I became very upset.

Becky stopped recording and came over to me and touched my hand. "That was great they're going to love this. Thanks for doing this. I love you."

"I love you too," I said as I grew a little more cheerful that a message from me was finally going out to them.

I had lost track of time so I asked Becky if she had shown the Babies the video the same day when she had not been home yet. So I felt like I was bugging her but I was very apprehensive that the message that I was still around was received and they would know that I had not disappeared. To go to school one day and come home that afternoon and find your parents are gone must have been very trying for them. They had gone through a lot.

Becky came in a couple of days later and she said, "The Babies saw your video and they were very excited."

Oh, I had so many questions about what they thought and what they said. Becky filled me in that they were happy to see me and to see that I was still around.

She said, "They wanted me to send a video message of them in return."

I was so excited that they were finally going to be speaking to me. I couldn't believe it. Becky produced the video camera, pulled out the screen and pressed play. The camera was almost eight years old and the batteries were running down quickly as if there were a gang of ghosts in the room trying to manifest themselves. I saw them on the back patio, all three of them. Phoebe and Henry looked pretty happy with what appeared to be dolls that looked lifelike. I had not seen these dolls before and they looked so real I became confused and wondered if we had produced more children while I was away with my experience. The memories of male birth having returned to me made me question which reality I could believe.

They yelled, "Hi Daddy."

Kate had her doll too. It was a Molly American Girl Doll with glasses just like Kate's. They were waving at me and playing in the backyard. As the oldest, Kate looked a little crestfallen knowing this was for me and I was not there. The gravity of the moment seemed to hit her and she would not smile anymore.

"Come on Kate, smile for Daddy," Becky said on the video.

Kate was not willing to cooperate and she began to ask questions. "You always say he's sleeping in the hospital and we can't see him. Why can't we see him? I'm tired of this." She then rolled her eyes as Kate can do when she gets flustered. I felt so bad for her, I wanted to touch the screen but I couldn't lift my hand still.

Becky replied, "Come on Daddy wants to see you be happy, he wants to see that you're OK."

Kate was still not willing to release her frustration when suddenly Phoebe rushed over to stick her Emily American Girl Doll into the frame and yelled, "Hi Daddy!"

Henry treated me to some of his tricycle-riding prowess. Kate began to cry and Becky stopped the video to comfort her.

The next scene was of them taking a walk around the block. I could hear the sound of the car that Henry was pushing on the sidewalk. Its plastic wheels giving that signature sound of activity. Kate was walking next to Becky as Phoebe and Henry stormed ahead.

"Come on Kate, walk ahead so Daddy can see you," Becky said.

Kate took a few steps in front and then came back by Becky's side. She began to cry and Becky stopped filming. I too began crying. I wanted to see it again but then couldn't. At least I knew that the life that I had was still there and the kids were in good hands. Even so, seeing the entire video, my life still struck me as rather foreign and I still could not fully believe that it had truly happened. I was confused and torn but filled with love for my family.

"What are those dolls? I asked, trying to change the subject.

"Your sister brought them for the Babies when we were unable to go to Atlanta to visit the American Girl Doll store the weekend you got sick."

I was so happy then that we were not with three new children, well, actually four since Henry got the Itty Bitty Twins. With my wet eyes I turned to the wall and began to stare again.

***

SICK AT HEART AND LONELY[103]

There are times when there was just no energy left. I could only be so funny for so long and entertain for so long, and I would prefer the wall for company. Obviously, I was conflicted. I wanted company and then I didn't want company. I believed it might have happened when I had to entertain my aunt and uncle while they stood there and just stared at me. They would give the entrée greeting and then there would be staring, staring, just staring. It was actually at times like this that I wished I were still intubated, not being able to talk did have its benefits. Instead I felt like I had to tell jokes and make them feel comfortable. That took a lot of damn work and it was very exhausting. I couldn't really complain, at least I could still see them and communicate like a human and not Bubbles the Chimp.

Friends of Becky's would pop in and talk loudly, and I really preferred that people not see me like this. I felt very exposed, very vulnerable. Becky needed her friends and I was happy they thought of us enough to drive from Charlotte to Winston-Salem to see me.

It was very nice for people to be thinking of us during our time of need except my thoughts would turn to something here by my bed. I always was looking for it, it was a magic thing but something I wanted, needed. My wall staring was being interrupted by these visits and while I liked visitors, after five minutes they became tiring and I needed to shut down again. Where was that confounded thing? I couldn't see it. I knew what I was looking for; it was the "Clear Room" button. When it gets pushed, voila! No more visitors! Quiet and Silence. Once they came in and stayed for more than ten minutes, the visitors became intruders.

Not to lay blame on the visitor, I knew the discomfort. I have visited others in the hospital and not known what to say but when the visiting becomes fidgeting and staring I could stand no more. I imagined out in the world when confronted with such an awkward situation and there was a silence then I could say, "It was great seeing you!" and be on my way. Except here, I couldn't walk away and I wasn't at the point of saying, "Get Out!"

It got to the point that after a while when I would hear someone coming in the room my eyes would shut and I would not open them until the person had left. At times I really didn't want the visit and I couldn't handle lying there anymore. The person that was me in the green shirt and shorts whistling while he walked out of the hospital, the person that was once me seemed to be further away every day.

***

CLOSE TALKER SALAD SAYS GOODBYE

After I had gotten my breathing tube removed and could thankfully talk once again Jenny, the close-talker nurse that I had early in my stay, made a surprise visit to come and see me as I was almost ready to leave the MICU. I was sure she wanted to finally get to talk to me and see how I was doing when I was awake and more lucid. Of course, I didn't have the deep meaningful thing to say again, words escaped me.

She said as she got real close to my face, "So you're about ready to get out of here Handsome?"

I said something to the effect of, "Yeah, I'm beat down and when I get home my kids, they are going to beat me down some more."

This was not the negativity that I intended to relay and she looked disappointed at my loss of appreciation for the life that had been returned to me. Especially when a young nurse, make that female nurse, just called me "Handsome" there should of at least been some joy. I couldn't really figure out a way to take it back and she replied, "Great." She did not get the sage words. I had nothing. There was too much in my head to get out in some meaningful way. I did not see her again after that encounter and I am glad I had her as a nurse. Becky had nothing but kind words to say about her.

***

OR TALK ABOUT THE WEATHER[104]

The Weather Channel was my new channel, of course. It became a habit to watch it in the morning since it had no political agenda, no bad news, nothing to make you want to stop what you were doing to watch, except for what the new fashion was in weather anchor attire. All of this spawned from the Elian Gonzalez coverage during the summer of 1999. I was fed up with the cameras just sitting outside a fucking house around the clock so we ended up turning to the Weather Channel in the mornings and it has been on ever since.

But perhaps this too was backfiring on me. It was a Sunday evening and I couldn't seem to find anything to watch. Sunday evenings were never my favorite time of the week anyway. I was feeling depressed and bored and the Weather Channel was not providing relief. Their Storm Stories segment had the Hurricane in Galveston in the early twentieth century featured. It was a rather depressing tale of death and destruction and my thoughts began to take a philosophical bent with the questions: Why did those people all perish? Why am I still here? Actually I was not out of the woods yet. I just needed to be vigilant to get out of here. I didn't know what else I could do to make that go any faster. At least I had been given a chance.

I continued watching The Weather Channel the next day when Dr. Rebefall came in for morning rounds.

"The Weather Channel?" he exclaimed. "You're getting too crazy here Howard."

I had to agree with that.

"Haven't you been watching basketball?" he asked.

"Not really," I replied. "I watch it sometimes."

"Who's your favorite team?" he asked trying to find some common ground.

"Don't really have one," I said meekly.

"What's your favorite conference?"

"I guess the SEC," I said without much relish.

I thought, *God I sound boring. Did I get some sort of boring bacteria from the body rebuild? What happened to the wit? Where ya at wit?*

"I'm a Marquette man," he said matter-of-factly as he began to examine whatever it was on my person.

I remembered always seeing Marquette back in the 1970s when Al Macguire was the coach on dark Sunday afternoons around the huge Sylvania wood cabinet TV in Brandon, Florida. The only place drearier than the MICU on a late Sunday afternoon was Brandon, Florida during the 70s on a late Sunday afternoon sitting around the huge Sylvania wood cabinet TV. My dad liked to turn off all the lights in the house for a doubly dreary effect. There I would be sitting on the couch eating chocolate chip cookies and drinking warm Coke with the obvious intent of improving my dental well-being. Of course this memory was not present at the time Marquette came up.

All I could say was, "Marquette, they're still around?"

***

WHEN EVERY LITTLE BIT OF HOPE IS GONE[105]

The music player that Becky had bought me could be both blessing and curse. It turned out Becky made a list for me called *Howard, Get Better* which contained my top twenty-five most played songs on Itunes. I realized instantly that I really listened to some dirgy music. At the top of the list was the Coors with Bono singing *When the Stars Go Blue*. If I could please make a suggestion, do not play this song when you are in any sort of critical condition or any state of sickness for that matter. It definitely opens the door for the blues to enter the room. I guess that's why the song as the word "Blue" in the title.

Once I started hearing the slow opening bars I began to tear up. And this was while I was trying to drink my Gatorade. My hands were shaking as I attempted to hold the cup and put the straw in my mouth with tears rolling down my face. I wanted for someone to notice me, the perverse need for attention. *Take pity on me! I'm listening to sad music!*

Becky looked at me and said, "If you're going to start crying listening to this dirgy music I'm going to have to take away the music."

Touché.

CHAPTER 26

My Room

ARDS occurs in approximately 55 percent of patients, generally developing after the onset of hypotension. Almost all patients with ARDS require supplemental oxygen, intubation, and mechanical ventilation.[106]

IN THE MIDDLE OF OUR STREET[107]

Mike was not here today, another therapist came in to work with me. As always it was painful what they did to me. My sedentary lifestyle made me dubious that my body ever twisted that way before. It seemed like an insurmountable task to get my shoulders back, to lift my legs, to lift my arms, to lift my head, and on and on. I had overheard from others in the room: nurses, doctors, and relayed through Becky that for every month in the MICU it took three months to get back to where you were before being admitted. While I was discouraged by this news I was relieved that the topic of returning to where I was had been broached. But three months? Who knew how long it would take. My body felt broken and I was not sure how or if I would be normal again.

I was still more shocked when I overheard a nurse asking Becky what the situation was at home in terms of stairs and access. Our bedroom is upstairs and we have stairs everywhere plus our house for all intents and purposes is on a cliff.

The nurse asked, "Is there a shower downstairs?"

"No," was the answer and I knew that my house would be a problem. I just had no idea that when Becky and I bought it four and a half years ago that I would be looking such a short distance down the road at such issues. The amount of money to make it handicap accessible was spinning in my head.

Help at home was also mentioned as in a live-in nurse, which I found rather depressing. I had visited old relatives with some sort of in-home care but it never dawned on me that I would be staring at such a proposition so soon in my early middle-aged life. I mean I hadn't even gotten to a mid-life crisis yet where my high school football jacket had been dusted off and worn proudly about the house. The only thing I could imagine or see clearly in terms of handicap access in my house was an air mattress or bed set up in the study downstairs with the powder room in which I found solace when all of this started.

So, this was it, I would be unable to get back into bed again in my bedroom? And another question: who would my nurse be?

I imagined myself in the study banging on the side of the bed with a metal cane telling my kids to shut up or I would call their mother. I had turned into some horrible monster in a hospital gown that no one wanted to deal with, a shut-in without a cause. And what was with the "their mother" business? What had happened now? I was already in such an estranged relationship that when I got home I would be referring to Becky as "their mother?"

Who would the nurse be for this unfortunate assignment? Of course, the only candidate that it could be was none other than Effeminate Curtis, the one and only. I could see him walking me up and down the street with me donned in a hospital gown and slippers and of course no underwear, pushing some IV stand on wheels and him in a white lab coat and those hands held out akimbo like an effeminate Frankenstein marching in some parade. What a pair we would make. How in the hell would I ever hope to make block leftenant with that image burned in my neighbors' minds? The jig was up, that was how it was going to be. So if I saw him again I had better be nice so that he would stoop to such a job.

Even with such a scenario in my head no matter how ridiculous, I had resolved myself to things being very different when I got home. That really didn't matter at the moment, as long as I was back there.

***

TASTING MUCH SWEETER THAN WINE[108]

My feeding tube was still front and center on my face, stuck there by some means I had yet to determine. That was how I had been fed all of this time. My weight was down, my mood was down and every time I was being weighed on the bed (not only did it provide ancestral records and flight information and bust nurses, it was a scale too!) I would fear the sight of my legs as the blankets were removed.

"Look at those chicken legs," one male nurse said. As if I needed to be reminded. There was no way those things were mine. The body rebuilding process had gone horribly wrong, the hair had fallen out and they were just so damn useless. Unbelievable, I was down to 170 pounds. There was nothing to me. I played football in high school at 165 pounds. How did I not blow away on the field in a mild wind?

Dr. Rebefall came in and said, "Once you start eating as we continue to unplug you, you'll start feeling human again."

I could not agree more but what was the first step? I really didn't feel very hungry at all. I was actually nauseous most of the time. Getting back to normal sounded very nice but wishful thinking, it was all wishful thinking. That eating thing felt like a world away much like the walking and talking without having to press on my trach tube. We talked to the nurse about this and she said the first step would be to have a taste test to make sure food could be kept down and that my sense of taste was still normal.

So who knew how this was going to happen? Did we need to talk to someone? Did I need to make an appointment? I just knew it was going to take forever to get in to see someone. I could not believe there was such coordination in this place that enabled them to remember all of this. It was simply amazing what they had done so far but I just didn't believe this taste test would come to be.

One day as I lay there staring at the wall a lady entered the room pushing a cart without any pleasantries wearing a white lab coat which in my mind made her official. She had curly hair and wore glasses. No one else was in the room at the time. She said some official title and from this I gathered she was the legendary taste lady with all of the different ill-tasting items she began to uncover from her tray and shove into my mouth.

Did anyone know that she was here? Was this test being recorded? Did the Yahoo Serious guy with the stickers put her up to this? Would I need to remember the results and pass them along to the powers that be? When I passed them along would they ask "Now what was your reaction? That it tasted like shit? Or nasty shit? This is important!"

I didn't really have long to mull this over since she was all business. "I'll be giving you a taste test to check your capacity to hold items in your mouth, check your swallowing abilities and your taste."

She shoved a dry cracker in my mouth which I held for a while. I tried not to gag on it. I concentrated but it was so difficult. She removed the cracker with seconds to spare from me gagging all over the place.

As if she was some evil taste magician putting on some evil magic show she said, "Now I'll have you try a heavy dose of bitter apricot jelly." At least I think that's what she said, it was the sharpest tasting jelly food I had ever had and I made a face. That appeared to be the correct response.

Some other tests were performed that involved me tasting other "nasty shit" and she left without saying another word. I hoped she was satisfied. It was one more step to get me back. I certainly hoped I passed. Also, I hoped someone saw her leave and that she recorded the results because I didn't want to taste that "nasty shit" ever again. Yes, that is what I would tell the powers that be. "It tasted like nasty shit."

***

I DON'T KNOW

As I slowly came into a more lucid state in the MICU, I felt I was being a ne'er-do-well by not earning my keep. The only thing really keeping me from getting out of the hospital was my own laziness. Dr. Rebefall still included me on his rounds but he was no longer giving me the silent treatment as he viewed my screen. He may actually have been warming up to me. I wondered what I did to bring on this change in attitude. Perhaps my behavior was getting a little more agreeable. Gladly there were no more of the silhouettes looking in on me in silence as I planned my schemes to escape.

During one round when he had finished examining me he said, "I'm going to be taking the next week off to attend a conference."

I thought, *how dare you, can't you see that I'm sick? I'm in a hospital for crying out loud.*

I was irritated that he would leave me. Then again, maybe the mouse could play now that the cat was away. As that thought rolled around in my head it dawned on me that maybe the mouse needed the cat, the cat needed to be here for the mouse! I became very concerned and thought I should be careful what I wished for.

I kept asking myself the outrageous questions: *Who would be watching me now? Will they know what they're doing? Am I not the only thing in his life? How can he possibly focus on anything else?*

***

DO MY EYES DECEIVE ME?[109]

The button on my trach tube that I had to press to speak still concerned me. It was a rather uncomfortable thing for me to do. I didn't like the idea of pressing on my throat when there was a hole in it. What if I was unable to get the button out or if I pushed it in too far or it fell into my throat, what then? I was quite nervous about it; so nervous that others on their visits had to press it for me.

One night my thirst came back in a big way and not wanting to disturb anyone and admittedly to show off my "wish I had these skills" skills I decided to do something for myself. As I was left alone with my thoughts I saw something on my tray that looked like a fruity treat that had been left for me, yet I couldn't figure out who would have left it and didn't tell me. My arms were not working; however my hands and fingers had some movement. Still, I was in a bad place. All I could do was move my neck. I kept eyeing this thing, whatever it was and I was certain that it was the cure for my thirst. It would solve all of my problems. I just knew it and I was going to get this thing.

It was a long night as I concentrated on moving my arms and my hands to try and obtain this sweet relief. I tried to throw my hands on it, just let gravity do its thing but without success. I knew I could do this and that fruity treat would be mine. It looked like a popsicle; so who left this just to melt away in front of me? Why would they torment me so? If I could have just gotten it on the tray, except my limited range of motion could only offer a limp wave from my hand. This went on all night. Right when I thought I had it, it would slip away. The thought of tasting sweet cherry something was overwhelming. What would I do when I got it? I wasn't even able or allowed to eat yet. Perhaps I could suck on it and I didn't care what I had to do, this thing was the key to relieving my discomfort.

The nurse would come in every now and then and I would stop my pursuit to show I could do it for myself, and then when she left I would continue. I felt like a child doing what he was not supposed to be doing. Out of the corner of my eye to my right I could see Becky sitting there. She had her head resting on her hand and her elbow on a table right next to the tray. How in the world was she able to sleep like that? Can't she wake up and see my utter torment? I mustn't wake her.

I'll just keep on with my determined pursuit and will get this damn thing myself.

As it grew light outside, my favorite time of day since the ghosts went away and all was good in my world, I looked to my right and saw what I thought was Becky in the darkness was actually some sort of stand that bent like an elbow with an attachment at the top. I had been fooled all night by this instrument and now it was just sitting there mocking me. At this point I gave up my pursuit and passed out. When I awoke once the hustle and bustle of the MICU began anew that day, I saw Becky sitting by my bedside.

I said to her with an air of surrender after tentatively pressing the button on my trach, "Please, please, hand that to me," as I pointed to the sweet treat.

"What, this?" she said as she picked up my sweet treat and showed it to me.

To my horror of horrors I saw that it was the plastic case for my trach attachment. I sighed deeply.

***

HOPE YOU GUESSED MY NAME[110]

The amount of time that I had been in the MICU was bordering on the ridiculous, even when I considered only the part that I had been fully awake. What had it been, three weeks? Four weeks? I kind of knew where I was, I thought, but this vampire lifestyle was really getting on my nerves. When I would get relative peace and quiet during the night, I could not sleep and when the place was a buzz of activity during the daylight I would nod off. These moments of relative peace were usually interrupted with my being awakened by someone trying to probe me or bring some news to me or the well-meaning visitors that stopped by that forced me to be in entertainment mode and it was exhausting.

My nurse's name on this night was Kim; she was Korean with an indelible American accent. As I complained of no one paying me any mind during the all-nighters, she was all about engaging me as I lay there in a state of sleeplessness.

She came in bright and cheerful when her shift first started at 7:00 p.m. and said, "My name is Kim, like 'Don't Kim Back Here!'" which I found to be quite catchy. She had great concern over my sleeplessness and decided to make me work as I lay there by talking to me, asking me questions, which I wanted during those dark hours. However I had gotten used to the silence and was not feeling too amiable at the moment. "What do you do?" she asked.

At that moment I was not quite sure, I must have done something prior to all of this besides hold the title of "Senior Executive Bitter Shut-In" and I didn't know if I had the energy to give her a long explanation, so I just said the simple answer: "Civil Engineer."

She then asked, "What kind of engineer's that?"

Since my simple answer was growing more complex it got a little frustrating having to think of the best way to explain it to her. I really didn't know how to explain it other than retelling a joke that I knew that sort of cleared it up but I couldn't remember the joke. As I recalled it was mildly amusing. She seemed to want to get this information out of me, so I said that I didn't really know how to explain it.

She shrugged her shoulders and said that she needed to get my meds which really did not brighten my mood anymore. She came back in with them and had her back to me as she mixed them up. She gave me a backward glance and smiled and looked back at what she was doing.

An evil thought popped into my head that with her back to me I could bonk her on the head and get the hell out of here. I realized even if I was that evil, I couldn't as the rest of the evening would attest I was in no condition or mood for such chicanery.

She gave me the meds one by one, and one by one I took them, and one by one they became larger and larger. They all proved to be so damn big. Who in the hell would be able to swallow these things? The action of swallowing was making me nervous, along with the fear of the choking. It was as if all of those old lady babysitters I had when I was little were crowding around the bed with their warnings which added to my trepidation.

I continued with my wakefulness, just looking around, all over the room. Kim returned periodically and finally said, "If you want to do something I have some weights you can use and we can start getting your strength back."

This was not really what I had wished for, and I could tell she was not going to leave me in peace. I found it to be a lot of work to be social during my vampire time.

I replied, "Sure," but what I thought she offered, what I thought I could do, and what I could really do were three separate things. What I thought she offered was for me to be wheeled into this gym which I imagined just happened to be on the MICU floor because all patients need time to exercise. What I thought I could do was be lowered onto the floor where I could do some mild stretching on a towel, then dumbbells would be provided for me to bench press off the floor. What was really available to me and what I could really do were none of the above. The discharge papers would be moved to the bottom of the pile once she saw this.

To my surprise she brought in a five ounce bottle of saline for me to hold in my hands and then I found out what I could really do. There would be no wheeling me into another room where straps would lower me onto a floor like a beached whale. I now knew that would probably kill me since my body was still not accustomed to the effects of gravity without the assistance of Instaflate. My arm could move, albeit with little control, but the saline bottle made the task seem insurmountable. I looked at my arm and it was like a piece of string. I could not believe that this was where I was starting from. What happened to my strength? It did not seem to respond to my commands to move. Kim needed to come over to the left side of the bed to get me started. She lifted my hand gently and I could get the saline bottle part way up to my face. Then, unceremoniously, it fell down on the bed since I was not able to keep my grip on it.

We kept working on getting the bottle off the bed until I could get it to reach my face. My arm was unable to get it to stop short of my face and I realized that I had a control issue getting the bottle to stop before the collision with Good Ole' Half Face. Kim wouldn't let me give up as I felt sorry for myself and annoyed at being disturbed, yet at the same time relieved that I was being acknowledged. She was spending time with me by helping me to continue my recovery.

She continued to talk to me about my family which I was still not really sure if they existed or not even after all the evidence that had been presented to me. I played along from what memory I had of them but the whole thing felt like a dream really. I couldn't have a family; I could't even lift this saline bottle off the bed on my own.

Finally, Kim said, "Your wife's awake, show her what you can do."

Becky had been sleeping this whole time, faithfully over by the window and I showed her my amazing feat of strength. My ham hands were lifting a delicate bottle to my face. A grand salute to the motor function.

"Great job," Becky remarked through sleepy eyes.

It dawned on me that the ability to lift such a small bottle was something I would never have thought I would ever try to use to impress her not even on our first date where my wit won the day, according to me, and lost the day, according to her.

The next night Kim asked, "What would you like to drink?"

I thought, *I know what I don't want lest my insides are ripped out again.* I replied, "I don't know."

She went down the list of offerings and mentioned Vitamin Water. "Have you ever had Vitamin Water?" she asked.

"No, how is it?" I replied.

"Oh, it's good, there are a lot of different flavors, want me to get you one to try?" she said like she was a spokesperson for Vitamin Water.

"Sure," I said not wanting to squash her enthusiasm.

She brought up the bottle. I still couldn't figure out where they went to get this stuff. My sense of time was still off so what was really five minutes felt like twenty minutes. She put a straw in the bottle and put it up to my lips. I took a taste and it tasted abominably bad. I didn't know what had happened to my taste buds and sense of smell. Everything felt "off." It was like everything had a plasticy sterile taste. My face showed fully my opinion of Vitamin Water.

"You don't like it?" she asked.

I shook my head and said, "I'm sure it has to grow on me."

I felt bad that I found something she spoke so highly of to not be so good. It would have cut me the same way if someone had said they were not that crazy about my cherished red Gatorade. Except that would be the talk of a madman.

The next night she said, "I asked my husband this morning what a civil engineer is."

I perked up and felt as if I was going to be tested. My hope was that she could relay to me what one was because I could not really explain it.

She continued, "Civil engineers design and build buildings, bridges, roads, things like that."

"Yes, Yes, that's what we do and I still cannot remember what that joke was I was going to tell you," I replied.

I never saw Kim again after that night so I never got to thank her for making my nights feel tolerable and constructive plus I never told her my joke.

Joke: An electrical engineer, a mechanical engineer, and a civil engineer were arguing one day about whether God is an electrical, mechanical, or civil engineer from looking at the human body.

The electrical engineer argued, "Look at the nervous system and the way it uses electrical charges to send messages all around the body, God must be an electrical engineer."

The mechanical engineer piped up, "You're wrong, God's a mechanical engineer, look at the skeletal system, the muscular system, only a mechanical engineer could have designed this, so God has to be a mechanical engineer."

The civil engineer then interjected confidently, "You both are wrong, God's clearly a civil engineer."

"How so?" the other two engineers asked.

The civil engineer replied, "Because only a civil engineer would put the waste line next to the recreation area."

Ba Dum Bum!

DR. REBEFALL SAYS GOOD BYE

I had that altogether familiar feeling that I used to get around December and June, especially at the Academy when finals were over and we could finally relax. My release from the MICU was imminent. There was talk about me moving to the Progressive Unit. I was going to miss my room and all the fond memories of rediscovery that I had experienced in here, but it was finally dawning on me that this unit was used to seeing death. People that came here were usually beyond hope and I was one of the new graduates that was literally about to make it out alive. As I chewed this over in my head I knew there was more work to be done. At least a first milestone had been reached.

It was late morning and my parents had arrived from one of their shopping trips. Becky was there and I was feeling a little more grounded and secure with things for once. Dr. Rebefall walked in for his last round. He knew I would be leaving since he was one of the many doctors moving me on out of the MICU.

He said, "I just wanted to say good-bye, you'll be moving on to Progressive later today so I wanted you to know that it has been great getting to know you and your family, and you're ready to move on to the next stage in your recovery."

He was more upbeat than I had ever seen him which was a really great sign and conveniently I was in a joking mood. Moves always excite me especially when they are so significant like this one. I recounted to him the tough times like the shaking head, when he first spoke to me and then I said, "I recall the time you checked on me and said afterward that you would be taking the next week off to attend a conference and I thought at the time 'How dare you, can't you see that I'm sick?'"

I got the best graduation present I could have imagined, I made Dr. Rebefall laugh. It was like the old *SNL* game show parody, *Make Joan Baez Laugh*, with me playing the part of Howie Mandel with the surgical glove around his nose. It was strange to see a face that I had known until this moment as only grave, serious, intense actually smile. For me it was like a dark room being opened to the daylight for the first time and that was the best present of all.

Dr. Rebefall laughed some more and said, "I knew you were in good hands."

Indeed I was, there always seemed to be some invisible force in play that always knew what was happening. We talked some more but he had to leave and that was the last time I saw Dr. Rebefall while I was a patient. The man who I thought was my Lex Luthor was my greatest advocate. Now if only all people that I am suspicious of were to save my life. He was the tough one that got me through to the next step to allow me to heal.

I felt bad about my attitude toward Dr. Rebefall. He was there when things still were not settled, when I was coming out of it, when I was at my wit's end, when I was at my most suspicious, my most confused and paranoid. He laid the road for me to get out. He was very modest and deferred the credit for saving me to Dr. Sherwood, but Dr. Rebefall got me out. I had a lot of people worried and what I was going through was serious, everybody was serious. When I saw him laugh that was the biggest relief to me. Thanks for the memories and I made a mental note to find a shirt like that.

***

ONE MORE FOR THE ROAD[111]

There was a lot of commotion going on, a young blonde nurse that I had not seen before was moving around my room, gathering things together. It appeared that today was the day that I was to be moved to Progressive. I was excited but anxious. I had been here for so long, so tormented at night that I still could not sleep, it was impossible. I tended to pass out from exhaustion in the morning just when the visits began. I felt safer in the morning like I had a lot of eyes on me. Everyone was awake and whatever might get me was no longer around and I could let my guard down.

So the nurse was going around the room gathering things and putting them on a cart. How much shit had I accumulated? I had just been lying here. Why does shit just accumulate with no action on my part? I felt bad that she was doing all of this on her own but I was in no condition to help. All I could do was watch her go around and around the room. I didn't know where Becky was. Did she know where I was going? I was afraid of the next step with no one around me. All of my thoughts and doubts simmered as the nurse continued to gather things. I was realizing what good hands I had been in in here and now my excitement about moves was waning. Now I had to get used to a new wall and a new hallway? This was going to be a difficult adjustment.

I felt like I would in college when I would move out of the old room for the year. All of the stuff that I thought was not there popped out of nowhere, and I ended up throwing out most of the crap I had kept all year and never used. Well, I guessed everything here was going with me.

My trip down memory lane was shattered as the nurse suddenly pulled up my sheet and hospital gown and said, "It's time to change your catheter."

Change my whatchama doodle? I thought.

My wang was in no condition for visitors. In fact a cocktail weenie would have put it to shame. So much so that the term "fun size" was even a hopeless, faraway goal for it. I looked to see if she was suppressing laughter over its appearance. No, professionalism saved the day as I began to feel rather uncomfortable and not from embarrassment. I supposed she was pulling out the old catheter. Holy shit! How much tubing was in there? I should have been able to feel that in my throat. That meant only one thing and that was something else had to go in.

The reality of realizing that my body was not as functional as I thought was a downer. She prepared my schmeckel for entry, and not the good kind either. I felt the most excruciating pain I had ever felt in my life. I could barely get a scream out. It was more of a low moan, like a goat would give while being mauled by a jackal.

"Sorry. Sorry." The nurse kept repeating just like the jackal would have done.

I could only think that there were only a few times in my life where it was proper to scream and this was one of them, just below the "Who is better? The Bee Gees or The Beatles?" debates from when I was in third grade. I was then taken back to a time during my coma when I remembered a pain that was not unlike someone breaking off glass in my rod. Through the coma I remembered it and I was sure getting it full bore now.

As the pain continued non-stop, I could only think when the hell this replacement was going to be in and the horror would be over.

"Sorry. Almost done," she said very apologetically. I was sure this was no fun for her either.

I had to muster the most discipline I ever had in my life not to move. I pleaded with myself to just let her get it done quickly in order to avoid any kinks in my dagger.

The misery had finally ended, she had finished but I could only think about the next time this would need to be done. Now whenever I hear the analogy of doing something fast like pulling a band-aid off, I will instead replace the band-aid with the catheter. I was just not clear why there had to be such a cruel parting gift and I am sure she let out a sigh when she saw "Painful Third Leg Tube Replacement To Be Done" in whatever doctors' orders she had received.

The time had finally come for me to leave. An orderly came to get my exceedingly uncooperative bed to roll into the hallway. There were nurses there that I remembered from my stay. It was comparable to the final episode of a really bad long-running TV series when all the former unemployed cast members returned for a final goodbye. Nora and Mr. Price were there as were some doctors or at least in my mind they were. I could barely keep my eyes open as the light in the hall was so bright. I saw a flash as if someone had taken a picture, but I had no idea if someone really took a picture or not. I heard someone yell, "And don't come back!" That was a fine how do you do. I guessed they couldn't stand the thought of seeing me again. Four weeks was long enough. I was on my way to the next step. I hoped they were nice in Progressive, and I hoped it went more quickly.

Part IV: I Thought I Heard "Pomp and Circumstance"

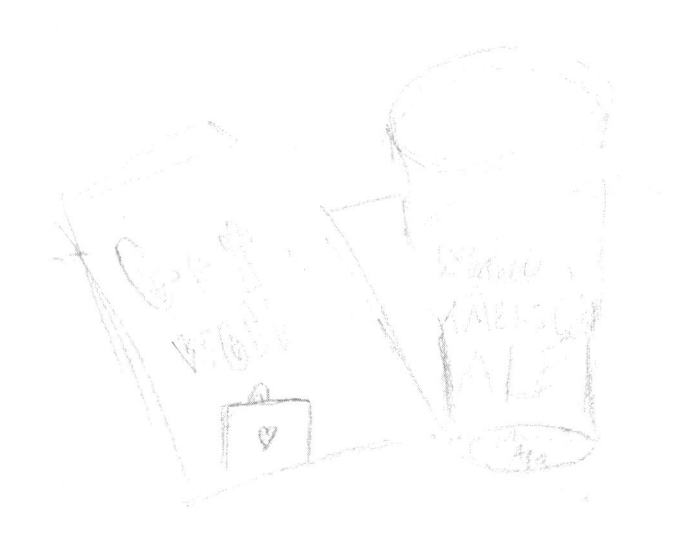

CHAPTER 27

Moving On

Supplemental oxygen should be supplied to all patients with sepsis and oxygenation should be monitored continuously with pulse oximetry. Intubation and mechanical ventilation may be required to support the increased work of breathing that typically accompanies sepsis, or for airway protection since encephalopathy and a depressed level of consciousness frequently complicate sepsis.[112]

FEBRUARY 9 - 18, 2009

WELCOME TO PROGRESSIVE, WE'VE GOT FUN AND GAMES[113]

I was rolled out into the hallway one last time in the MICU. It was like a gauntlet of slow claps from an 80s teen movie. I was moving on, and I could finally see behind the Wizard of Oz's curtain.

"Good Bye Mr. Hoover," a familiar face said to me.

I was backstage finally moving from my home away from home. I couldn't believe all of my stuff was going with me and I hopefully would not return. There were rumblings that a lot of patients that were moved to the Progressive unit were moved back to MICU because they could not adapt to the lower standard of care they were receiving. I hoped this would not be true in my case. I was very anxious about having a new everything, yet I knew it was the only way to get out. While the MICU nurses were outstanding, that place was making me crazy with its lights-on policy and its strangeness and death which always seemed to be around the corner. It was time for a change.

On the way to Progressive it was impressive to see all of these people walking around under their own power. It truly amazed and confounded me. Never again would I take my strength for granted. My physical abilities should not go unnoticed once they came back, I swore to myself. After what seemed like a fifteen-minute ride through the hallways, the thought of the bevy of activity that must have occurred around me during my stay was overwhelming. I saw more of the hospital, wherever it was, than I thought existed.

We finally arrived in the room in Progressive where I would continue my recovery. In terms of size it was much smaller than the MICU room I had grown accustomed to. There was really only room for one chair by the bed while the bed was fitted into the room at a bizarre angle so that it was angled toward the door. The TV was directly overhead and the wall was certainly not as entertaining as the MICU. Gone were all the shadows and doo dads that I knew backward and frontwards. I could even see that my parents and Becky who seemed to come out of nowhere were a little disappointed in the new place. I am sure they had grown accustomed to the MICU as well. At least this time I was facing the door so I could see everything and it was a change of scenery, nonetheless.

It was getting toward evening and the nurse shift change was already occurring. For the first couple of days I had two male nurses,

George and Peter. They both wore white pants and white T shirts with black shoes. It seemed the male nurses with the exception of Effeminate Curtis chose this outfit as if they were all in the Navy. The thought that I was on a Navy Base did dawn on me a couple of times having seen these outfits, which added to my already confused state.

"Hello, and welcome to Progressive," said George. He was in his thirties, wore glasses, and had a beard. "This is Peter and we're going to be on consecutive shifts with you over the next couple of days. We're changing shifts right now and Peter will be watching you during the night shift."

Peter reminded me of a Chief Mate on one of the merchant ships I served on during my stint as a cadet in the late 80s, so my suspicions were again raised with him. These guys seemed nice enough; it was just that my suspicions were still boundless. I just hoped they were going to stay nice. I missed my MICU buddies.

George returned to the room after a while. I guess he was getting acclimated with my chart when he said, "From your chart I see you've been through a whole hell of a lot. I imagine you're relieved to be getting through it. I can't believe all that you've gone through."

"Yes, so I've heard," I wasn't sure what the chart said but having a body rebuilt as well as giving a male birth can be a trying thing. I was hoping that we could get past my stupidity in the MICU and some of that would remain confidential.

While everyone was gone, the one thing that I really did not want to see, the dialysis machine, was brought into the room. I really did not want to get hooked up to that thing again. It just made me feel confined and made me feel weird with an awful tingly feeling. The young dialysis tech I remembered from the MICU had followed me to the room.

I said jokingly, "How did you find me? I thought I was rid of that thing."

"We always know where you are. We brought it just in case they need it," she replied.

I really was in no mood to see that thing anymore especially once I learned that it did not make Icees, At least its delivery brought a familiar face from the MICU. I missed them, but certainly not enough to go back.

During my time in the MICU I became accustomed to these different people coming into my room in weird garb checking on that machine. Eventually on those visits the tech would come back in and pronounce, "All done," and would unsnap whatever on my person. However, "All done" didn't mean shit to me. I was still just going to lie there like always.

***

CUM ON FEEL THE NOIZ[114]

I finally realized that what I was seeing through my peripheral vision coming out of my nose was a feeding tube. It seemed it was just hanging there and in a state of disrepair. George and Peter talked about how it looked kinked or clogged or something and that it needed to be fixed. Its current troublesome state was the first time I had become fully aware of it. Sure, I sometimes saw a bottle of something turned upside down by my bed and somehow I was not ravenous when I was awake, it just didn't dawn on me to ask what or why that was. The act of eating had been missed but it was by no means weighing me down.

Now I knew the reason, the feeding tube. Who had time to ask such questions? I had staring at the wall to do.

However, I felt that was the least of my problems, since my face was half missing. How could George and Peter even look at me with my disfigurement? The folks in MICU must have gotten used to my appearance like that Mel Gibson's surly *The Man without A Face*. That night I had finally been able to fall asleep. The lights were kept dimmer in Progressive than in the MICU so I was able to sleep a little better. During the night I was awakened by what sounded like a soda can being opened. My nose instantly caught the whiff of Pepsi. This did not dissuade me from keeping my eyes closed. I had never had a nighttime visitor come in and open a Pepsi under my nose like that so I lay still to see how this was going to play out. Would they pour it on me then release a jar of ants? I lay there as the visitor messed with the feeding tube. I wasn't sure what the end game was for the feeding tube, but I tried to let whoever it was finish and be on his/her/Dog Person's way since I really didn't want to confront anyone at this hour. After a while, with the fiddling complete the visitor left the room and I was left in peace.

***

THERE YOU ARE

The first night I had slept in a long time, my first night in Progressive and I heard a familiar voice come through the haze. "There you are. Finally moved him," the male voice said to Becky. I suddenly realized it was our good friend and former neighbor, John Landon, coming by.

After a few moments of hearing the chatter I woke up to say hello. "Hey, sorry for coming in the middle of the night, I just wanted to see how you're doing," he said.

"Thanks, come at any time, they keep moving me around to keep you on your toes," I said.

"I was on my toes, upstairs," he recalled. "I went to your old room and you weren't there. I got the shakes thinking the worst and went over to the nurse's station. They saw my alarm when I asked about you. You weren't in the system yet as having been moved. Finally, one of the nurses took pity and said she would walk me over. I went through hall after hall. It took forever to get here."

I was stunned that he would have seen an empty room where I could always be found. The thought of that was unsettling.

"Hey, as long as you're getting closer to the front door, that's all that matters," he said

That goal just seemed ridiculous, everyone knew this was my new place of residence and I would soon be getting my mail here.

***

WHEN YOU'RE DOWN HE'LL PICK YOU UP[115]

The next day I was able to get my bearings a little more. This was definitely a different looking section of the hospital. It looked older and my thoughts were confirmed when my parents asked about this area.

"This is the oldest tower in the hospital," George said.

So were they going to build them a new one? That didn't seem fair.

I could tell it was the start of the work day as my room faced out on two work stations that held two middle aged women pecking away at keyboards. They would also send and receive documents through a vacuum tube. How old was this place? They're still using vacuum tubes? These hospitals in Winston-Salem were so antiquated, in Charlotte we had much newer everything. I referred to a collective "we" as if I had anything to do with the advent of a new technology.

I would study these ladies as they were so focused on what they were doing. I couldn't see how they did it with all of this sickness around them and with yours truly staring at them. If my office had sick people looking out on me I think I might be a little distracted or tried harder to look busy. Work harder, not smarter! There they would work all day and as evening came the day would end for them and they would pack up and go home while I stuck around. I would like to go home but then again I wouldn't want to work here.

The mystery of the nighttime visitor with the Pepsi was revealed when Peter came back on duty that night. He said, "I had seen that your feeding tube was clogged and twisted so a solution I thought of was from something I read where soda has been a proven way of eating away at the obstruction."

I also had heard that and it was also a delicious way of getting rid of corrosion on the terminals of a car battery as well. What must that stuff do to your insides? I still remember the old wives' tale that I was told at the orthodontist when I was eleven years old of some lesson learned by an obviously bored person putting a piece of meat in a glass of soda one night. When said bored person, now excited with something to do, returned the next morning the piece of meat was gone. Perhaps a rat came in and ate the sweetest piece of meat it had ever had or the FDA had the wool pulled over their eyes all of these years. All I know is the bored impressionable eleven-year-old that was me tried the very same thing later that week and lo and behold the piece of meat was still on hand in the morning. Back then I felt relief not only that my insides would remain intact but we had a rat-free house as well.

***

HATE IS NOT A STRONG ENOUGH WORD[116]

With my new found consciousness I was beginning to realize that being in the hospital was a combination of long periods of silence, boredom, and panic as new faces came in wielding new instruments or opinions. I had to tell myself that each step was a step out of here. This made me feel better as a curtain would be drawn or I was asked to lie in this position or that position.

Becky now had to return to work for a couple of hours a day. I would become very anxious that she wasn't there to watch over me. Sometimes this task would fall to Big Daddy of whom I would hear his snores before I saw him. I couldn't blame him. The hospital was a place that I would like to sleep away my time in as well. It was quiet and time was all I had to get better.

Early during my stay in Progressive one of those moments of panic came to me. Big Daddy was sitting by the window with his paper keeping me company. It was late morning and George came in and said, "I'm going to have to change your catheter."

I thought, *but the young blonde nurse in the MICU gave me a departing gift of a catheter only a couple of days ago, how could this be?* I met George's statement with silence and dread. I knew the pain I had suffered there would be upon me again. I asked pleadingly, "Is there something I can get for the pain?"

George said no there wasn't, I just had to get through it. I knew of the catheter. The thought of a tube being inserted into the doodle made me cringe. At least I had valium before I got the Big V. The doctor then asked if I wanted him to do color commentary while he was performing the incision on my sac not once but twice and disappointingly for him not thrice. Of course I replied with a "Hell no!" As it turned out the smell of burning nuts was enough color commentary for me.

This time I saw George preparing the catheter. He had the box and took out a tray where he squirted some bluish goo onto it. At least he wasn't reading the instructions. While he was doing that he said to Big Daddy who was aware what was coming and was frozen in his seat, "He's going to hate me for this."

I thought this was pretty unnecessary; there was nowhere to hide from it. George then said, "OK let's do this."

I felt the tube enter my one-eyed monster and the pain hit me like an anvil. George threw a heart-shaped stress ball I had been given by the physical therapist and said, "Here, squeeze the shit out of this."

I began a low moan hoping that would take my mind off the situation, but it didn't seem to work so the moan grew louder and louder. Having finally thawed from his chair, Big Daddy made a quick exit from the room during the low moan portion of the program. My only hope was that my Johnson survived this and that I could piss again.

The thought entered my mind that I should have made a request to just let me hold it like the time I had to piss a bucketful at the old Tampa Stadium in 1991 when the New York Football Giants came to play the Bucs. Phil Simms gratefully passed the winning touchdown against the Bucs to avoid overtime and saved my bladder from entering another dimension since I feared stage fright in the antiquated facilities. There was also the time I drank my weight in beer to forget the ugly duet of girls my friend and I were out with one night. I knew this would only be considered for comedic value and while impressive was not medically feasible. Unrequired yapping would also have delayed the completion of the horror.

When I saw Big Daddy depart, I made my moan louder so that it would chase him down the hall. He knew what I was going through having been through it only a year before and he didn't want to be witness to it. I just didn't see how someone like famed 1970s porno star Johnny Holmes could survive something like this. He would have been approximately ten inches flaccid or so I heard. That's a lot of real estate to cover. His moans would have followed Big Daddy to the parking deck and back to his house in Georgia. Why Big Daddy would be on hand for the insertion of a catheter into Johnny Holmes is where the scenario obviously falls apart.

The seemingly endless pain finally came to an end but the feeling that something was in me made me uncomfortable as my awareness of such things grew.

George said, "Don't worry about the sounds, I always say to my nursing students that you have to experience something like this to know what your patients are going through." He continued to say, "That's why I've put a catheter in myself to understand that."

I didn't know if I had heard him correctly, when my pike and I are alone together my hot rod must know that it can trust me, not fear me.

"Anyway," George said, "women talk about their plumbing and all the hardships they have, well, their urethra's only about this long," as he held up his fingers only a couple of inches apart. "The catheter's in them in no time."

This was quite a pep talk and luckily my horror was over for now. I would now have a very weak comeback when the delivery of Phoebe without any pain medication is ever brought up by Becky again.

***

IT'S TOO LATE TONIGHT[117]

"Good evening, I need to know your name," the young female nurse asked me.

What happened? Did she lose my chart? She better know my name. I answered, "Howard Hoover."

"Mr. Hoover, where are you?" she then asked.

Call me "Sir" dammitt! I was in a fog, it was the middle of the night and I could hardly think. "General Hospital," I replied with some uncertainty.

Not looking satisfied she asked me, "And why are you here?"

I said immediately, "Strep throat," just to get her off my case. I knew the real reason. I didn't want them to know that I knew so I played along. Strep throat, indeed. Sure, I have been in the hospital this long when I could have just been at home with ice chips and bad daytime TV. Right. Wink Wink.

She seemed satisfied, turned off the light and left the room. I was relieved to have passed the test but the whole thing seemed implausible. There was no way I was in General Hospital, no way. I had not in any way been outside since I was moved to Winston-Salem and there was no way I took the eighty-minute drive south to General Hospital. Strep throat? There was no way strep throat rendered me this way, no way. It was the body rebuild, anyone could see that. My body was rejecting the parts those fuckers in Manhattan had inserted. This was not my body, no way.

In hindsight what I should have said was, "The rocking pneumonia and the boogie woogie blues." In any event who knows what would have happened had I replied what I really thought. Half of my face was missing! Why was I saying strep throat!? Let them know the real reason, they know! Enough of the charade!

Sometime later the light was on again. It was the same nurse, "Good evening, I need to know your name."

What was this now? A bed check? *Believe me, I have neither the ability nor desire to go anywhere right now. For the love of God let me get some sleep!*

"Mr. Hoover. Where are you?" The questioning continued.

In a place that's annoying the living shit out of me! "General Hospital," I said.

"And why are you here?"

"Strep throat," came the reply. She turned off the light again and left me in peace.

The following night the light came on again. "Good evening, I need to know your name."

It was the same nurse. I could see her smiling face above me. It looked like she was enjoying this, if she had to be up then I did too. I felt like having some fun with it and saying the alias I used when I was ashore during sea year, "James Tiberius Kirk," but thought better of it.

"Mr. Hoover, where are you?"

God Almighty, unless you beamed me somewhere I must be in the same place. "General Hospital," was my stock reply.

"And why are you here?"

"Strep throat."

She left the room satisfied. I was ready the next time. I felt like the grandparents in *Sixteen Candles* standing watch over the phone while that dreamboat Jake was trying to contact the overrated Samantha. Perhaps they won't be bothering me anymore now that I have told them what they wanted to hear.

The light came on. How fucking long was this night?

"Good evening, I need to know your name."

"Howard Hoover."

"Mr. Hoover, where are you?"

"General Hospital."

"Why are you here?"

"Strep throat."

Finally Becky who had been sleeping by the window perked up. "Is this necessary, to wake him up like this during the night and disturb him?"

The nurse explained that it was written in the night orders to wake me up to discern whether I was in my right mind or not by asking me these three basic questions. I couldn't believe this when more normal responses to her questions at this time of night would have been more questions such as: "Who am I?" Where am I?" Why am I here?"

When I was healthy and we had newborns in the house I could tell what time of night it was just by how I felt if they started crying. If it was midnight to 1:00 a.m., I was like a drunken eighty-five-year-old man that had no clue if he was in his house or sitting back sipping a brown liquid with Sinatra and the boys at the Flamingo in the early 60s. "Come join me for some Scotch!" I would scream as I would stumble towards the crying. "Lawford's bringing the girls!" Sadly, these exclamations never stopped the crying.

***

GET ON YOUR BOOTS[118]

I was always so hot, I couldn't take it. The covers were smothering me. I was thirsty and I could find absolutely no relief. It was right around dawn and I had spent a night with these damn socks that somebody put on me, obviously as a joke. They were driving me up the wall to no end. I couldn't handle them being on my feet anymore. I could barely move my feet so the usual practice of using the toes to remove them was not going to work like it always had in the past. The laziness I took for granted before this happened.

When presented with such a dilemma in the past I, like all other healthy people, could simply bend at the waist and reach with their hands to pull the socks off. What a cocky lazy relaxer I was with applying the alternative method of using my feet to remove the socks. What I would give to be able to bend at the waist and lift my arms and use my hands.

I was in a total supine position and I was going crazy. Instead of using my toes I was able to slowly press my legs together and slowly, oh so slowly, inch the socks down my calf inch by excruciating inch. My legs at this point were spindles and the calves I was using were just bone. They were awful to look at but they were my friend at this point. After several minutes one sock was down at my foot and with my other foot I was able to push it the rest of the way where it unceremoniously dropped to the floor. I continued this process with the next foot and it was another several minutes that passed before the next sock was off. I felt like a prisoner who had nothing but time to make his escape and no one could know.

During this time my paranoia was still high. I was afraid of being caught doing something that had not yet been approved and my time would be extended. As nurses came in I would stop, not even thinking to put in a request to remove the socks lest they scoff at me. If it were Polly I would have asked, since we had gotten through that whole nasty firing. Maybe not the Evil Clown face-making business but I would have asked anyway. These new nurses were going to have to gain my trust.

After what seemed forever for this slow process to end, my feet were finally free and I was suddenly feeling cheered up having accomplished such a feat that I always took for granted. There we go, this day could do nothing but be better than the last few. I was still in the hospital yet my legs were still moving.

As I basked in the glow of my achievement, exhausted but satisfied with a job well done, the physical therapist, who had a striking resemblance to Emma Stone, walked in and said hello a few minutes into my newly found foot freedom.

Then to my horror I watched as she bent down and picked up the socks off the floor, handed them to me and said, "Here, put these on."

CHAPTER 28

Reunion

Once the patient's respiratory status has been stabilized, the adequacy of perfusion (delivery of blood to a capillary bed in the biological tissue) should be assessed.[119]

JUST MY IMAGINATION[120]

"I'm thinking of bringing in the Babies if that's OK with you," Becky said one evening when she returned from the office.

"That's such a long drive for you. What would that be, ninety minutes or something one way?" I replied.

"Perhaps with the parking deck but no, we live right around the corner."

"I don't understand. Did you move everyone up here to be with me?"

"No, where do you think we are?"

"Well, we're in Winston-Salem at the well-known local university hospital of course," I replied. My confidence in our location was now becoming a little shaky.

"No, you have been here in Charlotte the entire time. You never left here. You have been just around the corner from our house the entire time."

My world had just gotten a lot smaller. I suddenly realized everything I thought, everything I imagined was not real. I was convinced that home was just a dream and I was in another time and place. This plain realization shocked me to no end. I began to cry with relief that I was safe and always at home. I couldn't believe it, I just couldn't believe it. The Babies had been just around the corner the entire time. I knew this place, General Hospital! I was here! I drive by here all the time! It was like the curtain had been lifted on the Wizard and I could now plainly see my life taking shape. It was not the abstract faint memory that I thought it was, it was here and it was real. I wept for joy and with embarrassment.

"I can't believe you really thought you were away from Charlotte this entire time," Becky said.

"I had to believe it, I couldn't think that I could be in such pain at home. I had to go somewhere else," I replied. "Everyone's really OK? Are they going to let me see them? Am I allowed? No one will stop you?"

She held my hand and said, "You're safe here, you have always been safe, and the Babies have always been safe, you must know that. You were under the best care just around the corner from our house and no one was going anywhere. The Babies have been going to school and have been getting along without you, it has been hard but they have managed. Lots of neighbors have taken them in and have given my mom a break. The Lavernes had them over for dinner and had a fire pit in the backyard, the Donner Noreens had them over for a movie night, the Joneses took Henry to Plaza Fiesta and then to their house, the Landons have taken them out to eat and had them over to their house. Everyone has been helping out. You mean so much and they were all willing to lend a hand."

I was in disbelief. I didn't know how to repay them except with my gratitude. I only hoped that I knew how to help when the time came. I was so proud of our friends and neighbors, it was an amazing feeling.

I stared at the wall with tears still in my eyes. My parents, aunt, and uncle had just arrived. Becky didn't tell them my revelation.

Changing the subject, Becky said, "The Babies are getting adamant about wanting to come and see you. I don't know if that'll be too much for you or not. It's your decision. My thinking was that I would bring Henry here since I don't think you could handle all three being here at once. I'll bring him in first to see if you could handle that because if he tells Kate and Phoebe that he visited you they'd never believe him."

That sounded good to me, I didn't have a better plan. I was just so excited and anxious to see the little guy. She then left. It felt like forever. I had to entertain my parents, aunt, and uncle with one-liners that I thought were funny.

My dad said, "What a wonderful feeling it'll be for you to sit and watch TV with your son on the bed with you." That sounded like something I thought would never happen. I still wanted to leave; I was feeling more normal nevertheless it was not going as quickly as I thought it would.

Finally without warning I saw Becky round the corner and she said, "Someone wants to see you." Then who should round the corner but Henry. I never thought I would ever see him again. I thought he was gone or never existed. At that moment I knew that the life I had left behind was still there and a sense of calm and relief just came over me.

I said, "There he is! My little fella!"

He looked a little confused walking in and was silent for some time realizing that he was on stage with all eyes on him. He had on the familiar blue windbreaker with yellow stripes running down the sleeves. Everything was coming back to me; it felt like years since I had seen him. My life was still here, it was really still here. I was so thankful. I felt so good about it all.

My parents being there with my aunt and uncle confused Henry a bit. Big Daddy spoke first, "Do you know who that is, Henry?" Henry looked up at me.

I said, "It's me, Daddy!" My appearance must have been shocking to him. He only glanced at me and looked away. He just could not believe it was his daddy. I agreed that I did not look myself with half my face still missing, at least I could have put on the *Marvin* mask before his arrival, but I was not to be swayed. All I cared about was that he was here and I had not dreamed his entire life.

"You want to get on the bed with Daddy?" Becky said.

Henry looked indecisive on this count. He definitely thought I was a stranger and he didn't answer.

"Come here with Daddy!" I said choking up a bit.

He sat on the bed reluctantly looking at Becky, my parents, and then he would look back at me but he would look away quickly. It appeared he found my feeding tube alarming. I had lost forty pounds and my body was rail thin and I had the trach tube still sticking out of my neck not to mention half my face was missing. He was mulling the scene over in his head. This certainly was not what he had expected when he was coming to visit Daddy. We turned on some cartoons for him and he watched while keeping an eye on me like I was Frankenstein ready to pounce on him. He didn't say much and usually he can't keep quiet.

Becky then said, "Talk to Daddy Henry, you were saying so much on the way here."

"How have you been Henry?" I said. Not really sure of what to say myself. I didn't want to scare him and it was getting late.

"Good," he said.

"You know that I'm Daddy right? I've been here the whole time and the doctors and nurses helped me get back," I said

He nodded. I tried to move my arm to touch him but was unable to. Probably better since I didn't want to alarm him too much.

"OK Henry, we're going to leave now," Becky said.

Henry looked all too willing to go.

"I'll be back, Henry. I'm coming home. It's just me," I said as he left. "Thanks for coming and I love you."

The two of them left and I began to cry silently for joy. He was still here.

***

ANYTIME AT ALL[121]

We were talking about Henry's reaction to my feeding tube but of course I thought that was silly since I was a Two Face wannabe and the real reason was my missing face. As if the night could not be fuller of surprises, Kate and Phoebe rounded the corner. While Henry didn't know what to think of the atmosphere, the situation, and if I was indeed his daddy, Kate and Phoebe were bundles of shrieks as they saw me for the first time.

"Once I got Henry home I just had to bring the girl Babies," Becky said about her plan taking shape as she went along.

Kate and Phoebe immediately came to my side and began whimpering like puppies, giving me googly eyes and smiles.

"I'm so glad you're here!" I said. "How are you!? The girl Babies! I love you so much!"

They were straining to jump into the bed with me. "Hi Daddy!" came their reply. "We miss you so much!"

My world was coming back together. I couldn't believe my fortune, I had to get out of here and be their Daddy again. I was a little leery about them getting too close since I was still under no contact but I wanted to hug them so much, they were so cute. Ever since that dark day when I didn't know where Kate was or if she even existed, now there was a great big light shining on my life.

"I have been here the entire time sleeping and getting better," I explained.

"We wanted to see you so much," Kate said, "Mommy and Grandma said you were sleeping and that we couldn't bother you. It has been so long," she said with her voice shaking with excitement. Phoebe was quiet, standing right next to her.

"How are you Phoebe?" I asked.

She said "Good," in her Phoebe way with the answer belying more meaning than she was willing to let go of. "How are you Daddy?"

"I'm doing much better but I'm weak and I have to stay here until I'm strong enough to go home," I replied.

"Are you glad to see us?" Kate asked.

"Happier than I have ever been. You don't know what a relief it is to see you guys. I have always been here. Sorry I left without saying anything," I said trying to explain yet not say too much. I was at a loss for words. They were so cute and innocent. I just hoped it wasn't too trying for them.

We sat in silence. They were staring at my feeding tube. Answering the question before they could ask I said, "That's Daddy's feeding tube, it keeps food coming in and all that time before I came here I had been eating like a sucker."

"Does it hurt?" Phoebe asked.

"No, the only problem is since it's on the tip of my nose it gets in the way of watching TV," I replied lightheartedly.

They looked full of questions that they didn't know how to ask and I was full of reassurances that I didn't exactly know how to give. I cried so much over them, and this moment was draining me. Becky, seeing my energy dissipating said, "It's a school night so we need to get you guys home and Daddy needs to rest."

"You do look tired Daddy, do you want us to come back and visit?" Kate said.

"All the time," I replied.

Becky left with the girls and my parents, aunt, and uncle also took their leave. I was left alone with my thoughts. So much had been revealed, I was back in Charlotte and my kids were healthy and really existed.

George walked in the room and said, "You have a beautiful family."

All I could say was, "Thanks."

***

TUBE REMOVAL MACHINE[122]

An old friend was about to be leaving me today, George made the announcement when he came in to check on me. Yes, the feeding tube was going away. The next step to recovery but the more prominent, I thought. The thing had been troublesome, but the least of my problems, from the start. Late night fixes, the view blocker, and it reminded me of a wad of old chewing gum that some prankster had stuck there.

"OK, we're going to remove this now, I'm sure you'll hate to see it go," he said.

"Not a problem," I replied.

"Would you like to do the honors or would you like me to do it," he asked.

I could only imagine the horror of ripping this tube out of my nose which God knows was how far down into my body. "You do it," I said quickly.

Then with one motion he pulled on it. The sensation of something moving through my insides came over me. The end traveled from my stomach, up my esophagus, up my throat and suppressing a gag reflex was out of my mouth. It was not as uncomfortable as I imagined but it was not pleasant either.

"You'll slowly be eating solids, I think they'll start you on a liquid diet," he continued, giving me the benefit of knowing what I had coming.

Let the unplugging continue.

***

STRAPPING ON THE FEED BAG

At first I thought I was seeing things once again. The tray was put in front of me; on it was the light liquid dieter's dream come true. Beef bouillon, that was it. Warm too. Big Daddy was the only one in there with me. I had not been feeling very hungry with the no solid food for over four weeks, my stomach was not there. Big Daddy took the cup of hot liquid and sat me up in bed. My hands were too shaky and weak to hold the cup. I didn't know if this was the recovery that the hospital had envisioned with my father feeding me. However, when the choice came between having him do it or having hot soup spilled on my dangling participle I chose the former. The latter perhaps later but not now.

"Come on, you need to have some of this," he said as he tilted the cup and I drank it.

It was like nothing I had ever tasted before. I could not believe this was beef that I tasted. It seemed my taste buds were a little out of whack; I was trying to get this metallic/plastic taste out of my mouth, but at least the beef bouillon I could tell was beef bouillon.

As I finished up the bouillon I was relieved to taste something that wasn't water or a sugary drink. George took the mug away and said, "You did well. You should tell them you're ready to move on to other things like ice cream and such." He then left the room.

"Who do I tell if I'm not telling you?" I wondered. "Am I ready for such a big step? Ice cream?"

***

WE STILL HAVE A CURE WE THINK YOU'LL APPRECIATE[123]

The smiling nurse not only kept waking me up at 3:00 a.m., she was the next torch bearer of the shots in the stomach. They still hurt like hell and there was no way I was really getting used to them. Every eight hours like clockwork I would be awakened with the dart being thrown at my abdomen and it was getting tiresome.

I finally asked, "Is this really necessary every eight hours?"

The nurse said "This is the eight-hour dose that has been written down in your chart, so we need to give it to you during that timeframe. There's however a twenty-four-hour dose if you prefer."

"There is? Yes! Please!"

The nurse looked a little stunned at my reaction perhaps a little embarrassed that she had not thought of that. "I'll see if I can get that changed." She left after having shot me one more time. Life was a little better without what I called "The Eight-Hour Countdown."

***

LADY IV, GET AWAY FROM MY BIG INSTAFLATE BED[124]

I was told one night that my IV needed changing and that the IV lady would be around at eleven to change it. A late night IV change? Now I had heard of everything. I still could not explain my fear of needles and pain, considering what I had been through so far. Why this wasn't old hat by now was anyone's guess. Once a puss always a puss.

Becky was with me that night and the room was silent. I just wanted the IV lady to get there so I could finally go to sleep. I couldn't relax knowing that she would soon be on her way. The dim lighting was not really helping the mood in the room but slowly as the hands of the clock showed the moment of truth as 11:00 p.m., my anxiety grew to a crashing crescendo not unlike the one that any Barry Manilow song reaches with the sound of a cart slowly squeaking down the hallway.

My first thought was, *Quick! Hide!* That skill, however, was not in my toolbox at the moment so I just lay there. We soon realized that the reason for the slow squeaking of the wheels was due to the age of the IV lady. She was a slow walker slowly pushing a cart full of lots of goodies such as tubes, rubber bands, leeches, and needles.

The sound of the wheels announced her appearance long before her creepy shadow was projected on the wall just outside my room. Finally, the moment was here, *Ladies and Gentlemen, I give you Lady IV!*

She came into the room rolling the cart ever so slowly, until it mercifully came to a stop. The silence left in the room was by no means comforting. Lady IV was no spring chicken and it appeared as though she could use an IV herself, it must have been a long day.

"Hello, I'm here to switch out your IV," she said as she slowly came around to the side of the bed.

Do your damndest Lady IV, I fear you not! I thought with the utmost bravado. Instead I muttered an ever so modest, "OK."

The bright fluorescent light came on in the room. She looked at the IV in my left arm and took that one out with a flick of her wrist. She then sat next to the bed and looked at my arm. Lady IV studied it for a while and finally said, "I can't really find a good vein to put this in," she said to no one in particular and certainly not for my benefit.

Hush your mouth Lady IV, let me not hear your discourse over my veins, can you not tell that I am squeamish by nature? And if you are looking for other veins there might be some guy down the hall who I heard might be a troublemaker. Go after him.

"I guess we'll try this one," she said in a tone of surrender.

All this time Becky was sitting in her chair not saying a word. Her fears of Lady IV were surpassed only by mine as we both waited for this to be over. The rubber band went around my left arm. I felt the cold swab of the alcohol and then the poking commenced. Usually unpleasant things like this take no time and I am able to open my eyes with no problem. I mean I had just had a catheter stuck in my instrument! Certainly I could handle this but that was not the case at the moment. Further struggles occurred as she withdrew the needle and tried for another stab. The second stab didn't go as well as the first as I gritted my teeth waiting for the horror to be over.

She took out the needle again and said, "This vein is troubling, it keeps flipping out from under the needle."

At this I thought, *Vile Lady IV, keep your commentary to yourself. I care not to hear your confabulation over my vein. Hey! I sound pretty smart!*

I could sense Becky's discomfort as the grueling torture occurred for a third time. I was about to call the whole thing off when finally after the fourth time we had success.

"I hope that stays in, your veins are hard to find," She said with some relief.

What the hell was I supposed to do about that? My arms were string with no fat, there was no fat in there to provide any leverage. I was so glad that it was over and I really hoped I was not damaged in any way by this. I said, "Thank you," and added in my mind, *Please return from whence you came.*

She smiled pleasantly and the slow squeak of the wheels began as she rolled slowly out of the room. The sound took a while to fade away as she found her next victim. Maybe it was that troublemaker guy down the hall who I totally fabricated in my head.

***

HEY Y'ALL PREPARE YOURSELF FOR THE RUBBERBAND MAN[125]

"I'm here to remove your pic line," said the young nurse with the face shield.

It was around 10:30 p.m. and I had just turned off the TV. Why, when I am tired and am ready to retire after a long day of staring do I have people coming in wanting to mess with me? What I had turned off was not about to keep me away from sleep since I was getting more and more onto a regular sleep cycle. It was another meaningless college basketball game that was boring me to tears with the symposium on masonry occurring before my eyes.

The nurse came in in her white lab coat, mask, and face shield so she may have been something other than a nurse but it was hard to argue with the lab coat. I could barely see her face. I figured she looked like she knew what she was doing so I just said, "OK."

Her phone began to ring. I could see her pocket begin to glow. She answered, "Hey there, I can't really talk right now." It sounded like a personal call to me. "Because I got to remove a pic line, baby!" came her reply to the obvious question, "Why?" on the other end.

"OK, I'll talk to you later." She put the phone back in her pocket, put on some latex gloves, and took my left arm. I wasn't sure what this all implied so I consented to the arm giving. I couldn't look since I was dumbfounded that she would need my arm for anything. It was a skinny string bean that I couldn't move and I hadn't really noticed anything different about it so I was waiting to see what would happen.

The next thing I knew she was fiddling with an instrument and using it to remove something. She knew the exact spot where it was, I don't know how. Out of the corner of my eye I could see her remove it like a magician removing the endless string of handkerchiefs from his sleeve. It just kept coming, she kept pulling and lo and behold she was holding the dangling line that looked like a small snake in front of her face. She dangled it there, studying it. All I was waiting for was a "Ta-Da!" I was confused as to how that got in my arm and what's more how it stayed in it. There was silence coming from Becky's corner and I couldn't see her since the nurse was standing between the two of us. Needless to say both of us were speechless. I knew what I must have had, if someone could please explain it to me in a way that would stick in my mind, had to be pretty serious; and I was glad to be unplugged one more time, but then again I was worried about whether I would need that tube again. Removing was one thing, putting that mofo in again would be something I would not savor.

And like that she said, "Have a good night," and left. I guess the unplugging that Dr. Rebefall had mentioned had finally started in earnest.

CHAPTER 29

Temper

Critical hypoperfusion (decreased blood flow through an organ) include cool, vasoconstricted skin due to redirection of blood flow to core organs (although warm, flushed skin may be present in the early phases of sepsis), obtundation or restlessness, oliguria or anuria, and lactic acidosis.[126]

I WANNA GET OUT, I WANNA GO HOME![127]

The nurse set the tray down in front of me; she was not my nurse. She was a young brunette with olive skin and heavy eye shadow, and appeared to be either coming from or going to the clubs. George and Robin's watchful shifts had ended that day. It was lunch time and I was alone in the room. With a flick of the wrist the nurse took the cover off the plate like we were at Fleming's Steak House and I was about to savor some of their kick-ass French Onion soup. Once she got no response from me she said, "OK?" I nodded weakly. Then she turned on her heels and took off like she had a bus or a drink special to catch. As a matter of fact I was not OK, but my ability or notion that I could say otherwise was not in me at the moment. I guess she would have brought it up had I not been OK, so my deferential attitude at this time led me to believe that I was OK. OK?

The tray was about two inches in front of my face. I was practically eye level with it. Now I was under the questionable eye of Nurse Half Ass. She was an older lady with glasses, skinny and with curly hair. I had seen her maybe once during this shift and that was during a passing glance. I had not seen Nurse Half Ass in a while and I was scrunched down in my bed in a very uncomfortable position. There was no way I could pull myself up to any semblance of a place where minimal comfort could be found. I took a fork gingerly and tried to lift my arm to get some food. What time was it? 11:30 a.m. Where was everybody? I know I bitched about visitors but God could I use some now.

Usually my nurse checked in on me after the meal was delivered to see how I was doing. There was nothing. I saw Nurse Half Ass out in the hall getting a tray with a cup on it and returning to a room down the hall on my right. I swore the Royal Family must have been in that end of the hall, I had not seen her go anywhere except there, certainly not in here. When I actually needed my footboard to fire someone it was nowhere to be found. Damn returning sanity. I waited patiently, just waiting for someone, anyone to come into the room or ask if I needed help. Time dragged on and I was unable to lift my hand anymore; I gave up trying to lift myself. I just sat there helpless.

I did see one person, one of the middle-aged ladies I had seen working so feverishly directly across from my room at the computer and putting things in vacuum tubes to send whatever to remote portions of this immense place. I wondered how long it took for her to know what the hell she was doing in that particular job. I watched her for a while just envying her freedom of movement. *Look how she can sit in a chair and lift that tube, those were the days.*

I finally collected my courage, cleared my throat and said, "Excuse me," rather weakly.

She won't help me, I thought. *she's too focused on what she's doing with the vacuum tubes and how utterly cool they are to help. She can't be interrupted.*

But once I heard my own voice I felt a little emboldened and said again, "Excuse me." I didn't want to create alarm. Actually it was alarming since I was trying to enter this other dimension, pierce that fourth wall. Then I said louder, "Excuse me."

She suddenly looked up with alarm, looked around as if some inanimate object around her had spoken and then looked right at me. She looked surprised that I was talking just as surprised as I was that the fourth wall had been pierced. I must have looked like a piece of furniture all this time.

She got up from her chair and walked into my room very uncertainly. "Yes, what do you need?" She sounded more helpful than I thought she would, I was so relieved I said something.

I said, "I need help. Do you know where my nurse is? I can't sit up to eat."

She said, "I'll see where she is, hold on." She left the room; a short time later she returned and said, "She said she's busy and she'll be down in a minute."

After forever Nurse Half Ass came back in the room and looking exasperated said, "What is it?"

As if the situation wasn't plainly obvious, feeling like a child I said, "I need to be lifted up in bed, I can't eat."

"You'll need to hold on while I get someone." She then left.

My situation was now known so I would need to hold on longer but I was so fucking uncomfortable. Even with the power of voice, relief still seemed far off. I was working myself into a temper tantrum. I was angry, aware, and anxious. I needed to be seen. Where were my parents? Where was Becky? I felt abandoned.

My parents came in and I said with undisguised panic, "Where have you been?"

They seemed stunned that I was upset. I guess with being out of the MICU the immediate alarm had passed, therefore constant visits were not required. I was scared. Scared about tripping up in the middle of the race and I needed someone to be here.

"It's OK, we're here," my mom said.

My pent-up emotions were falling out now, uncontrolled. "I want to sit up, and no one was here, and I can't eat, and I'm shaking! No one will help me!" I wailed like a spoiled child. "I'm being ignored!"

"The nurse will be coming back shortly, I want to wait for her and not move you right now," my mom said.

All of a sudden like a ray of light I saw Becky round the corner. I was a damn mess by this point and felt like a failure. She took one look at me and without saying a word, slammed her purse down into the chair by the door, turned on her heel and left the room. How it must have felt for her to see the man she married, the father of her children looking like a tearful pile of goo. I heard her say immediately out in the hall, "I need to talk to you." I knew it would be OK with Becky here and was relieved but with the relief came the tears. I couldn't help it. The realization of the shape I was in was hitting me full on.

"WHY! WHY! Why did this happen! I can't do anything and I'm in this fucking bed that won't fit!" as I yelled and kicked the foot board.

Then I saw the lady from across the hall come back into the room. I yelled my appreciation overzealously but I meant it, "That lady saved my life! She saved my life!"

The lady grinned sheepishly as if that was really untrue; I didn't care, she was helping me. I then yelled as a couple of nurses came in without Nurse Half Ass, "I Want my life back! I want my life back!" I yelled over and over again. I thought it was a bit overly dramatic to be screaming this when indeed I did have my life back and by all miracles I was lucky to be here. The vent was overwhelmed and I had to let it go. The uncertainty, the fear, the pain, it all came out in one glorious outburst at all those nightmares, all those bastards that tormented me in those other worlds. The road was getting too long and I wanted out.

Becky came back in with another nurse who was very apologetic. I felt easier now. Grim silence was not going to do it this day, sometimes wailing like a two-year-old was the only way to get things done.

***

FOOD, GLORIOUS FOOD[128]

Progressive was as its name suggested, progressive, it was full of transitioning. I could feel the constant attention of the MICU was gone, either you progressed closer to the front door or you regressed back to the MICU. In any event a judgment call would be made about a patient's situation, and I was hoping I was providing a hopeful outlook for whoever was doing the decision-making regarding my status.

Add on to this the anxiety I felt about my appetite since it just didn't exist. I thought that this certainly would raise concern and send me back a few steps. Whatever the reason, I just could not stand the sound of food, the thought of it, the sight of it, especially the smell of it. I felt helpless. The anxiety felt by a neophyte going on his first date or the grand expectations of how a big moment would end, one you had thought about for the longest time was what it felt like when meal time would come. My stomach was in twists and turns. I began to fear meal time. When 5:00 p.m. came, I would see those food-tray carts rolling in the hallway and the fear would build inside me.

I would think, "I can't eat this, I can't do this, I won't be able to touch it and the feeding tube will go back in and I'll be taking a step back in getting out of here."

I would almost panic when that food tray would hit my table. I relayed my concerns to the nurse that brought in the tray once and she said, "If you're going to get better then you have got to eat."

This sent a wave of fear and guilt through me. I thought I was failing and I was being given a wake-up call. I really couldn't help any of it. My body just did not crave food. I really feared what the next step was going to be if I continued my non-eating ways.

But it wasn't only the challenges with my stomach or the mental aptitude to actually desire food it was the physical handicap that I had with my hands. It seemed they would shake uncontrollably as they began to wake up. I was not sure if this was a side effect of the paralytics I had been given during the dark days in the MICU or not, I just did not want to call attention to it. It was hard not to do this. Attention over this was implicit when I was trying to eat. It would take an hour for me to eat a few mouthfuls which I could barely stand to put in my mouth. I would ignore it but I could feel the concern on my parents' faces and on Becky's. I must have looked pathetic, a half-faced weirdo with his hands shaking uncontrollably trying to steer food in his cake hole. I wondered how long it would be before they came back for the tray and would monitor what I had. I obsessed over this fear, my stomach was not cooperating.

I said again to another nurse, "I can't eat."

She said, "You're going to have to, that's the only way to get your strength back! Or we'll have to put the feeding tube back in you."

I was overcome with pity, fear, anxiety that I was failing and failing with what should be something easy to do. I survived all that had come before and now it was going to be prolonged because I could not eat.

To add insult to injury, I was given a chocolate drink of Nuprin with every meal that I could not drink much less look at. The can would usually remain unopened as the nurse would ask whether I wanted it or not as she took away my tray. One had a confused expression when I replied "no" to her query regarding the untouched Nuprin as she left the room with the still full tray. I thought I was an hour away from that feeding tube being shoved back in.

***

SPONGE BATH

Without a shower for the last month, the occasional sponge bath was my only outlet for hygiene. Early during my time in Progressive while George was still my nurse there was a morning when a young blonde girl came in with a plastic basin, pitcher, washcloth, and towels. She was obviously a rookie, perhaps a Nurse's Aide, and said little to me except, "I'm here for your sponge bath." Big Daddy gave me a wink from the window and left the room. George came in to do something and see if she had everything she needed.

"Do you want me to chart this?" she asked.

I didn't hear his answer but he looked like he wanted her to give him a sponge bath.

How young and eager she was. I remembered being like that.

She was all business, made no small talk and put in a yeoman's effort. I was a little embarrassed by the exposure of my Big Ben and with a tube hanging out of it no less. She left no stone unturned and although I wanted a little more gentleness at the same time I was thinking that I should be enjoying this. Even if I was watching myself on camera going through it I would have looked at my condition and seen that getting better and getting out of here was more important than any joy that could be derived from the moment.

As someone said to a room full of revelers when I was in high school, "There's a fine line between pain and pleasure." I wasn't sure if this is what he meant but this was the ideal situation for that quote. However, in my situation there was only the fear of pain. Pain, if I felt pleasure and that fear was between me, the peace maker, and the catheter, if you catch my drift.

She finished quickly and was gone without saying a word. With half my face missing she must not have been able to stand the sight of me.

On the other end of the pain/pleasure spectrum, a couple of days later two big women came in and worked me over like a washrag. I was flipped this way or that and was unable to provide resistance even if I wanted to. There was no pain vs. pleasure debate here, only pain and the forecast called for more. As they ripped the sheet off me they started to go after my bishop with relish. They scrubbed the tip like they were removing the rust from a '74 Pinto and similar to the factory recalls surrounding the Pinto's fuel tank I was afraid that my hickey would explode from the pain.

I finally had enough with the rubbing and said, "At Ease." I thought they were going to break off the tube in my bazooka.

One of the nurses said, "There's this scab here that we should remove."

Scab? On the tip of the percy? That's the last place you want to remove a scab and I should know because I'm enduring the process right now!

But they relented and my business was saved for future adventures.

A young Hispanic nurse came by another day to shave me and give me another bath. What the hell was going on here? It was like someone was testing me behind the curtain. "The young blonde nurse, the sadism of the big nurses, now send in a little international flavor," somebody would say in a growly evil voice.

Was this some sort of devious arousal test similar to the taste test? I wondered.

She reminded me a little of Salma Hayek but then again I was still delirious. She had a very soothing demeanor about her and a great voice asking me, "Is OK?" I was anxious when the shaving began, those hospital razors were unforgiving. Thanks to her skill, I received no cut whatsoever and the shaving was thankfully conducted well north of the equator. She was done and left and I felt much better that the fear of pain was gone for the time being.

***

PHYSICAL THERAPY

Mike was in and out and would send in other physical therapists in his place. One came in, a young brown-haired girl. Big Daddy was there once again which I found odd and highly coincidental. The one time he wasn't there I got the big nurses working me over. It always seemed like he was there when a young something would come to see me so while his snoring could be annoying I couldn't argue with the results. Once again she interrupted my stories on the talking picture machine.

She said, "You ready for your therapy? I'm going to work you out."

Big Daddy then piped up inappropriately as expected, "You poor sap, she certainly will work you out," as he left the room.

The therapist smiled sheepishly. I nodded trying to cover my embarrassment pretending like I didn't hear him.

***

ABOUT LAST NIGHT

I was awakened by Nurse Half Ass talking to my mom who was sitting by the bed early in the evening. She seemed to be telling her what had gone wrong earlier and why she was unable to get to me in a timely manner.

"I'm on light duty right now. I had to help this overweight man get into the bed and my wrist was badly sprained. I've been put in Progressive and I've been playing catch up the entire time with this brace on my wrist," she said.

I felt bad for my outburst, but I didn't show that I was awake. I was still angry about the whole incident and wondered why they had a nurse watching multiple patients who was supposedly on light duty. I wasn't in the MICU anymore.

***

FLY BY NIGHT[129]

The move came suddenly. I was told after dinner that a room had opened up and I was to be moved that evening. My new home was about to be my old home. I thought of what John Landon said that it's good if it gets me closer to the front door.

At 11:30 p.m. I couldn't wait any longer and right when I was about to turn out the light, a two-man crew came in to move me. Big orderlies they were and they began to move all of my stuff onto the cart. It was not as entertaining as watching the blonde nurse in the MICU and it had a very secretive feel to it but at least this time I was confident that a new catheter would not be my parting prize. I could only assume that these guys might have split my serpent down the middle had they been called to do that painful deed. The cart was loaded and Becky was frantically looking for all of her things to put on the cart as well because it would be hopeless to be left behind and lost in this maze. I felt like crap and was tired. I had to convince myself that the next step was the next step and I was ready for it to happen. At least I didn't have to walk or move anything. Being helpless as a small kitten does have its benefits.

The bed was moved out into the hallway. Once again it provided a great comedy of errors to all of those who tried to move it with the current moving crew being no exception. I had heard it all before as I told them, "You guys aren't the first to curse this bed."

I could finally see behind the curtain of this stage and all of the hallways that I had not seen since the last move. I took in the sights this time, all of the rooms, all of the doctors and nurses working through the night. The place just astounded me with its constant energy, with life and death passing through these halls every day. I felt like such a veteran to have avoided the latter. As they walked me past a door that must have opened to the outside, I could feel a cold gush of wind hit my face.

Closer to the front door. Getting closer to the front door.

CHAPTER 30

Awakening

After initial assessment, a central venous catheter (CVC) should be inserted in most patients with severe sepsis or septic shock. A CVC can be used to infuse intravenous fluids, infuse medications, infuse blood products, and draw blood. In addition, it can be used for hemodynamic monitoring by measuring the central venous pressure (CVP) and the central venous oxyhemoglobin saturation (ScVO2). [130]

ROOM 7XXX OR HEAVEN ON THE SEVENTH FLOOR[131]

I was moved into my new room. It seemed newer, a little more out of the way and it had a bathroom much to Becky's delight. A male nurse was on shift when I came in. He had a shaved head, glasses, a dark goatee but more amazingly and strikingly was that he had more metal hanging around his neck than Mr. T.

I thought, *better not piss this guy off, you never know someone's mental state when they're wearing that much crap around their neck.*

It was amazing the amount of monitors that I needed to have plugged in and moved along with all the tubing, the process seemed endless and tiring for my prone self to watch. I was impressed with how seamless it all seemed and how they all knew what everything was. There was never confusion about this part going with that or anything. Nurse Bling and another male nurse were putting a puzzle together in the middle of the night in a room that only had light coming from the sink. I also was amazed at how quiet it was in this part of the hospital. Was there anyone here? It seemed as silent, as still as that place they took Jamie Lee Curtis in *Halloween II*. I was at their mercy but I felt more comfortable than I ever had. The best thing of all was that after an hour of effort when Nurse Bling finished, he turned out the light and closed the door. Complete darkness, complete stillness. I could not believe that after the open door policies of the past four and a half weeks that I was finally in the dark. I felt human and suddenly I fell asleep.

***

WHAT RHYMES WITH BLAGYL?

Once my taste test was done, I was able to start swallowing some medicine in earnest. Maybe I should have failed on purpose to avoid the awful pill they called Flagyl that I renamed Sir Flagyl because one has to show respect for a wary adversary. Sir Flagyl was another of my meds that I feared as much as the blood builder shot into my stomach. Sir Flagyl came into my life when I got the flexi-seal attached to my kazoo. So it was the most glorious or ominous, depending on your point of view, two-for-one deal in the history of my life.

I asked my bedside doctor, a lady who was about my age, wore glasses very well, had straight brown hair, and was quite petite to clear up the confusion that surrounded me about Sir Flagyl. She began to come in later during my stay in the MICU. She said that she knew my primary doctor but hell if I didn't keep forgetting her name. I would ask her and my parents, who were as forgetful as me, would ask as well the never ending question: "Why? Why? Do(es) I (he) have to take this awful medicine?"

I recalled from my Swiss-cheese memory her explanation of there being a test to see whether or not there was an intestinal infection or parasite present and the test that proved this was only seventy percent accurate so the only way to make sure that the parasite was no more was to give me Sir Flagyl. And it appeared I would be taking this for two weeks to ensure that this was the case.

What was the reason I hated and respected Sir Flagyl with such a passion? Let me count the ways. First, in its tablet form it's shaped like some sort of dog biscuit and close to the same size. My swallowing skills were not exactly up to snuff since my trach tube was still hanging out in my throat so swallowing things was not really a skill that I had at the moment. I tried and tried to swallow it but I kept gagging and throwing it up. This would happen not only as I tried to swallow it but even when I envisioned finally swallowing it. Success was not guaranteed once I thought it was down, and no amount of water would make it go down.

Second, Sir Flagyl got into my head playing its dangerous mind games. Anxiety would overtake me when a new nurse would come on shift. She/he would introduce themselves and then say, "I'll go and get your meds and I'll be right back." The fear would then seep in and I would feel that this was when I would finally choke to death. The body rebuild may not get me but that goddamned dog-biscuit pill would.

After the umpteenth incident of being unable to swallow this horse tablet Becky piped up, "Is there any other way he can take this? It just isn't going down and it's causing him quite a bit of anguish."

"This is the smallest dose it comes in," came the reply.

"Can't you split it up at least?"

"That really isn't a good idea, the broken ends would be jagged and that could tear something on the way down."

I certainly didn't want that and that was the third reason I hated Sir Flagyl.

The nurse continued, "We can break it up into some applesauce or ice cream, would you like that?" She spoke to me directly.

Applesauce or ice cream? Yes! Yes! came my thought yet my actual reaction was a more subdued nod.

It seemed my problems were solved, just eat what I enjoyed and have the medicine. Win Win for Howard! The nurse left and came back in with some sort of implement to crush the medicine that looked like a big ordeal. Then the powder was put into a bowl of ice cream. Since my arms were useless, especially my hands and fingers, she fed it to me. The ice cream was a heavily anticipated event. I took my first bite of ice cream in weeks and the taste that came through was the fourth reason I hated Sir Flagyl, the taste was one of bitter asphalt. It was as if I was forced to lie on a parking lot and lick the oil-slicked surface. It was the worst damn taste I had ever experienced and I grew up in the 70s when liver was served to children for dinner on a regular basis.

I was livid. How could they besmirch the good name of this yummy ice cream? It was so nasty. I don't know what I would have done had the Taste Lady included this in her bag of tricks.

"You must eat all of it," the nurse said.

I knew I was going to have trouble with this, I had unwittingly spread Sir Flagyl to a volume that now I really didn't think I could handle. I struggled to finish enough to get the nurse the hell out of the room. I quickly discovered after I tried to get through the last of it that the only thing worse than eating powdered Sir Flagyl was the aftertaste that powdered Sir Flagyl left in my mouth. It left a trail of destruction of the taste senses all the way down the throat. I never got used to it, and I even tried to swallow it again but that powdered form stayed with me for quite a while. I can still taste it today, and if I ever think something tastes horrible I just think back on those days with Sir Flagyl and shake myself out of it and know that things were worse.

***

NO MORE, NO MORE[132]

That night I was treated with a nurse that gave Effeminate Curtis a run for his money only this guy gave a shit. I liked him, he was less annoying. He was a small guy with a goatee, receding hairline, dark hair, in his early thirties and he wore a dark blue top, white pants, and white nursing shoes. He also had a pretty effeminate voice with a Southern twang. I really thought about the myriad of cultures and lifestyles I was encountering on this journey so nothing was really surprising. It all fit with the international and cultural parade of nurses I had on my long flight in the MICU weeks ago.

We had a good shift together that night. Toward the end he asked if I wanted a popsicle or something like that since I was still quite thirsty at this point. I said, "Sure." The shift change came and there was no popsicle. I said nothing about it because I didn't really want the popsicle anyway and figured I only would have wasted it.

The following night when he came back on shift he said, "First I want to apologize to you, I was getting into bed today when I suddenly realized, 'I never got that poor guy his popsicle.' I'm truly sorry about that."

"That's OK," I responded, "I was fine without it." I was actually impressed that he remembered it but felt weirder about the vampire-like hours that this guy must have. How did he get anything done outside of work? When in the devil did he sleep?

That night my slumber was broken when he turned on the sink light. It was time for the dreaded meds. I always hated this time and I'm sure it was not the favorite part of their shift either. Waking up sick people in the middle of the night was a mean thing especially when sleep was the only freedom they got. Still that cursed light went on.

When this happened Becky would sometimes move and sometimes she wouldn't. She was still staying with me during the night and leaving during the day and getting back to a semi-normal work routine. On this night she was here but she wasn't moving.

The nurse looked down at me and whispered, "Mr. Hoover, it's time for your meds," as he held some water and the plastic cup of vile pills that I knew I would never be able to swallow. Plus, I knew my buddy Sir Flagyl was skulking around in there.

I replied in a matter of fact voice, "No." That's right, I said it, I am taking a stand against all of these middle of the night disturbances that ruin slumber.

The nurse's expression was one of shock; he had not been expecting this rejoinder. He then said, "Sir, you have to have these, you must take them."

With his firm voice hanging in the air my courage quickly dissipated. My mind went to a huge orderly coming in and prying open my jaw like a carp and getting those damn pills down. I then said with a sense of resignation, "Fine."

He raised my bed, gave me the pill cup and the water cup. I nervously took it, my hands shook, he watched to make sure I was taking them. Each and every one. Now, I think of situations like this and wonder in disbelief how adult patients quickly become children in the hospital. It sometimes has to be that way in order to get better and I was going to see these pills through whether he was there or not. I was that disciplined.

I opted for the small pills first in order to rev up my courage for that monstrous horse pill Sir Flagyl that was certain to be the end of me. The small white one I took and it went down with a lot of water, in fact I may have drank over half the cup to get that bastard down. Next was another small one. I took it and the water ran out before I could actually get it the majority of the way down my fuckin' throat. Why didn't I just ask for more water? Beats the shit out of me.

It just sat there in my throat. As the nurse watched me, the balance between a patient with quiet dignity and one in the throes of discomfort shifted to the latter as I began to gag on the little fucker. On the butt end of this gagging I began to power boot. In shock I saw the nurse run around the room a tither as to what to do. He then left the room and returned with a large blue basin from somewhere. He shoved it under my face and then ran out of the room. His running hither and yon had actually got my mind off the gagging but I do believe I heaved the pill up.

The activity had roused Becky from her slumber, "What's the matter?" she said.

"I can't swallow these fucking pills!" I lamented.

I sat there with the blue basin under my face for quite a while until the Yorking episode passed. Becky removed it and set it on the floor and I fell back to sleep. I don't think I saw the nurse again after that. My rebellious vomitous attitude I guess was too much for him. I was disappointed because even though flashing had always bothered me, I thought I would be over it with all I had been through, I just wasn't. The potential for laughing at the carpet remained but at least it kept me from Sir Flagyl for the time being. However, having a nurse acting like the world was going to end when sick was about to come didn't make me feel too comfortable either.

***

AN UNCERTAIN VOYAGE

Physical therapy continued during my time in Progressive. Mike appeared one day with a large walker that he said would allow me to walk while I was strapped in securely. I was very anxious about standing on my own two feet. The few times I had been upright in a sitting position were altogether terrifying and knocked my confidence down a great deal. However, I was starting to feel like the bum that won't move out of his parents' basement and the time was now for me to start moving on my own.

With two therapists and Mike in the room they slowly got me to a sitting position and rolled the walker in front of me. I immediately began to feel faint. They applied the straps to me, tightening as they went. The time that I was sitting up was wearing on me quickly. There was utterly no energy and I felt that they were asking me to levitate the chair in the corner with what they were asking of me. With me gripping the handles of the walker and my forearms resting on the pads they took off the brakes and I was standing in front of Becky. It appeared that she couldn't believe her eyes; however, I do recall walking on our first date.

Mike said, "Now take a few steps."

Gingerly like the ice wizard in *Santa Claus is Coming to Town*, I began walking like a Rankin/Bass character with the "put one foot in front of the other" rhythm in my head. I began to walk and began to panic after the first couple of steps unlike the ice wizard. I felt exposed and utterly helpless like I was about to fall into a dark crevasse.

I asked urgently, "Where should I go?"

"Wherever you want," came the reply.

Really? Anywhere? There was conflict over that three-word answer with the spirit being unsound and the flesh being quite not up to snuff. I really just wanted to get back in the sack. I quickly marched toward the foot of the bed. I felt like Magellan plotting a bold course to find a new passage to the wall of my room. That was it for me. My legs were done, my body was done, I was exhausted beyond words and felt like I was going to technicolor yawn. I couldn't believe how weak I was but at least everything worked if not for very long. I felt bad about all of that strapping and preparation that was done to send a man to the foot of the bed and return him safely to his pillow. Whatever the effort that went into the five-foot walk I thought they were pleased, and I hoped I had satisfied Mike. Perhaps they had seen enough horror to know that something good was happening, even though it was slow.

Then Mike said, "That was perfect, we'll leave the chair in here for the next time."

I lay back in bed and it felt so soothing and comfortable. I was sorry that I had been so angry with good ole' Instaflate. I felt like a bum giving up but that was all I could give.

***

FULL OF URINE

I got some exciting news one day. I was lying there during the daylight hours and could hear Big Daddy over by the window snoring away. I was just staring at the wall as usual. Suddenly a tall doctor poked his head into the room and introduced himself, "Hello, my name's Dr. Johnson, your nephrologist, I haven't had the chance to meet you yet."

"Hello," I said. "Good to meet you." I was trying to suppress an expression that we had met before. Then it dawned on me that it was Dr. BMOC himself of the "get out of hospital when you're better" bill joke. It hit me like a freight train. A blast from the past standing before me. Holy shit, I hoped he wasn't really a regular viewer of *Patch Adams* and thought himself a thespian. I wondered what gags he had up his sleeve now.

He continued excitedly, "I bring good news. We have a liter and a half of urine!"

I looked around to see if he was talking to anyone else and if this was one of his damn dirty gags. This must have been ordinary news around here but not for me. What did that mean? I looked at him blankly and said, "Really? Where?" I swear I hadn't pissed myself. A liter and half would be like Harry Carson, Hall of Fame linebacker for the New York football Giants, throwing a cooler of urine on me. That is, if my knowledge of Coke bottle sizes that lose their fizz quickly served me correctly. Besides what was this "we" business? Did he add a half liter of his own? Also, why was he sticking his head in the door like he had just visited my urine? Was I passing liquid remotely to some other room?

He said, "Really. This is exciting news."

Then like that he was gone. If he was smiling, then I knew things were going OK and one cannot argue with good news when it has to do with urine. I still had no idea what it meant. I think I would have noticed had a volume of liquid that large been exiting my body. After he left I looked around the room to see where in the hell this liter and a half of urine could be hiding and I still didn't see it. Maybe that's why he didn't come into the room. It was a huge puddle on the floor. *That man really knows puddle sizes*, I thought.

***

MY FUNNY VALENTINE II

It seemed Valentine's Day was constantly approaching for what seemed like an eternity. I kept seeing commercials for it on TV. The NBA All Star Game kept being advertised with the note that it was going to be on Valentine's Day. I couldn't get away from it, everyone was talking about it, and I sure as hell couldn't get to a store.

The countdown was so damn obvious, like in *Sleepless in Seattle* where they were constantly mentioning that Empire State Building rendezvous. We went from Christmas to Valentine's Day in a flash like in the movie. When the showdown comes in the restaurant where Meg Ryan tells Bill Pullman that she would rather be with some dude she has never met than be with him, Bill Pullman just accepts it. I remember thinking at the time, *Dammitt Bill Pullman! This is 1993 Meg Ryan when she was at her peak, this is unacceptable. Fight for her you dunce, she sure as hell has been fighting through getting over you!* So with that she was gone and now I was still approaching Valentine's Day and it just wouldn't stop approaching. Plus I really know too much about *Sleepless in Seattle*.

But I was not the only one feeling the heat, Becky was telling me about having to go into Kate's classroom to decorate her desk for Valentine's as the teacher had requested or actually ordered. So I witnessed with paralyzed body, Becky cutting and preparing the decorations over in the chair by the window and me lying there unable to help. This lent even more proof to us having kids, because who in the hell would be cutting up construction paper hearts in a hospital room except a parent?

I also noticed that my sense of time was way off as well. Whenever anyone left the room it felt like an eternity before their return. They could be gone for an hour or five minutes, it didn't matter, to me it was forever. I was now reminded how I would feel as a young child waiting for something to happen. This was how I felt when she was gone the next day to decorate the desk.

Later, my parents came in and said that they were going to get some flowers for me to give to Becky and then brought a card for me to sign. This was going to be interesting but at least I had an excuse this Valentine's for not being able to get to the store or to be creative for creativity's sake. I did feel like I had shortchanged her yet perhaps, just maybe, still being here alive was enough even though it was my fault that I was here.

My mom held up the card for me to sign. At this point I was barely able to move my arm so my dad held it up and I scribbled what I thought was, "I couldn't have gotten through this without you. I love you. Howard." It may have read "MMMjjjdddfff jjjjj sss purple monkey dishwasher." I was grateful that my parents thought of this even though my handwriting was more of an illegible scrawl, it was the thought that counted.

CHAPTER 31

Community

Once it has been established that hypoperfusion exists, early restoration of perfusion is necessary to prevent or limit multiple organ dysfunction, as well as reduce mortality.[133]

SAVE IT FOR THE DIALYSIS AFTER[134]

After the exciting urine news from the day before, Dr. Johnson topped himself on this day and said, "We're going to get you off dialysis soon so you'll be coming down to the dialysis center where we can get you done quicker and I can keep an eye on you. This will probably happen tomorrow."

I thought, *keep an eye on me? Was news of my temper tantrum in Progressive spreading like wildfire through this place and now I was viewed as a problem child? Shit, I knew the attitude would screw me over sooner or later. How much had this set me back? Hold on a second, he did say this was the last dialysis.* That was certainly good news, I had grown weary of the dialysis machine and was ready to get back to life without it. It felt like progress and the unplugging would slowly continue. Also I felt kind of popular as if I were being called to hang out with the cool kids. "The Troublemaker with the Attitude of Unknown Goals" would be my nickname. Sort of rolls off the tongue.

Early the next morning, just like Dr. Johnson said, my trip to the dialysis center began. Two orderlies brought in a more traditional bed to the room. I was to be moved off the Instaflate? This was certainly big news. The two male orderlies slowly slid me and my assortment of tubes and bags onto the new bed. After feeling this new bed I instantly knew how hard I had been on Instaflate. The gurney mattress had hardly any padding and my bony ass immediately felt the effect. Plus I missed my crawler at the end of the bed that said "Instaflate Activated." Even though I still searched for those long lost family names that appeared on it, they never returned.

I was really road tripping now. If they felt free to move me more and more then I must be getting better. I was excited about movement. Again, I could see behind the curtain and saw the Wizard as they rolled me out of the room. It felt freeing. They rolled me down somewhere in the hospital into a room filled with dialysis machines. Other patients were all over this dorm-style room. It was more open than anything I had experienced in what felt like ages. The openness was a little unnerving and I suddenly longed for the more reassuring confines of my room. The dialysis tech came over and greeted me and then proceeded to snap lines to me like I was a car in the shop.

I saw Dr. Johnson over talking to an older doctor. So this is where he resided when he wasn't traipsing around the hospital measuring urine puddle sizes for volume with his eyes. Man, how tall was Dr. Johnson? Eight feet? Nine feet tall? He had the height of that amazing colossal man in that movie *The Amazing Colossal Man* with his head almost touching the ceiling. I just hoped he didn't go mad like Mr. Colossal Man, excuse me, Dr. Colossal Man. I wondered how the relationship between the older doctor and the younger doctor was. Did the older doctor think they were equals? How much of the "show your stuff" attitude did Dr. Johnson have to endure until he was accepted? He waved to me but didn't come over to talk to me. *That's strange; I thought I was popular now.*

The tech then said, "We'll be bringing you breakfast soon."

I was again in no mood to eat; my stomach was a wasteland of non-hunger. I spoke to a jolly nurse on the seventh floor who didn't seem to worry about it too much. She said, "When you're ready to eat, you'll eat."

That was the attitude I needed. I just wasn't ready yet.

The tech turned his attention to someone against the wall that I could not see. I was absolutely the youngest one in the room. I supposed these were the souls that made it this far and they were holding on here. It sounded like there was an old woman in the corner to the left of me complaining in a mumbled sort of way.

"I don't want to hear it, you still have another hour," the tech said half angrily, half playfully. It sounded as if this banter had been going on for some time to the point where the tech was comfortable talking to whoever it was in that fashion.

I could see the wheels spinning in the machine and the "Everything's OK" alarms were not going off so far. By this time I had realized that it was no longer an Icee machine but I sure as hell wished my ignorance was prolonged. Seeing my blood get scrubbed because my body was incapable of doing it on its own was quite an eye opener. I always took my health for granted. I just hoped to God my recovery would continue unabated.

The usual process of body slippage in the hard bed once again commenced. I was not very comfortable and had only one sheet on me. I could actually pick up a magazine but I could not really focus on the words, they were just going in one eye and out the other. It was a magazine a rung below People, not exactly a technical manual. Captions comparing/contrasting the cleavage of this starlet with that one were akin to studying differential equations for me.

My eyes turned to a guy who appeared to be in his fifties sitting about thirty feet across the room from me. He had a long beard and was balding on top. He had a plate of scrambled eggs and he was eating sausage. I don't know what was wrong with me. Seeing this guy eating eggs along with all of this blood turning around in the machine under the heavy fluorescent light was making me feel a bit queasy. Actually, nothing was wrong with me that would make anyone queasy. I was struck by the nonchalance of the guy like he had come in off the street and was totally used to this as if he were getting a haircut.

I couldn't believe I was in this situation. I was still so stunned by it all. How did I get here again?

The breakfast-tray cart returned. I could wait on breakfast; I just knew that breakfast could not wait on me. Usually I could stare at the wall and be comforted but this wall had a guy eating eggs in it, so that wasn't going to work. The guy's appearance was merciless in increasing my queasiness yet I couldn't take my eyes off him. I was just surprised that he didn't return my gaze with a scowl. Then happily I saw the talking picture machine was on above me. Yes, the talking picture machine would provide a diversion from my insane judgment of this guy eating breakfast.

The moment of truth had arrived when I saw the breakfast trays slowly being distributed around the room. *Stiff upper lip Webbie* [Webster is me middle name], *those eggs won't kill you*, I said to myself.

I knew I was going to be in the dialysis center a while; it always seemed to take forever upstairs. Usually from ten in the morning to three in the afternoon for a usual round of dialysis, then the tech would come in my room and say, "You're all done," and start unsnapping all of the lines.

At the time I half believed that "You're all done" meant I was about to go home but it just meant lying there for eternity. At least here I could see others going through the same thing I was and it sounded like they were enjoying it even less, if that was possible.

The mumbling continued against the wall.

"I have about had it with you. Are you going to eat your breakfast or not?" said the tech in an exasperated tone.

"Mumble, Mumble." was the reply.

"That's all we have right now. You have another thirty minutes."

"Mumble Mumble."

"It's thirty minutes, and that's the last time I'm going to say it,"

The tech then brought my breakfast. It was the same plate of stuff that the guy sitting across from me had. I eyed it suspiciously to make sure they had not given me his plate. I couldn't even look at it. I picked up a biscuit and attempted to put it into my mouth. My hands were shaking so badly I could barely get it into my bazoo. It tasted like cardboard and I could barely get the bite that I managed to keep in my mouth down my throat. I felt like I was seasick, the nausea would not go away. This was Eating 101 to the extreme. I had to learn this shit again? I attempted some eggs but after watching the bearded guy eat my insanity quickly shunned them. I kept trying and trying for ten minutes, twenty minutes, thirty minutes, forty minutes, all the way to an hour. It just wasn't happening and now everything was cold.

I was watching CNN and they had parked the newscast in the Lincoln Museum in Springfield, Illinois. There was this insane comparison they were grabbing at between Obama and Lincoln. I thought the whole report was preposterous. Until Obama works with a McClellan then there was really no comparison. I congratulated myself as I remembered a historical tidbit. Fortunately or unfortunately, no one around me could read my mind and therefore was not on board with my happiness.

The report kept going on and on. Valentine's Day and now Presidents Day was tormenting me, all of these cold weather holidays were simply too much. Is it traditional to exchange gifts on Presidents Day as well? Refer to my *Sleepless in Seattle* rant.

"You have hardly eaten a thing," the tech said as he took away my tray.

"I know," I said fearing a tongue lashing like the one Mumble Mumble had received.

"Anything wrong with it?" he asked.

"No, just not hungry right now." I just wanted him to get the food away from me so I wouldn't insanely start pointing fingers at the scrambled egg guy for my eating woes. And I mean all the fingers.

My comfort level was getting lower and CNN kept going on about Lincoln and Obama. I was really getting annoyed with the whole thing. I have nothing against him. He is the Commander-In-Chief. Was he really Commander-In-Chief? In those first primary debates he was one of those afterthought guys that was placed at the very last podium….on the left. I was in a really irritable state where even airing the newscast from the museum of Snuggles, the Fabric Soft bear would have been met with derision. On second thought, the concept of a Snuggles Museum was already met with derision. There was just too much gushing. Enough already.

I asked the tech, "Can you please turn on ESPN."

Yes, the obnoxiousness of those witty sportscasters would save the day. The graphics might kill my eyesight but I was willing to take that risk.

The tech said, "Certainly," as if he had nothing better to do.

He got the remote and the channel would not change to ESPN or he couldn't find it. After a while, I figured the search was fruitless and everything else looked so bad I didn't want to take any more of his time. I did plead in my head, *please don't turn it to anything with a studio audience!*

"CNN's fine, just leave it there," I said.

"Sorry about that, I don't know why we can't get ESPN."

The mumbling once again began over against the wall.

"Yes, you're done," The tech replied curtly. "See, that wasn't so bad."

"Mumble, Mumble."

As I slipped down further in the bed and my discomfort grew I thought that I could lie there with my legs crossed like I used to at home just to put a brake on the slippage. I crossed my legs and of course with my Navajo, sans undergarments, condition I was shooting the room a great big *Penthouse* Monster Shot. It was the only way I could stop the slipping and get some comfort. After a while I kept shifting from one leg to another and that was not doing it. I was beginning to feel really antsy as if I had ants running through my veins or having the tuna-fish story explained to me with power point slides for visual accompaniment.

The tech came over to cover me up saying, "Your modesty's showing. Please cover up."

I didn't care, I was ready to leave and now I understood what Mumble Mumble was talking about. I began to get tingly in my extremities and I felt like jumping out of the bed and running far away. I was very antsy, almost panicky.

More Mumble Mumbles from the wall. I tried to calm myself down by just closing my eyes but that didn't work. Again I crossed my legs. I was now on the side of Mumble Mumble! I thought, *fight the Power! Don't take no shit! No motherfuckin' shit!* Perhaps they could prescribe dialysis for my inner dialogue.

"You're showing the world everything. You need to cover up." The tech was being a little more direct this time.

At this urging, I flattened my legs out. I didn't care. Let the room see my undercarriage, I had nothing to hide. Everyone else had seen it.

As I began to look back around the room waiting for this whole ordeal to be over I heard a voice say, "I remember you."

I looked up and saw a woman in blue scrubs with short hair, glasses, and in her late forties walking across the room by the scrambled egg guy. "You were in the ER last month, you're the father with small children."

I waved weakly kind of shocked that I was pulled from my world of insane judgment and said, "Yes, that must be me."

She continued, "We just kept saying 'We have to save this one.'"

This really stuck with me and bothered me a little bit but as I began to think more about it, I got really bothered by the thought. At one time I was on a thin line. It was really hitting me hard at the moment. That word "saved" really dug into me. *I almost died here and now I am complaining about some discomfort, slipping in the bed, and the potential of my doctor going mad from being both amazing and colossal? Get ahold of yourself Webbie! Cleavage and the scrambled egg guy ain't so bad and you found a new compatriot in Mumble Mumble. There is good in this moment.*

Mumble Mumble was finally wheeled out. I hoped I would be next. How long had I been here, five or six hours? No? Just a little over two hours? So in the meantime I switched from the Obama gushing to the magazine and its compulsory cleavage where viewing was compulsory to the position of showing the room Mr. Happy to thinking about what the nurse from the ER said to keeping tabs on Dr. Johnson's sanity. Scrambled egg guy was finally wheeled out, when the hell was it my turn? *Quick, get me out of here before they wheel some fat guy in eating a gyro with extra tomatoes and taziki sauce!*

The tingling was getting worse and worse. I thought I was going to die right there in this room. I was beginning to get panicky. I thought, *Shit, I made it this far and here I am at the finish line about to finish dialysis and I have developed some sort of unknown condition.*

As my worry grew and the tingling followed suit, the tech came over and said, "You're all done."

He began to unsnap me. It was the sweetest words I had heard in the past two hours with the exception of whatever the hell Mumble Mumble had been going on about.

Should I mention the tingling to the tech? What would he say? What would he do?

My thoughts were interrupted as I crossed my legs again. The sheet fell off as the tech began to wheel me out. "You can't do that while we're in the hall," he admonished me. I could see his point. The generous view of my pylon would indeed raise a few eyebrows, even mine.

I thought, *I'm here to rattle some cages you damn dirty filthy prudes.* When in reality I was a card-carrying member of the Prudish League of Gentlemen.

As we left I saw an old lady sitting up with an uneaten sandwich in front of her that looked just huge and might be capable of eating her instead. The sandwich just sat there knowing that the old lady wouldn't be very tasty. The older doctor was sitting by her bed trying to comfort her. I heard him say, "We're not trying to kill you." I could only assume he was talking about the sandwich which would have looked intimidating as hell to me at my healthiest. So I felt for her, being confronted with a huge sandwich that could not be eaten even if dunked in water for a half hour, but then who would want to eat that soggy mess?

I was wheeled out and taken through the maze of hallways. The tingling was not subsiding and I was too worried to say anything. As we got back to the room Becky was there. I was so upset at the tingling and the length of my time away I just let out my frustrations to her. I relayed to her what the nurse said to me downstairs about saving me. "Why would she say that?" I asked through my sobs.

"She was just trying to make you feel better. A lot of people here were and are pulling for you and the fact that you made it is nothing short of miraculous."

I wasn't convinced. Everything was beginning to annoy me and I wanted out. Now.

Later that day Dr. Johnson came in to see how I was doing. "We're going to do some tests. If everything comes out well that'll probably be your last dialysis."

I couldn't believe my good fortune. My kidneys were almost back. I had been so ignorant of my condition for so long, this was a huge development. I couldn't believe that what I came into the world with I could still use. I had to confess to him the tingling sensation in my legs and arms that were sending me through the roof with lightheadedness. I was reserved about celebrating and I still thought that I was not out of it yet. I was worried about the reaction to my question of why this was happening.

As I relayed the issue to him he understood exactly what the problem was and said, "That's probably from the high-efficiency dialysis machine you were on. It speeds up the process and your blood's cleaned much faster. The tingling sensation's normal. It should dissipate in a couple of hours," and with that he left the room with his white cape flapping behind him and I had taken one more step.

CHAPTER 32

Failure/Success

The focus on the ScvO2 derives from a clinical trial in which 263 patients with severe sepsis or septic shock were randomly assigned to therapy targeting a ScvO2 >- 70 percent, or conventional therapy that did not target a ScvO2. Both groups initiated therapy within six hours of presentation and targeted the same central venous pressure (CVP), mean arterial pressure (MAP), and urine output. Mortality was lower in the group that targeted a ScvO2 >-70 percent (31 versus 47 percent). This approach is known as "early goal directed therapy" (ie, administered within the first six hours of presentation).[135]

REHAB TIME IS HERE AGAIN[136]

They always seemed to come in when there was something good on TV so of course I would have to get used to them turning off my stories, which I still felt was rather rude in a get-down-to-business sort of way. Simply ignoring them was not going to be acceptable. Becky was there with me on this morning as we got used to the normalcy of a normal room. The TV was great, the equipment and furnishings around me were less severe than Progressive and the MICU, and the best part was the door could be closed. It was just beautiful.

Today, two big ladies came in to put me through physical therapy. I was used to Mike and his young assistants so this threw me. Not to say I was disappointed, variety is the spice of life, but it was different.

One of the ladies cheerfully said, "We're going to get you out of the bed and get you walking today."

Oh, I thought I was done with all that. Hadn't I showed them enough with my four steps a couple of days ago? Couldn't we leave it at that? I knew I had to take more steps to get further on my way to the front door and get out of here. Was I going to disappoint the 1995 me in shorts and the olive-green T-shirt whistling his way the hell out of here? I thought not. I was going to be that guy soon in spite of the fact that I was weaker and more helpless than a small kitten. There was nothing here to guide me except my attitude.

"OK, we're going to lift you up into a sitting position on the side of the bed," one of the ladies said.

I said, "OK." Not really having anything prophetic or humorous to say. I just hoped I could replicate my recent success from earlier. Drumming up the courage to once again leave the safe confines of Instaflate that I had grown to love after my horrifying four-step journey, I took as deep a breath as I could.

As soon as the two ladies lifted me up I began to grow faint like a wilting prince. I reported as nobly as I could, "I think I'm going to pass out." It was indeed the head rush from hell. My Jamaican nurse was there and she was called in to hook up the blood pressure monitoring device to make sure I was not really faltering. They quickly continued to strap me in to the leather walking device Mike had procured for me, but my strength was waning fast. So fast that I didn't think I was going to last much longer just sitting upright.

While the ladies were waiting on my nurse to check my blood pressure, needless to say it seemed like a fucking eternity, I kept asking myself, *what the hell's taking so long?* Had I yelled this I might have toppled over, my energy didn't allow me to be pissed off. I just sat there hanging in this seat, strapped in like a puppet. My feet were dangling on the floor feeling the hard tile through socks that were too damn warm. That floor felt unforgiving and I didn't like it. I was unaccustomed to the "ground."

As my body slogged through this painful re-introduction to normal human movement, I thought that I didn't care what that blood pressure machine told them. I knew I felt like shit and unless there was a miracle I was not going to be able to sit there two seconds longer.

"OK, your blood pressure's looking fine," said the first rehab lady.

Tell my head, my legs, everything that, but I only nodded silently. My spindly forearms were rested on the leatherette arm pads, my hands gripped the handles. My feet dangled nervously off the bed. I stood up. I couldn't do it. I couldn't even hold my head up in a convincing fashion. All of my normal movements, strength, stamina, and agility had gotten on a bus and headed the hell out of town and I felt alone as if I were on an island. I was not going to make it.

To encourage me one of the rehab ladies said, "Come on, there's a pretty lady over there that wants you to walk over to her."

I could feel Becky's encouraging gaze on me. I could tell that just seeing me like this must hurt her. I wondered back on all that had happened so far and how I got to this point but quickly snapped out of it and turned my attention back to the task at hand. However, the task at hand was about to make me sick

"I can't do it," I repeated, "I can't do it." I said it in such a convincing fashion that I believed it myself and began to weep as it dawned on me how easily I had given up. I was inconsolable. I felt like I had let down everyone and was just a damn bum. I had a vision that these ladies were going to give up on me and storm out of the room. They were going to tell Mike that I was hopeless and I should be tossed out like an ingrate. Before that happened they would include their own editorial on me with, "Look at you, we save your life and you can't walk five fucking steps? Shame! Shame!" Then when that was over we could just see where it went from there.

Somehow after all this time I had not yet learned that there was compassion here, and instead of shame I got a big dose of encouragement. Thankfully the encouragement was nothing like Mickey from *Rocky* would give, nonetheless it was with a kind word that they spoke to me slowly and caringly.

"That's OK," one of the ladies said. "You'll make it, maybe not today, but you'll make it. I know it. I have seen some people try this and there's simply no hope for them but we still help them. You'll be walking in no time, I just know it."

The other lady added, "MmMMMMMHHHMMMM!"

I didn't believe them. I never could take a compliment cleanly and thought they were just being nice like my guitar teacher. I wanted to give it another shot but I couldn't. They spent fifteen minutes strapping me in for nothing and now they had to put in another fifteen minutes unstrapping me.

"I'm sorry. I'm so sorry," I kept repeating as I tried to hold my head up.

"Don't worry about it," they kept saying.

They laid me down and lifted my legs back up on ole' Instaflate. Instaflate felt wonderful yet there was a shame in my sudden comfort. I cried and cried and thought, *what a shitty start to the day.*

***

EYES WITHOUT A FACE[137]

Recall that I was in a half-faced way or so I thought. Obviously everyone had become used to my distressed appearance. My wife and children still loved me even though I looked not unlike Councilman Harvey Dent. I would and could accept a lifetime of deformity if I still had them in my corner.

However, the truth showed itself in the reflection of a framed picture hanging on the wall facing my bed one morning. The shroud was lifted on my deformed appearance when my bed was raised for lunch to be served. I had my glasses on, who knew how they were supported with half a nose, and I caught a glimpse of myself in the reflection. My relief was so heartfelt, I gasped with joy that I was actually whole. I had not become Two-Face, as I had feared this entire time but was myself. I was still Howard Hoover, well, even without half of my face I still would have been Howard Hoover. Albeit, I still had lost quite a bit of weight, was unshaven and had a trach tube hanging out of my throat that looked like a bizarre necktie but I could work with that. I was still me. I was very encouraged by this.

I exclaimed to Becky, "I see myself."

Becky was apologetic for letting me see myself. I had changed so much since I was in the hospital. "I'm sorry you had to see that," she said.

"Are you kidding me, I'm ecstatic! I have my face. My face is whole with no disfigurement," I said like a kid on Christmas morning.

Becky was shocked at my reaction. "You mean you thought you were really that disfigured?"

"Yes, I thought half my face was gone and I would be leaving here wearing a *Marvin* mask," I said with unmeasured relief.

"Oh, I'm so sorry that you thought that. No, your face was OK the entire time," she said reassuringly.

I didn't care if I was sounding vain. I wanted my face back. The discouragement of not walking was eased a bit, I had my face! Alleluia. This was a good day! The guy in the olive-green shirt and tan shorts had something to work with and I could sense he was pulling up his socks, ready to go.

***

FREEDOM FRIES IS MORE THAN JUST A NAME

My nausea had been relentless, my aversion to food led me to believe that I would waste away and they would lock me away here. Once again dinner time came and went and I could hardly eat a thing. I was just depressed by this continuing saga. This night would prove to be different. I didn't know how it popped into my head but it just did. I started thinking about French fries. Yes, French fries with lots of ketchup. Was this a dream? Was this a trick? Was this intended to shock? I sat there and thought about them a while longer. I wanted to make sure that a sudden wave of nausea did not overwhelm this pleasing thought. No, the French fries were still there with lots of ketchup revolving around my head.

I then thought I would finally go for it and I would speak up. It was about 7:30 p.m. and the dinner hour had long been over with my appetite having once again been invisible. Luckily Becky was here.

I said, "You know I suddenly have a hankering for some French fries."

"Really? Are you sure?" She asked in a pleasantly surprised voice.

"Yes, French fries with lots of ketchup," I said as confidently as I could.

"I'll see what they have downstairs," she said and without a beat was off to find what I had not had joy in for weeks.

I waited, anticipating the moment food and I would be reunited in a non-adversarial way. What would it feel like not to fear those trays being stacked in the hallway? The feeling of failure of not having eaten being just a memory? Would my stomach follow suit and be able to handle this fried bonanza? *Don't fill yourself with worry*, I kept telling myself but the stomach had a mind of its own and mine especially needed coddling during tense times or at least it used to.

Becky returned twenty minutes later; she was carrying a huge Styrofoam container. The odor filled the room as my appetite remained unabated. She set the container down and opened it. There it was, a full-ass container of French fries with more packets of ketchup than I could count. I asked her to open a few packets for me. My hands and fingers were not yet equipped to handle some tasks. I took my first bite with a full dose of ketchup. That was good. I felt like Homer Simpson beginning to eat his first slice of a hundred slice pack of American cheese in the middle of the night except there was no Mr. Burns or Flanders on the ceiling above my head. I continued on, patiently eating, knowing that to rush this joyous event would invite an overwhelmed stomach that had just welcomed nibbles, Nuprin, some liquids, and that Fucking Sir Flagyl over the past few weeks.

My wonderful journey to the bottom of the container continued without hesitation, however. The hunger continued and I was slowly finishing. The entire damn container was finished. I could not believe it. Through my shaking hands and tender stomach, I did it. I never thought that at the age of forty-one I would be so proud of myself to finish an entire container of French fries and the wonderful feeling it instilled in me. It was a wonderful, delicious, prideful step.

***

PAJAMA/HOSPITAL GOWN PARTY

We had a tradition in our home, not as serious as a *Fiddler on the Roof* tradition, mind you, but a tradition nonetheless, and that was a pajama party on Friday nights. This included pizza and a movie and if we were truly ambitious homemade pizza with homemade dough. The Babies looked forward to it all week and when Friday finally came the pajamas were brought down and the evening was set.

The pajama parties had been missing Daddy for long enough, Becky surmised. They were just not the same without me, especially when she would go back to the house on Friday nights and would give her mom a break from watching them. The making of the pizza and the other things that made that night special were just empty with me away. I knew I sure missed it and she decided this Friday to bring the pajama party to me.

First I asked, "Can you do that?"

"Sure as long as it's visitor hours, kids are allowed here. What movie would you like to see?" she asked.

I said, "Better keep it short, I don't know if I can take a full movie."

So of course this left out *Cars* and its uproariously long courtroom scene. *And Justice for All* spent less time in the court room. Also, the pajama party would mark the first time I saw all the Babies together at one time since this all began.

The sun was still setting early so it was dark outside by the time they came in around six. They all marched in one by one and Phoebe held aloft a DVD exclaiming, "We brought *Iron Man!*" which I was a big fan of but would not be watching now. We finally settled on *Lady and the Tramp* which I pushed for since I know it doesn't break eighty minutes. Becky, God bless her, made it a double special pajama party night with homemade pizza. I couldn't believe the amount of work she put into it. Just amazing; I had just had dinner so with my awakened stomach I only had room for one piece. It was like I remembered it. Home had made its way into the hospital. The Babies took up positions all around the room. Eventually they preferred the foot of my bed which was just fine. The bed and I had been through a lot together and I was happy to have visitors, especially this type.

While I enjoyed *Lady and the Tramp* I must admit there came a time that I really just wanted Tramp to kill that fucking rat and end it already. I started fading and Becky was watching me.

"Are you OK? Do you want us to stay?" she asked.

There was no way I was going to send this lovely bunch away no matter how tired and weird I felt. "No, I'm fine," I said as reassuringly as I could. I wanted the Babies in here with me but I was so damned tired and Lady still hadn't been rescued from the shelter and they hadn't met some of the other animals which I still get confused with the animals from the *Aristocats*. And I hadn't even gotten to the Siamese cats and that bitch babysitter, the thought of whom just puts me over the edge. Even thirty minutes in I knew there was a lot of stuff to go through before we got to the rat killing. I had trouble paying attention to the screen, I wished the images would go away. I longed to stare at the wall. I felt terrible about this, the pajama party not being enjoyed as fully as it should. I was getting upset at my discomfort and sadness yet I stuck to it and the movie was finished.

Becky said quickly, "OK guys, say good night to Daddy, he needs his rest."

It was true, I was going to go to sleep, I did need my rest. Felt like I was eighty-years-old. They argued, especially Henry who said, "But we haven't seen *Iron Man* yet."

"Sorry, not tonight, he can watch it later," Becky said.

Phoebe left *Iron Man* reluctantly and kissed me on the cheek, Kate gave me a kiss and a reassuring tap on the hand and smile. Henry climbed up to kiss and hug me. "Good night Daddy Waggy," he said.

"I love you all," I told them.

Becky took the plate and ushered them out but before she left I said, "Thanks for doing all this, I love you."

"I love you too," And she closed the door and I closed my eyes.

***

I'M JUST WAITING ON A FRIEND[138]

An old friend was coming to town. He had heard from my sister what had happened to me. Bob Larson was coming. I have known him since the fourth grade, September 1976 to be exact when we used to cut up in English class making crude remarks about sentences in our workbook that we thought had extra bawdy meanings such as "Jenny is watering the lawn" and "Tom is brushing his hair." With the carnal knowledge of nine-year-olds we would pore over these sentences looking for hidden meanings.

Then Mrs. Tiller, our teacher, would eventually scold us telling me once, "Mr. Hoover, exams are in four weeks."

I'm sorry but four weeks to a nine-year-old was like four months to an adult and to a guy in the MICU it was like four years. She wasn't getting through to me that way. In any event from that moment on we became good friends and this was one of those seminal moments I guess when friends were there for each other. I so looked forward to his arrival and my bedridden impatience had no limit. It seemed my mom was the point of contact for giving up to date announcements on where he was on his journey. My mom doesn't mind talking loudly on the cell phone in front of other people no matter what is going on or who is in the room so I was able to hear one half of the conversation.

Hours would seem to go by and her phone would ring "Oh, you're at the North Carolina/Virginia border now, you're about four to five hours away," she would say loudly.

Holy shit, I thought, *is he in Cinderella's carriage? Why's this taking so damn long?*

For as one should have been aware by now, time had no meaning to me. Twenty minutes would go by and it felt like three hours. My whole internal clock was off so he could have been walking from the parking deck and I still would have been impatient. I awaited his arrival because finally a link to my past was coming and I could really have my spirits lifted from a different angle. My mood was like a muscle;

it needed to be worked out in different ways so the usual visitors were not getting it done at this point.

My mom reported that since it was Valentine's weekend he was going to just stay until Sunday morning (Valentine's Day) and be on his way. I thought, *damn Valentine's Day ruining my fun. Hasn't it gotten here yet?*

Ever since Mike made his Kennedyesque statement about having me walk across the room to Becky *Mimic II* style and hopefully return safely I had been waiting for this day to come. Needless to say I was no closer to doing that very thing. I was starting to believe that that gigantic *Mimic II* bug was going to be giving Becky that flower before I ever could.

What seemed like a day had passed. My parents were even wondering what had happened to him, and I was amazed when they reached any destination. I had my own theory, perhaps he got confused and went south to the fifth Stuckey's north of the Florida/Georgia state line on I-75 to soak in the atmosphere. Inside joke that I don't even get.

Another call came, "He's reached Charlotte." Then I got the wonderful opportunity of hearing my mom give directions over the phone. I was about to say something, what, I don't know, maybe a, "Just tell him to fucking get here already."

The annoying updates were getting to me. After the virtual reality directions she gave I thought I could have found the place and I was just days from thinking I was in the mountains fighting the Dog People. After she got off the phone we waited some more and then lo and behold he had arrived. Holy crap there he was. We hadn't seen each other since October 2007 when we toured Gettysburg, conflict by conflict.

"It took me a while, but I've arrived," he announced.

"Bob Boy, how are you?" Big Daddy exclaimed. The time would come when he would mock Bob for his past romances but this was not the time.

After donning the yellowish gown and gloves he came over and shook my hand. "Good to see you." My shake was weak and I was surprised to be able to do it.

"Good to see you too, glad you're finally here," I said croakily.

"I have been swimming in the ether on our e-mails. No replies were forthcoming from you. What the hell happened? I swear I was just talking to you about that Panthers loss to the Cardinals in the playoffs and then you were off the screen. I couldn't believe it," he said.

"I know, I know, that seems like another life ago. A visitor came into the room some time ago and I swear I thought it was your mom and I spoke to her candidly about my disappointment in the game and the defense that I dubbed the "Fabulous Flying Larry Fitzgerald Escorts,"" I said.

"Liz (his wife) was in tears when she heard what was happening to you. She sends you her love and best wishes," he replied.

"Thanks so much."

"Your condition has been spread like wildfire by Chad on Facebook. It has gone viral, he's letting everyone know about it." Chad was a mutual friend we had known since seventh grade. It seems he was getting updates from my sister and he was passing it on.

Suddenly I didn't feel so alone. I felt energized as we continued to talk about nothing and everything. I lamented about how I had thought I had lost everything and that my family didn't exist and how Becky had been through everything with me. I then said, "She has meant so much to me through this whole thing, I love her so much. I still remember when we got into the limousine after we were married. She turned to me and said with a big smile on her face, 'Now we're a family.'"

Being overcome by the memory I began to weep. "Becky's such a quality person, we all know that, we knew you were in good hands with her by your side. I think our lives have been improved tremendously by our wives. You're lucky to have her in your corner."

I agreed and then as if on cue the Babies came running into the room. I said to Kate as she came to the side of the bed, "Kate I want you to meet my good friend that I have known since fourth grade."

Looking unimpressed and willing to accept the unintended challenge she replied, "So what, I have known some of my friends since kindergarten."

A challenge really wasn't my point but I laughed as the Babies made themselves at home and Bob was left standing by the wall for the moment saying hello. My dad then came over with such pride and brought Becky over with him, "Have you met my daughter-in-law." As in, he knew Bob knew Becky he just wanted to re-introduce her out of pride. I was thinking as I lay there how lucky I truly was.

***

THE RETURN OF DR. HOWARD, DR. FINE, DR. HOWARD!

After the kids had left Bob said, "I'm going to sit over here and read for a while to get out of your hair. I'm here to talk to you if you like."

I guess it was obvious I was getting tired. Dr. Fine returned while Bob was there. For some reason I thought he looked like a college friend of Bob's and the two of them would hit it off but they didn't seem to know each other at all. I found this rather odd.

My mind was taken away from this awkwardness after Dr. Fine looked at my trach tube. He said, "It looks like this can be taken out now. The smaller gauge seems to have done the job and you look healed enough around the hole to have it removed."

I was so excited, another notch, another step closer to leaving but I didn't want to be overly exuberant in case he wanted to keep me further for being too excited. So I just said as calmly as I could, "Really, that's great news," except the excitement in my voice was plain to hear.

He then proceeded to remove the trach tube. I was caught off guard. *Really, right now? This is happening right now?* Why was I still surprised by this? Every time an announcement was made I should have known by this point that shit was going to happen

Dr. Fine had a humorless bedside manner that was all business and he meant what he said so I didn't say a thing and played along. It felt like my throat was being twisted with the tube. It was a very strange feeling but there had already been quite a few of those so why not just throw this into the collection? I just hoped he knew what he was doing, which I suppose he had proven on his prior visit.

I began to think about a time before all this happened, I would see a hospital and think to myself, *that place knows what it's doing.* What I didn't add to that thought was that the place had faces and people just like me except I hoped they knew what they were doing. When I saw a face it could be hard sometimes to give myself to them and put my fate in their hands. I would have liked to have at least seen a diploma.

Dr. Fine's demeanor appeared to be, "Nothing shocks me and this is all expected in the course of what I do." So I let him go to town. The tube was removed and dressing was applied and with that he was gone. I was a little insecure about having this all done without Becky here but at least it was over. I don't think Bob was up to speed on the watchdog program like Tori had been so it was just between me and Dr. Fine.

Bob got up to see what had happened and I said, "Look, you arrive and I already have progress. You're quite the good luck charm."

As we talked longer I noticed that I was laughing more and more, which was good except that when I was exhaling there was a hissing sound and the tape over my throat was rising. It was not a sensation that I was accustomed to. In fact it made me freak out a little, I just played along with it like it was supposed to happen. Bob didn't say anything about it. I was very aware of it and it made me feel like I was breaking wind through my throat in church during a graduation ceremony while I was receiving my diploma from Vice President Dan Quayle. I suppose four inches higher and I would have been considered an ass face.

It was now dinner time and my food came. My parents returned and Bob accompanied them to the cafeteria. When they returned my parents left after a few minutes and left Bob and me. Not being able to join them really hurt.

***

PLEASE ALLOW ME TO INTRODUCE MYSELF[139]

This was my first totally conscious experience with them, I had heard about them. It was a program at my church that Cooper was in charge of. I guess I was now on the list for visits from these members of the congregation that would go out and comfort those in the congregation that were in need. This day was Sunday, finally it was Valentine's Day, and Bob came back for his final visit. He had to leave and be back in Arlington by tonight. I felt bad that he was going; it was good to catch up with him again.

The church member that walked in on this morning was a guy a few years older than us; I always sat behind him a few pews back during the services but had never spoken to him. Since I had the knowledge of seeing the back of his head for ten years he had no knowledge of my face and it was obvious he didn't know who I was.

He came walking in while we were talking and he said, "Hello I'm [Insert Name] and I'm with the [Insert Name] Ministry at Local Episcopal Church here to visit with you."

I was caught unawares on this one. I supposed the lady I mistook for Bob's mother was the first [Insert Name] Minister back in the MICU. This was the first visit when I had my wits about me. Bob introduced himself. I said, "We have known each other since fourth grade, he came from DC to visit."

"That's great," he said sounding unimpressed. "Mind if I turn this off?" as he went over to turn off the TV. "So what happened to you?"

I really shouldn't have discussed it with him and I was surprised he didn't know. I guess Cooper had decided it was best that I tell if I wanted to tell. So I went through the story and it was just fucking exhausting to do. Even though I was still not fully convinced that was how it went down.

"That sounds bad," he replied. Then he added, "So without further ado, I want you to continue your visit, but I did bring communion for you so we can get started."

I said to Bob, "You didn't know you were going to get some churchin' in when you came in here, did you?"

It was an abridged (much abridged) version of the regular service and took only five minutes, which was good since I was barely able to handle *Lady and the Tramp*. Any longer would certainly have taxed me even if a dog killing a rat in front of me was part of the ceremony. [Insert Name] did the readings, we did responses, I was actually able to hold the paper, and he did a small homily then it was time to give the wine. I took it since I didn't think there were any limitations on my diet except if I had requested a fifth of scotch I might have been denied. Once he was done and the wine was given he was off.

During lunch Bob departed again with my parents and when they returned I was sound asleep. "Howard," my mom said, "Bob's leaving now."

I was groggy but I managed to say, "Thanks for coming, it meant a lot to me. Give my best to Liz and the kids."

"I will, and I'll remember to send you that list of football books," and then he added, "As the day is long, thy will be done." Just adding some spice to the narrative.

"Thanks." I was a little sad, however my parents were still there and Aunt Grace and Uncle Barry would be around to stare at me in a little bit.

***

MY FUNNY VALENTINE III

The day was finally here, Valentine's Day finally had come and Becky came back from school the Friday before and showed me what she had done with the decorations for Kate's desk. The heart with the stern face, the confetti and the name Omega, the fictitious international soccer star I came up with to taunt Kate and Phoebe when I played them in soccer just to let Kate know that I was still around. And of course the Babies had prepared Valentines that Becky laid all over me. I was so happy, I guess I was a Scrooge about Valentine's Day but I could not argue with the result. Needless to say Mike's plan for me to walk to Becky did not come to fruition. My actual limbs were not up to the task so my one contribution to the day was not to be.

That night the NBA All Star Game was on which was a relief since I wouldn't have to see it advertised anymore. I was exhausted from it. I tried to watch it and all I was given for my anything but rapt attention were over-the-top player intros. Shaq came out to do some weirdo dance with the annoying expressionless masked people from the Gatorade ads. It was not an exaggeration when I say that this dance went on for five minutes, he wouldn't go the hell away. I thought they were going to have to turn the lights on him like they did to Ted Nugent when I saw him open for .38 Special in '86, he just wouldn't leave the stage. Actually after seeing the first three songs of .38 Special's set we all wished Ted would come back, and I understood how he must have felt opening for a lesser Van Zandt.

There were more player introductions and finally to put icing on the over-the-top celebration of a league that had seen better days. I saw, and I shit you not, sideline reporter Craig Sager wearing a pink suit complete with pink leather shoes. The camera was on him as he watched the action, his very countenance seething with smugness and self-satisfaction. I thought, *put me in a suit like that and watch me get my ass kicked however I would rather kick his ass while wearing the same suit.* How would that have looked? I think he would have taken me.

The action on the floor was terrible so I turned it off after the second quarter to stare at the wall. Even though I was immobilized and had nowhere to go I felt like I had better things to do, so I stared at the wall. It may lie, but it was never smug.

***

I'LL KNOW YOUR NAME, EVENTUALLY

She came to see me on the seventh floor again. I still didn't remember her name and I felt ashamed because every time she came in I would say, "I'm sorry I forgot your name." She was once again very patient with me; I just had a road block with her name. She was still a little younger than me and wore her glasses just right. The strangest thing was she came during daytime rounds when Becky wasn't around. Becky never met her but she was a big part of my remaining time in the hospital. When she came in the first time she said, "Mr. Hoover, I'm Dr. "I Forgot Your Name" and I work in the same office as Dr. Phillips, your primary doctor."

"Ah yes," I replied, "how is he?"

"He's fine, he wanted me to come around to see how you're doing," she said.

"I think I'm better than when he saw me before," I said. He had come twice that first weekend to visit me in the MICU when I was unconscious. He saw that my name had been removed from his appointment list on January 15th so he did some checking and look what he found.

"I would agree with that. He has been keeping up with your status remotely and I'm here to check in for the office," she said.

I was totally dumbfounded that they would go through this much trouble to look after me. Whenever the nurse would come in she would stay out of the doctor's way. I thought maybe Doctor "I Forget Your Name" could get me out of here by getting a message to Dr. Phillips to free me from this place. I guessed I was still looking at all of this the wrong way.

One thing I was not thinking about in the wrong way was Sir Flagyl which or should I say who seemed to enter my nightmares at every turn when I had to take it or him twice a day. I still asked her about that as I did on her first visit and the stomach shots and the "why?" of each. She once again explained that the purpose of Sir Flagyl was to fight off a type of bacteria that usually shows up in the intestines. During my entire stay at the hospital it was beginning to become clear to me that not only was I being unplugged but infection was a significant concern and I was in no state to endure another bout with one. Dr. "I Forget Your Name" went on to explain again that the test used to detect the bacteria was only seventy percent accurate so instead of risking that other thirty percent they gave Sir Flagyl instead to cover all of the bases. It would be a two-week course of deliciousness and gagging and it just started a few days ago. I saw no light at the end of that tunnel upon hearing this. She then explained that the shots in the stomach were a blood builder since my blood had become so depleted of everything these shots were crucial to getting me back to normal.

Of course, I listened to this as if I had heard it for the first time. I was just hoping that by asking repeatedly perhaps a different answer would be given that was to my liking. After this explanation I thought, *OK, I see*. I knew I would be asking again and my parents were around too so they would be asking as well. I didn't mind her visits. She was nice and patient with my repeated questions.

***

HERE COMES THAT INFECTIOUS DAY FEELING AGAIN[140]

The English Patient was a film I viewed years ago and it was obvious at the time that the purpose of making the film was to test a viewer's endurance with the running time. I still can't remember if Ralph Fiennes' character, the English patient, died in it or not, but I felt like I had when I saw it. In my current condition and with all of my theories I now jokingly referred to myself as "The Ignorant Patient." Notwithstanding the pretentious cinema that I have seen over the years and my shaky vow that the Ignorant Patient would not succumb to a similar fate, there was one thing I was not ignorant of and that was infection. Although the hated yet revered Sir Flagyl was there to protect me, he couldn't do it all. Everything that was in me was a risk and I wanted it all out, now. Prevention was the key ingredient to my survival and I was worried like hell, especially with the maypole catheter which had to be re-inserted every three days.

The end to this hated three-day ritual was nigh when finally Dr. Johnson came in and said, "Your urine output's going great and your kidneys are now functioning properly so we're going to remove the catheter."

I couldn't believe it, just when I was going to throw in the towel on ever having a properly functioning dong again I was provided this wonderful news. Those puddles must have gotten enormous.

Dr. Johnson continued, "We're going to try you out on a urinal." And with that he left with his white cape following obligingly.

I was to try to start peeing in a urinal? Once the catheter was removed? I didn't know how this was physically going to happen since I was unable to really sit up or get to a toilet. I learned from the nurse that the urinal was a plastic jug, and not the familiar piece of porcelain that in my mind would be ripped from the wall of the bathroom and brought to my bedside. I had not used one of these since I had my appendix removed at nineteen years of age. Sure, no problem.

It was time for the catheter to be removed. There was no fanfare or royal guards blowing horns except in my head as the nurse pulled the catheter out of my tortured cucumber. The removal still hurt like hell but I didn't care as long as it wasn't going back in.

The ultimate question when the urinal was presented to me was, "How?"

The nurse not very sympathetically said matter of factly, "Just lie on your side."

Getting on my side was an adventure in and of itself. Combined with trying to produce and control a steady stream of urine from a prod that had been asleep for weeks was akin to demanding that I shoot sparks from it. Gamely, I took the nurse's advice and tried the suggested maneuver. Sadly it felt like all of the bullies that tormented me throughout my childhood were standing there watching me and poking me in the back. I hoped those were just fingers. I couldn't do it. I kept pushing myself asking, *why's this happening?* It just wouldn't work. Ultimately I would halt the effort before I blew a gasket. *I can deal with this another time*, I would say to myself for comfort.

But what comforted me was not good enough for the nurse on her return to check on my volume. My efforts produced just a few drops and she would say with shame in her voice, "That's it!?" and would take the urinal away. Once again a new fear began to set in, this time about my questionable pissing abilities as I tried to think piss-inducing thoughts. The threat of the feeding tube was nothing compared to this threat. The goat felt the eye of the jackal.

CHAPTER 33

Back

Earlier studies of critically ill patients that used similar targets (ScvO2 >- 70 percent found no mortality benefit. This might be because these studies were not conducted during the crucial initial hours.[141]

ROOM 3XXX -NIGHT MOVES[142]

I was moving closer to the front door just like my old neighbor said I would, but the moves occurring during the evening hours were a little unnerving. Although this move was not as extreme in the time of night it occurred as the move from Progressive or as monumental as the move from the MICU it was nevertheless one more step. I was going to miss heaven on the seventh floor with its great TV, DVD player, cleanliness and all the good news I seemed to receive there.

Becky was thankfully with me on this move because quite frankly I couldn't have gotten through it without her. My trusty Instaflate, I, and the growing items that had been collected over my days in the hospital were transported by a separate cart. Believe me I had no idea how one person could collect so much when they were doing nothing in the way of collecting stuff. It just began to breed around me.

After a somewhat shorter trip than I had grown accustomed to on my previous moves the caravan came to a very familiar looking hallway. I remembered it as looking very similar to the postpartum wing where they took Becky after each of the Babies was born which shouldn't have been a surprise since all three of them were born in General Hospital. I had no idea we would be back so soon but for different reasons. However it was a different floor from the postpartum wing, and the relief that my male pregnancy was not a reality still stuck with me. Even though I looked, I fortunately did not see a baked bean in a bassinet anywhere.

Although the hall looked familiar it didn't seem nearly as clean as my other stops. Equipment littered the hallway, paint was peeling. It appeared that some sort of improvements had started and were now at a stopping point. I was wheeled into the room which had a very used feel to it as if it had been a bus station waiting area in a former life. I was disappointed in the digs but I still had a private room and you can't say enough about that in a hospital. The no-contact rules still applied to me it seemed. The bed was put into place and for the first time the door was to my left so I could work on those neck muscles.

Finally the night nurse popped her head in. She was Japanese, so I think I had covered all of the continents and cultures on my journey. English was her second language it seemed and it appeared humor was not a top priority in her culture.

"Hello, my name's Asahi. I'll be your nurse on this shift. First, I'll get you your meds and a urinal so you can void," and she left.

So now I not only had Sir Flagyl but also the pressure of the world's worst stage fright hammering on me. She quickly brought in the meds along with Sir Flagyl. I had gotten used to the shot in the stomach since I was getting a little fatter around my midsection thanks to the Freedom Fries and I was impressed with how less it seemed to hurt each time. My compliments were given to each nurse that did it exceptionally well. She then gave me the other meds and I had learned finally that I needed lots of water for the misery of swallowing. Finally, I requested the delicious Sir Flagyl in apple sauce or ice cream as I had been offered on my other stops. She seemed a little inconvenienced by this but agreed. She asked me how long it had been since I had drained the lizard. I said I didn't know, actually I hadn't at all since they took the catheter out the day before and all of my attempts were failures. I sure as hell was not going to say that. I lied to save the integrity of my hammer. She said then it must have been a while and handed me the urinal unceremoniously and told me to get busy.

I lay on my side very dubiously and attempted the impossible, nothing came out. I had officially arrived at the conclusion that I was in no uncertain terms being told to wet the bed. The problem was that the mind/urinary area connection wouldn't allow me to do that. It just wouldn't. After a few minutes Asahi returned to check on me and with her return there was a bit more of an attitude. Maybe she was still pissed about the serving of Sir Flagyl in the ice cream request. At this point I felt it was best to be honest so I claimed my problem right away and suggested that if I could maybe sit up in a bedpan?

"No. No," she replied. "We need to measure your output and we can't do that in a bedpan. You can't go on your side?" she asked incredulously.

Excuse me, I thought, *I have been without the use of my sword for the past four and a half weeks, it's going to take a while. Besides you don't need the urinal to measure, Dr. Johnson can tell the volume just by looking at a puddle.*

But I didn't and uttered a shamed "No" and she left. I sat in stunned silence waiting for her to bring back a Doogie Howser to make a bigger opening in Ole One Eye.

Asahi did come back to check on me a few minutes later, "No luck?" I grimaced and shook my head. It was like standing at a stadium urinal and having two drunk guys on either side of me yelling in my ears.

She said gravely, "If you can't go in the urinal then I'm going to have to put the catheter back in."

My spidey sense tingled so much at this suggestion, actually normal human sense would have worked fine, that I thought my head was going to explode. And after saying that she left but she didn't take away the fear and agony she had left behind. Not only was I thinking of the pain of the catheter but the absolute setback I thought that it would represent. I could not accept this.

I immediately begged Becky, "I don't have much time, please help me."

We set out on a quest, a quest to make the ultimate stage fright disappear and produce a frothy stream of urine that one would be proud to hold in a chilled mug. I changed up my position first by lying on the other side, that didn't work. Becky turned on the water to make my mind let go of what it was holding back, that didn't work. Then we both remembered the infamous camp prank that I may have seen last in *Meatballs 1* or was it *Meatballs 2*? Anyway it couldn't have been in *Meatballs 3 – The Revenge of the Kid that Looks like Sarah Connor*. Becky immediately got some warm water from the sink for me to put my hand in. I lay on my side with the urinal at the ready. I was ready for Niagara Falls to come out of my charger that was how sure I was about this. Lo and behold nothing happened. I couldn't believe this was not happening, the feeling always appeared when I was healthy and there was no pressure but it sure wasn't on board when I needed it the most. The water was getting colder, I was getting more upset, and that nurse was coming back with that tube to stick down my divining rod. I was in a panic, like I was about to be given a death sentence.

"How much time do you think I have? How long has it been?" I knew my time was finite; the forecast was calling for pain. Then it dawned on me, a thought, *You have had the power to void the entire time.* Except it wasn't the Good Witch from *The Wizard of Oz* that was in my head, it was that glorious porcelain thing staring at me through the open door to the bathroom.

I said, "That's it, I have to go to the toilet." We were past measuring time. I had to get this out now. Screw reading the urinal to the point of taking the meniscus into consideration for pure accuracy.

Becky said, "I can't carry you in there by myself, I'll need to get the nurse."

I was a little suspicious. "Do you think she'll go for it? I think she really wants to stick me in the root."

"The only way it's going to happen is for me to get her help."

Asahi, as if on cue, came back in the room and Becky asked the question and the answer would either crush me or lift me up, "He wants to use the bathroom if that's OK. I need help getting him in there."

"Sure," the nurse replied, "let me give you a hand."

Her answer was bright and cheerful so perhaps she didn't want to stick me after all and I didn't want to get stuck so we were going to get along just fine. They got me into a sitting position which was a miracle in itself. I hadn't really moved since my failure to walk over to Becky. I guess I was still pretty heavy when they struggled to get under my shoulders. My legs were like jelly, my flexi-seal was following me around like a tail. I was really unable to help and without the multitude of straps that I usually had accompanying me I was just worried I would drop on the floor. My sympathies and feelings went out and still go out to anyone who has lost the use of their limbs or ability to walk. I never thought at this age I would be in need of such assistance to get to the bathroom. Simultaneously I was happy, sad, amazed, and humble.

They both got me sitting on the toilet and I was able to hold myself up by the railings. The tail somehow looped out of the toilet onto the floor providing an interesting conversation piece for the proceedings. Before they left, the nurse gave me the urinal to pee in so they could measure it. At this point my hands had no power to lift anything let alone my piccolo so instead it just sat in between my legs. I sat there without the ability to hold my roto rooter down so I was at the mercy of gravity at this point. My bladder was full, I just knew it, I needed to go, I had to go. I had to get this body working again. There was no one in here but me, my tail, and my dingus so I just had to do it. I got them to move me in here so this had to work.

Suddenly, as if a faucet had been turned on it happened. I was dumbfounded that this one function that I had taken for granted brought me so much happiness. I shivered with excitement as it came out as if I had just had two pitchers of beer. Only twenty-five percent was able to go into the urinal for unfortunately I was pissing up in the air, onto my gown, and the rest was getting on the floor. I was crying, I was so happy as the puddles formed on the floor around my bare feet. I didn't care, there was no embarrassment, there was no fear of what I had done, there was just joy in being able to do the most basic of human functions and do it very poorly.

After a while, Becky opened the door and asked, "Are you OK?"

Through tears I said, "I did it! I did it! It still works, I still have it."

Asahi came in and I had a sudden pang of fear that she would stick me anyway rather than clean this mess up every time I had to go. Instead she was very understanding. I said as if I were a guilty four-year-old, "I made a messy mess in here." I then added in my head, *and quick get Dr. Johnson in here, this puddle is still full of information.*

She said, "Don't worry about that, I'll clean it up, and stop talking redundantly."

I was so grateful to her as I thought, *Thank you nurse I once feared. I shall now call you Asahi Ichiban.*

I was now the happiest and most fulfilled person on the planet. I was back baby, sitting in a pool of my own urine.

***

LONG TIME WAITING TO FEEL THE SOUND [143]

The next morning I was feeling good about my urinating success from the night before, my appetite had returned and I was rather chipper. The breakfast lady came by to take our orders. She asked, "Would you like some coffee?" Such a normal, everyday question made me feel so human I had to reply yes, so she brought some bitter-tasting stuff to me and Becky, which I drank heartily even though its taste was a little off-putting. My breakfast was coming soon and I continued staring at the wall and talking to Becky. Life was good because I was free from the fear of the jigger tube.

After about thirty minutes with no breakfast having yet arrived, a tech came unexpectedly with a more mobile bed and said, "I'm here to take you down for some X-rays in Radiology."

My first thought was that my breakfast would get cold although I didn't know where it could be. I said, "Fine." As if I really had a choice in the matter. I was still in a good mood, and nothing could get me down right now.

Becky asked, "Do you want me to come with you?"

The tech said, "It's just a routine X-ray; he'll be back in no time."

I added, "Just enjoy your breakfast, I'll be back."

He put the mobile bed alongside mine and I was able to slowly slide across onto it. And with that I was gone. Through the hallway I went with all of the backstage production passing me by. Then onto an elevator; it felt like I was going down and then I was out in a hallway that was rather dim with translucent glass tiles along the walls that let in some natural light. The tech rolled me into an alcove in the hallway and said, "Someone will be by to get you in a minute."

So there I was in a waiting room in the hospital just cooling my heels before I finally ate. A man then opened the door across from the alcove. He was large and had a strong resemblance to retired defensive lineman Mike Rucker of the Carolina Panthers. He said, "How are you doing today?"

I said, "Fine, just fine." Thinking that any negativity would lead to him snapping me in two like a twig.

"I'm going to take a few pictures of you," as he rolled me into the room. It was a dark windowless room with a lot of X-ray equipment in it.

"Can you stand?" he asked.

"No, not really," I replied. I couldn't remember when I last sat up much less stood when I wasn't peeing all over myself or sobbing uncontrollably. In Mike Rucker's world this would not stand.

"OK, then let me get something to support you." He then returned with a wheelchair.

I don't remember how it worked. I just remember being in an upright position and the sitting at that moment was killing my ass. He raised my arms one at a time as he got both profile and front views of my chest. I thought my shoulders were going to snap off they were so stiff. I was in a great deal of pain, but I wanted to impress Mike Rucker with my toughness. He really didn't seem to care about my stiffness, if I was to be bent into a pretzel he would have done so. I really missed the rolling X-ray unit that confounded me so in those days in the MICU.

"Just need a couple of more pictures of your lungs," he said, "and we'll be done."

I was sweating from all of the posturing; this was really taking a lot out of me. The final pose where I held my arms up on my own had to be taken a few times since they kept falling. This was really impossible. After a couple more attempts, finally he said, "All done." He helped me get back onto the mobile bed, and wheeled me out to the same alcove. "Someone will be by to get you shortly."

I was glad it was over and that I was soon to be in my room with my breakfast; what did I order? An omelet, pancakes, frittatas, crepes? I was getting hungry as hell now but was still the model of a patient patient. Mike Rucker returned to the X-ray room and shut the door. There was no clock anywhere so I had no sense of how long I had been there.

I waited and waited. The novelty of being done with the X-rays had quickly worn off, and I began to feel a bit stranded. Certainly someone would be coming by to get me. I tried to calm myself down. The alcove was offering no sense of comfort and felt a bit confining. There was a picture to my left of a natural landscape with a setting sun. I stared at that for some unspecified period imagining I was there witnessing it in person on a beach far away. Then I stared out at the hall and the reality of where I was came back. I was beginning to get a little crazy because the curtains were obstructing my vision. I couldn't see anyone coming. I could only hear their footsteps and saw them only when they were right in front of me. I thought each time they were here to get me, but they weren't.

After some time of this silliness I felt a bit embarrassed by my stranded condition. I thought I had to have a reason for being here, some explanation if someone asked or perhaps soon some of the "in" group of hospital workers would walk by and say, "Look at that stupid guy sitting there like a dog until someone gets him."

Maybe this was meant as a prank to let them see how long I could sit here unattended before I lost my mind. Well, it was working.

The mobile bed was making me miss my Instaflate. My ass was hurting, I was sliding down in the bed, the sheets were too smooth. What I would have given for sandpaper sheets. There was no one around to help me, and I was getting a little worried. I then made myself try to forget my hunger and fall asleep. I saw Mike Rucker leave the X-ray room again. Throwing caution to the wind I asked, "How long have I been here? No one has been to get me."

He looked at me like I was crazy and said, "It's only been twenty/thirty minutes. Someone will be by soon."

Shit, twenty to thirty minutes sitting like this felt like an eternity especially without a periodical with compulsory cleavage where viewing was compulsory. He didn't realize I had the patience of a five-year-old. I needed to be moved now. I hadn't felt this jumpy since the dialysis center. Maybe I should have formed my own complaint department like Mumble Mumble did, then there would be action. Again, I tried to force myself to go to sleep. I was awakened from a fitful sleep some time later by voices. I had no sense of the time; I was totally disoriented. I didn't know how long I had been asleep. Twenty minutes? An hour? The voices were coming from an office next to my alcove. What kind of hallway was this with an X-ray room across the hall, an office next door and me sitting in an alcove with just my thoughts?

It was two men and it seemed to be a patient/doctor conference. So much for confidentiality; I was the human fly on the wall.

The first man said, "Mr. Jones, we have the results of your tests."

The other man who sounded pretty young said, "What are they?" with a hint of anticipation in his voice.

"It's cancer," the first man said, his voice sympathetic with a hint that he had relayed this news many times before.

I felt horrified to be listening in on this conversation. Other than a sigh the patient seemed to be taking it well, as if he had been expecting the horrifying results.

"Has there been a history of this in your family?" asked the first person who I presumed was a doctor and maybe should have known the answer to this already.

"Yes, my parents, my sister." I couldn't believe this poor guy's family medical history. How could cancer have its way with one family like that? He then asked, "What's the treatment?"

"We'll have to start you on chemotherapy very soon and surgery might also be an option."

I really didn't want to hear anymore but I couldn't shut my ears, I couldn't walk away. Where the hell was someone? I certainly didn't want to call out to anyone and certainly not them since they would know I had been listening. What the hell was going on here? Doesn't this guy know how to close a fucking door? I felt guilty that I felt uncomfortable. I could see some light at the end of my tunnel, but what of poor Mr. Jones? He was at the doorway to a horrifying unknown and must have felt terrible. No, let's get back to me. What about me? I just got through hell, and I was here now listening to this horror that had bad juju all over it that I feared would follow me when someone did finally come and fucking get me! They kept talking about cancer, the test results, the chances of survival, the uncertainty of everything, normalcy in his, Mr. Jones's life.......

Finally it dawned on me that this was how someone found out about something so life changing, right here in this hallway; either that or getting thrown in an ambulance to battle Dog People at a moment's notice. I felt really, really sad about everything, just everything. My "up with people" attitude from this morning had gotten on a plane and left town at that moment, and there were no delays for that flight. I felt very lonely and very afraid. Thankfully, the door to the office finally closed. Perhaps this was best shared in privacy. Perhaps my shifting around had alerted them to my presence. I must have sounded like a caged rat or maybe it was my over-the-top throat clearing or perhaps Mr. Jones was finally breaking down and he was feeling his world shake. I didn't know. I was so depressed thinking about having a job where I would have to impart such bad news in a windowless room. I implored no one in particular, *please get me out of this hallway.*

Opportunity came once again with the sound of footsteps in the hallway, so I turned my attention to hearing those signs of life coming toward me. Waiting for anyone to come down the hall and summoning the courage to call out to them was my self-imposed duty at the moment. I felt like that weird guy at the mall with the strange kiosk that everyone glances at but doesn't want to make eye contact or, heaven forbid, have a conversation with. I had to be quick because these people were walking by like I had a load of Blue Oyster Cult cassettes to unload. It was easier to track down an orange apron in Home Depot than this place.

Finally a young woman wearing scrubs, so she had to know what she was doing, was walking at a slow enough gait where my voice could catch up to her.

"Excuse me," I said. She looked around like the walls were talking to her. "Over here," I said. She looked over and rather hesitatingly came over.

"Can I help you?" she said reluctantly as if I had a time share to sell her.

I was nearly in tears that someone actually stopped. I said, "I was supposed to be taken back to my room a while ago after my X-rays but no one has come to get me."

She said, "I'll find out what's going on." I felt relief that finally I would be taken away from the miserable hall.

Sometime later, perhaps five minutes, thirty minutes, an hour, I have no idea, I heard footsteps coming. Suddenly a man in dark blue scrubs and glasses finally stopped in front of my alcove. "Yes?" I asked imploringly.

"Mr. Hoover," he said in a thick accent of unknown origin, "you can't go to your room yet, you're waiting for someone from Specials to remove your catheter."

This did not register with me at all. I was struck dumb with the thought that I was not done with this hall.

I said, "What?"

"Your catheter, sir, it needs to be removed and someone from Specials will be here to do it; they're on another procedure at the moment and will be here in a little bit."

"There must be some mistake," I said thinking of this Specials term as something I have only heard at my kids' school and was getting irritated at him for throwing around hospital lingo as if I was supposed to know what the hell he meant. "You had better double check because my catheter was removed two days ago, and I don't know what elementary school classes have to do with my health."

He grimaced not knowing really what to think of either of these two statements. "Really?" he asked suspiciously, "You're down to have it removed; I see none of that in your records."

"I'm telling you it was removed!" I said agitatedly, "Why don't you believe me?!" The Ignorant Patient was getting some teeth now. Of course I was thinking of the catheter that had been removed from my banana just days ago. The thought that something else was in me was totally out of the realm of possibilities. Couldn't he see that this had to be wrong?

"You must calm down sir, you're to have the catheter in your chest removed," he said pleadingly.

"No, there's nothing like that in me, I want to go back to my room now!" I said incredulously. There was no way in hell I had something like that in me, no way, I would have noticed. I know it wouldn't have escaped my notice.

"Please sir, the catheter has to be removed to guard against infection and you have to wait here." His accent was becoming thicker as he became agitated, and I was having trouble understanding him so I became more agitated. It was a vicious circular reference.

Where the hell am I now? There are too many foreigners in here that I can't understand, I thought as my attitude became a little less tolerant with each passing moment and a little more Archie Bunkerish.

"Please get someone here that I can understand! I don't believe you! I don't understand!" I screamed. I was now kicking the mattress without fear that I might be disturbing Mr. Jones grappling with his life changing moment next door let alone that Mike Rucker might tear out of the X-ray room and prove his potential for snapping me like a twig.

He said, "You must wait, you must calm down. Please sir."

I was about to lay into him again when he said, "Someone will be by soon." And like that he was gone; he knew I couldn't follow him. I was in a panic. Some butcher was coming to get me. I had heard about this before, patients having limbs amputated by mistake or having their sword turned into a sheath, who knew what horrors awaited me? I was trying to go over my options. There were none. Becky was probably wondering what the hell had happened to me. What would I be missing when I saw her again? Would we be a Mrs. and Mrs. by the end of the day? I was alone, I was scared and the butcher was coming.

I heard footsteps and talking. I got really nervous when around the corner came Dr. Cold Case and another female with glasses wearing a mask. She had dark curly hair. Dr. Cold Case, who I had seen last in the MICU, said, "Mr. Hoover, we have been looking all over for you."

I was angry but I couldn't decide if I should piss off the people that were holding the instruments of torture with a misguided tongue lashing. I said as calmly as I could, "Yes, I need to know what's going on from someone I can understand."

Dr. Cold Case then said, "This is Ms. So and So, PA from Specials who'll be taking out the permanent catheter in your chest. It has been there for dialysis and other intravenous needs."

Things were becoming clearer to me yet the horror was not abating. "We need to have it done and out of the way right here, otherwise it could get all blocked up and become messy," she said as she made a squeamish gesture. I was surprised to see a doctor make such a gesture. I was still not feeling comfortable with the proceedings, and there was no way I could argue my way out of it.

I asked, "How long does this take and how invasive is it?"

Ms. So and So, PA answered, "Not really invasive at all. It's below your skin about this long," she held up her hands about six inches apart, "and it will take about twenty to fifty minutes to remove." Even though she had the most soothing and calm voice that was still longer than I would have liked and I would have thought that even if Barry White in his sultry voice had delivered the news.

"Why so long?" I asked nervously.

"Well, you never know what can happen, but without any complications it should be only twenty minutes. I do a lot of these so don't worry."

I still could not see her face, and I nodded letting my resistance lessen. After a few more questions from Dr. Cold Case, she left and I was left with Ms. So and So, PA.

I said, "You're doing this here?"

"Sure," she answered. "There shouldn't be a problem."

I felt like I was being operated on in a waiting room. No, I was being operated on in a waiting room because I had been doing the waiting! This was making me more than a little nervous, there was no one else here except us, what if something went wrong. Dammitt!! I swear I was healthy last month, what the hell happened?

She said, "You look nervous."

"I am, I don't get this done every day," I said.

"I'm just going to put a numbing agent on your chest where I'll make the incision. You may feel a sensation in your chest but you shouldn't feel anything," she said.

"You mean you won't be knocking me out?" I asked shakily.

"Not for something this short and routine," she said patiently.

"Will there be a scar?" I asked. Beach season would be here before I knew it, and I liked to impress with scars.

"Only about the size of a dime and it'll only look like a red bump," she replied.

Although I was disappointed that the scar wouldn't be bigger, I wanted to get this shit over with especially since I was being opened up in a hallway. My fear of infection was becoming more and more heightened, and I didn't think this was the cleanest of places to be having this done.

She then asked, "Would you like me to tell you what I'm doing as I do it?"

Like I told the doctor during my big V, "No," I said.

She said, "Just relax; it'll be over in a little while."

I sure as hell hoped she knew what she was doing. I felt less and less sure and that I was just hanging around now for the second wave of infections to get me. I looked to my left and found solace in the sunset picture on the wall. Trying to imagine that I was standing on a beach far away, my thoughts were ruined when I realized that even in the daydream someone was cutting into my chest.

She broke the silence, "I know being calm's the only way to get better. I was in a bad accident once. I was out running and a car hit me in the crosswalk. I broke my back, dislocated my hip, broke an arm and a leg."

With this I took my eyes off the sunset, looked at her and exclaimed, "Oh God!"

Looking like she had said more than she should have she replied, "I'm OK now, I'm only telling you this because I had to stay calm and still to get better and it'll happen. You'll get out of this hospital and be back to normal. I had to give it time and be patient and you're going to have to do the same."

I must admit I had never had anyone put it to me like that and I was dumbfounded by her honesty in sharing that with me. I was not seeing the light at the end of the tunnel before this, but I knew that I was going to have to take it slow and take my time and it would happen. I had already come so far, don't give this up. I nodded in agreement.

She said, "There, all done. I'll clean you up and you're good to go. Remember what I said, you'll get better, just give it time and good luck."

She finished up the procedure, packed up her stuff and was gone. I never did see her face.

CHAPTER 34

Sharper

Relative intravascular hypovolemia (a state of decreased blood volume) is typical and may be severe. As an example, early goal-directed therapy required a mean infusion volume of approximately five liters within the initial six hours of therapy in trials. As a result, rapid, large volume infusions of intravenous fluids are indicated as initial therapy for severe sepsis or septic shock, unless there is coexisting clinical or radiographic evidence of heart failure.[144]

ONE MORE TRIP AND I'LL BE GONE[145]

With my unexpected surgery completed, now was the time to finally have my ass back in my room. I was hungry, I was tired, I was spent, I was scared, and I was annoyed. Getting back to the room, my little fortress of solitude was what I was looking forward to most. After a few minutes of being relieved that I had all of my limbs, my skull, and my sword I heard footsteps coming down the hallway. An older man came bopping along that had a strong resemblance to Big Daddy. He had a golf shirt on that made him a volunteer I supposed.

He said, "Taking you back up," as he consulted a thick dossier. He maneuvered the bed out of the alcove and into the hall. We were off and I was away from that awful alcove. We were back in the elevator and we came out in a hallway which looked sort of familiar but did not seem to be the one that I had been in that morning. My slight sense of worry became a little more pronounced as he wheeled me into a room that really looked familiar but certainly did not feel right. I swore the door was to my left this morning now it was on the right. What was this? Had I gone crazy? And it was clean as a whistle. This was not the room I left this morning. Where was the Instaflate bed, where was Becky, where was all of my stuff that kept following me around?

I was spent after my tumble downstairs so I was just trying to accept it as the nurse came in and helped the Big Daddy guy get me from the mobile bed to the one in the room. This bed was hard and uncomfortable and short.

Mighty and Forgiving Instaflate I'll never speak bad about you again!

I was trying to figure out what the hell had happened this morning and if my move was just a dream, when I realized that the nurse was the same stern humorless Jamaican nurse I had on the seventh floor. Shit, I am moving back or maybe I never moved at all. Like Patton I was not into paying for the same real estate twice. She began to disrobe me without a word; then began to scrub me with my keister being her primary target.

I thought, *yes, without a doubt this is my old room. I'm in my old room, what the hell!* This was no longer heaven on the seventh floor.

I decided that I finally had to say something. This shit had gone on for too long. "Does my wife know I'm here?" I uttered without the greatest confidence, not knowing if my move had happened at all.

The Jamaican nurse stopped scrubbing my exhaust pipe and paused. Finally, a statement that pierced her emotionless exterior. She remembered me, I should not be here she must have realized, and she said, "I'll go check."

She left the room. I felt better because I was not supposed to be here and wasn't crazy but also pissed off because I was here. She came back in and said, "You're right, I thought you looked familiar and you shouldn't be here. We'll have someone to take you down right away."

I thought, *familiar? You don't remember my sobbing episode?* Maybe it was better she didn't, she might have made me stay to toughen me up. I was still mad. I was happy, but mad.

A different guy came in to get me this time a few minutes later. I was transferred back to the mobile bed and taken away. My thought at that moment was that someone would have to clean up again after my thirty-minute stay. We got back on the elevator and my anger was brewing still; I felt worse than I had before we left the alcove. I was wheeled back in the room on the third floor; it was still crappy but it was where my furthest advance had taken me. I had not been dreaming and a great wave of relief came over me. There was my stuff, Instaflate! How I missed you, and Becky was standing there and asked, "What happened to you?"

At this question I once again became teary man as I asked, "How long was I gone?"

"About four hours," came her response. "Where were you?"

"It was awful." As I recounted the waiting, the ignorance, the not knowing about the procedure, the wrong room, being bumped even though I had a first-class ticket and getting put in coach and now having to sit next to Del Griffith.[146] The entire thing.

My nurse came back in and I said, "Is my breakfast still around?"

She said, "No, you were gone so we sent it away. Lunch won't be for another half hour."

I yelled like a small child learning there was no more chocolate milk. At that moment, as if the timing could not be more perfect, a young girl came in and asked, "I 'm coming around to take a survey of how well we're doing with a patient satisfaction survey, so I wanted to ask you a couple of questions of how you have found your stay with us. On a scale of one to five with five being the best."

I don't usually raise a stink and I know people are trying to do their jobs and I appreciate that, but if I didn't speak now they would never know the utter hell I went through this morning. This place saved my life but they had to know. So seizing the opportunity I said, "I don't need to hear the questions, I give you a one for all." Unless the question was about them pissing me off, then I would have given them a five.

The poor girl looked like I had grown horns and a tail right in front of her. She stuttered, "R-Really."

"Yes," I replied.

"Why, what happened?" she said nervously.

I said, "I don't want to talk about it right now. I just feel sick about it."

With that Becky went through the whole story even adding a "Purple monkey dishwasher" to add confusion like in that rumor game. The girl left the room and almost immediately a more senior person filed right in to get the story.

"I got no breakfast, I thought I was going for just an X-ray and then I'm getting something pulled out of my chest I didn't know was there and then I get taken to the wrong floor. Then, to top it off, I'm given the keys to a car that isn't even there. I have had it!" I recounted, each word getting more emphatic.

I had an audience and I had a voice and I was finally using my new-found power. I could see why patients are cantankerous. Being sick sucks even if everything is going perfectly, and when it doesn't that's when panic and frustration sets in. I was not of my right mind but I was irritated and so was Becky.

The lady in charge was very apologetic about everything. "I'm so sorry that the room list was not updated, and I don't know why you wouldn't have been informed of the catheter procedure. It was just bad communication. We'll definitely correct these problems so they never happen again."

That was all I wanted to hear, that someone said, "Sorry," and showed some empathy toward me. I considered the matter over especially after lunch came. So I made a mental note to add "Have catheter removed from chest" to my list of things not to do before eating with "Go to Home Depot" still at the top.

***

BE HERE NOW [147]

It may have been the long hours in the chair, the restless nights, the winter season, or just the hospital wing itself and its unclean state, whatever it may have been Becky came down with a bad cold that she couldn't get rid of. Fortunately for her and for me, I just didn't feel that way at the time, she was off to Miami for a conference for three days. I missed her being around especially at night, since there was no one there to watch over me. I felt a little exposed but I was beginning to adapt. My parents would arrive around lunch time. They obviously thought the worst was over so their shopping trips went on as usual; however, I was still in quite a weakened state.

One day I was sitting there just staring at the wall, although the wall in Room 3XXX was not nearly as interesting as in the MICU, when this lady wearing a white lab coat appeared. She didn't fully enter the room. She just stood at the door. She was in her forties, had brown shoulder-length hair like the mother from the overrated *Home Improvement*. She didn't bother with opening pleasantries; she just began to talk about how it was important that I start getting into a daily routine so I would be able to adjust to life outside the hospital more quickly.

She went on to say, "Also, if you use a computer, you need to type or write or do anything to get your mind moving and re-develop those habits you use when working. If you have work to do, then it would be a good idea to do some now so that your body and mind can adapt. You have been through a lot so you need to start staying busy so your recovery will be quicker."

Her attitude was one of shaming me and was one of "you're being a bit lazy and we have had enough of your ass being here watching *Family Feud*, so start working or get the hell out."

I sat there dumbfounded and slack jawed just staring at her blankly thinking, *first of all Family Feud sucks and besides they're interviewing Fucking Octomom in a few minutes.*

The rant in my head however became a little more serious, *work? I just have a trash show on, because this TV here stinks, minding my own business when you just show up. I have thrown myself many parades for learning how to eat, talk, piss and now you want me to start working here like I am some sort of bum getting by on my flexi-seal and oily good looks?*

She stood there as the rant in my head finished because I didn't want to piss her off whoever she was. She stared at me some more as I had my mouth agape still wondering if she was real and said, "Do you understand what I'm saying?"

Without saying a word I nodded compliantly. And with that she closed the door. I then looked around the room to see if anyone else was in there that could agree that what had happened had really happened, but no one else was there. I feared her return, and thought constantly from then on of my status of looking "busy," like getting a screwdriver, and tightening something on Instaflate. If she returned I could just be getting on with whatever tightening needed to be done.

***

I KNOW YOU FROM SOMEWHERE

It was the whole Clark Kent/Superman thing going on. Dr. "I Forgot Your Name" came in once again, and Becky was nowhere around. Was it Becky disguising herself as a doctor? Actually Becky was still in Miami which sounded so great and so out of reach to me. I knew she was at a fancy hotel but since she was under the weather I knew not much fun was being had. Poor thing, it was good for her to get away from me feeling so sick. I missed her and felt alone.

But my parents were around, and just like clockwork Dr. "I Forgot Your Name" came in. She exclaimed, "They keep moving you around. It's getting harder and harder to find you. You'll be so well, that they'll have moved you out of here the next time I need to see you."

I always liked Dr. "I Forgot Your Name." She was patient, and answered any and all questions, and with my parents and me, "The Ignorant Patient," around I knew she was going to have her hands full. The Sir Flagyl situation had not gotten any better, and I was still counting down the forgotten number of days I had left until the curse of licking concrete was over. "It's almost there," she said "Just a little longer."

Again we all asked as in chorus, "Now why do/does I/he have to take this again?"

She would adjust her glasses I noticed before she gave the long often-repeated answer to this question about the test for the infection being only seventy percent accurate so to cover all bases the delicious Sir Flagyl was administered to combat it.

We sort of would stare while we digested this information once again. It was seeping in a little bit at a time, it truly was, and we asked some more questions like the condition of my feet which were still a ghastly purple color especially in the toe area and the trach dressing. She patiently answered all of the questions. My body was feeling like the broken down 1970 Sedan Deville some friends bought from an old man when we were in high school. The litany of problems with the car was great, but it and I still had some cross country trails left in it to burn. She then updated me on my condition, and she remarked how everything looked promising. I always had a difficult time believing good news, come in with any uncertainty, and it was curtains for me.

With that she left but not before I could ask about Sir Flagyl again, and why I had to take it.

***

I BELIEVE YOU'RE MISTAKEN

I was becoming more and more alone, and while this time increased, the likelihood of fucked up shit happening also increased. One evening

I was lying there staring at the TV which slowly began to replace the wall for entertainment when an orderly walked in, and gave me my dinner of sauces and liquids.

What the hell is this? I thought, *first they're trying to force feed me when I don't want to eat, and now that I'm ready to eat they're trying to starve me.*

I quickly reached for the nurse button and pushed. I was told someone would be in there. When they arrived I said, "Yes, there must be a mistake. I have this when I should be getting real food."

"Oh, no, there's no mistake. You're on a liquid diet before tomorrow's surgery," came the confident reply.

"No, I'm on a comfort food diet, and there's no surgery, you need to check again," I said as my voice began to rise. I was committed to crawling out of here like a legless zombie if they were going to cut me again.

She looked at me dubiously thinking I was pulling a fast one but I had my dander up after my four-hour disappearing act two days ago. What did they have buried in me now, a gerbil? She argued with me for a little longer but I held my ground.

"No. No. No," I said emphatically, "no one has told me anything I am having done tomorrow, and until I hear from a doctor that knows my name and condition I'll not be agreeing to that."

She said with an air of finality, "OK." and left. Soon she was back, and said, "I apologize. That meal was meant for next door, we'll be bringing you in a full tray momentarily."

I was beginning to lose confidence. I had to get out of here and quick.

***

THE MAN WHO SAVED ME

Once again, I was alone in the room. Everyone was either in Miami or out shopping/returning/exchanging things. I didn't feel out of the woods, yet I didn't blame them. Being stuck in a hospital room when you aren't sick and visiting is only second behind being the sick one. Going to the hospital for a visit feels full of purpose but once you get there it's, "Shit, this is depressing, and there's a sick person. I must leave now." There is a need to be free and out, I would certainly agree to that except I was used to being alone. My thoughts, the wall, and Fucking Octomom were all I needed.

The door opened, and in walked a young-looking guy with blond hair that hung boyishly over his forehead and a dimply smile. Well my deary my, I sound like a blushing school girl. I guessed that reaction was proper for someone that saved your life. However I differed with Becky on the resemblance to Doogie Howser. Instead I found he had a strong resemblance to Alex Lifeson, guitar wizard of the Canadian musical trio, Rush during their *Grace under Pressure* days. "Howard, you haven't met me. I'm Jeremy Sherwood. They said you wanted to meet me, they've been moving you around I see."

I had of course been waiting to meet the man that made the correct changes to me in the ER, and turned around my prognosis to not only live but to get to where I was right now. I couldn't believe that he was in the room. They actually let this genius in this part of the hospital? I had heard so much about him, and the things he did for me when I was under in my journey into other worlds. He handled many things from Big Daddy's crying binges and pleas to save my life, family-called meetings, to a "family friend" aggressively challenging his treatment of me. I heard that he said back then I was ten minutes to ten minutes when he really meant I was minute to minute. I was in his hands, and now I was meeting him.

"My Gosh, hey!" I exclaimed. "There's the man, I have wanted to meet you." Like a frat boy meeting his favorite fantasy football player, I almost dropped my invisible screwdriver in the process.

He grinned sheepishly over my enthusiastic greeting. "I have been meaning to get down to see you, but I was off shift from the hospital after I saw you in the MICU, and now I'm back on."

I didn't understand the strange schedules of doctors and still don't, what an interesting life. I replied, "No problem, I have just heard your name so much I wanted to get to meet you, and thank you for everything you did for me."

"That's part of the job, and I'm extremely happy everything turned out great," he replied.

"I wish my parents were here to see you, they spoke of you glowingly throughout. After I woke up I learned all the troubles that had occurred, and I hoped everyone behaved," I said.

"Everyone was fine, I just loved your family, they were always in your corner," he replied.

"I have just been unsure of what I had for so long, it has taken me awhile to even take in what it was, and I still don't understand it."

"Your body went through a one-in-a-million event, it was like a nuclear bomb went off inside it. Not many people get as far as you did but it started when the bacteria that causes strep throat got into your lungs and from there into your bloodstream. Your body over reacted to this, and it began to shut down one organ at a time. You weren't in good shape when we first met," he said.

I was nodding. The Ignorant Patient was beginning to understand the ramifications of this. No body rebuild, no male impregnation, no protest at a historic site that nearly killed me. I had questions but saved the Sir Flagyl talk for Dr. "I Forgot Your Name." I wanted to know about the trach incision and how long it would take to heal, how long it would take for my lungs and kidneys to return to normal. We talked and laughed like we had been through a war together, but he was going to need to leave in a little while. I just couldn't believe my parents weren't here to see him or he never would have been allowed to leave. Where were they? Actually his time in the room would have tripled had they shown up. They were so appreciative of everything he did. Those must have been some dark days in January. With all the questionable things that had happened of late I wished he were available to hand hold me the rest of the way out of here.

"I'm very pleased with how far you have come; I have been keeping up with your progress remotely, and I'll continue to do so. It was great to meet you," he said.

"It was great to meet you too, and keep watching," I said.

"I have one favor to ask."

"Anything," I said.

"Here's my card, in about four to six months if you wouldn't mind calling my office for an appointment, I would like to check on your lung function."

"Of course, thanks to you there's another four to six months for me," I said.

With that he left. God Bless this place.

***

BAD BOY HEARTBREAK

I really didn't know who my doctor was at this point. I would have a flurry of them come in and visit. Where it was Dr. Rebefall for so many days in the MICU I had trouble putting a face on who was pulling the strings on my recovery now. I couldn't believe they knew what the other was doing. Dr. Cold Case would come in periodically. I was not really sure of her role, perhaps the "Dr. of All Talents."

One day she came in, and I had playing on my Ipod some hair band song from the 80s. As she was checking me she said, "My gosh, I remember this song, what is this?"

I replied, "It's Warrant [or insert some other name like Kix, Mr. Big, Rice Chex, Fruit Brute] I have this greatest hits album from the 80s called *Bad Boy Heartbreak*." Unlike me, those bad boys caused a lot of heartbreak.

"Where did you get it?" she said expectantly.

"In Target, in the CD section there's a discount rack, it only cost eight dollah cheap cheap." For some reason I was conjuring some past visit to an overseas bazaar.

Then another hair anthem came on, "I remember this one too. What did you say this album was called again?"

"*Bad Boy Heartbreak*," I said. I must admit I was beginning to enjoy saying the title; whoever thought of it was a genius. No, Dr. Sherwood was a genius, whoever thought of it was a very capable person. Finally I had some information to impart even though it was worthless. I didn't even go into how I bought it for a white elephant gift exchange a couple of months ago and how luckily I came away with it because who knew? It could have been a one of a kind.

She was very interested, and after she once again made sure where she could find this memory lane soundtrack in Target she left me repeating, "*Bad Boy Heartbreak.*" I just hoped that wasn't all she remembered from her visit and the only thing she wrote in my chart. It must have really brought back memories. She probably could see herself dancing to it at some frat party long ago with her Cold Case Hair swaying in the smoke-filled dimly lit room.

I was so glad I was able to add a non-medical highlight to her day.

***

WALK ME TO THE DOOR[148]

My physical therapists kept finding me. The one that looked like Emma Stone was mostly around with Mike I guess having time off. I hadn't seen him in a while, since Progressive which seemed a long time ago. Emma came in with some large rubber bands and began to show me some exercises I could do with them. There was a blue one which was for my strength level at this point, and the much harder-assed orange band which was definitely more advanced. Emma showed me the tricep exercise, then the chest pull exercise, and one other. I couldn't possibly remember this basic list so I had her repeat them to me. Becky wrote each exercise down, and diagrammed the movement before she had left for Miami. After so long without movement, the idea of movement was sounding challenging.

My one ounce of input into the conversation was my observation that the bands smelled like wedding cake. Emma, with a puzzled look on her face, said, "I hadn't heard that one before."

"Just think of the money you could save on a wedding putting a couple of bands on the table at the reception," I said to a blistering laughter onslaught and applause that I heard in my head, the kind given by the suspiciously overly appreciative studio audience from *Happy Days*.

My mettle was being shown in other ways as well. With the helplessness of my disappearing act a couple of mornings before having faded, the physical therapy once again delved into my walking. I had not tried this again since my journey to the toilet so I was a bit apprehensive at another setback. As a gift for my new forays into walking I received two pairs of brand new slippers, one pair from my parents and one from Becky's mom. Big Daddy referred to them as "bunny slippers."

The therapist came in, and helped me into the walker, the big leather one that I failed so miserably in on the seventh floor. My head was getting a bit clearer by this time, and I wasn't so faint while they strapped me in. I actually survived the strapping in, and now it was time to put my feet on the floor. Once again the floor seemed so cold and unforgiving. Growing wings and taking flight seemed to be just as possible at this moment. Eventually my feet felt a bit more solid underneath, and I just began to put one foot in front of the other. This time though I didn't feel rushed, and I didn't feel as helpless. My neck was still weak, with my giant head feeling like a lollipop, but I was able to finally withstand the stress of my own weight even though the harness was providing much of the support. I did have to get my feet moving to actually move the wheels.

As I took my first step I realized what I took for granted every day. The ability to walk was indeed a miracle of evolution, and the way the muscles go to sleep if not used just confounded me. The entire movement seemed alien to me, even though I had been walking since I was a toddler.

Under the watchful eye of Emma I was able to walk staggeringly to the foot of the bed. "Do you feel OK?" she asked.

Surprisingly I did. "Yes," I replied.

"Can you get to the door?" she asked hopefully.

I nodded as sweat poured off my head, and shame was coming out the rear of the hospital gown. I felt a little like I was stranded on that island again. The comfort of Instaflate was calling to me but I had to break the surly bonds of fifty-thread-count sheets, and touch the face of the door handle. I was almost there, I couldn't believe it. Emma couldn't believe it, I couldn't believe it. I already said that.

"You did it!" said Emma. "Are you done or do you want to go out into the hall?" she asked.

I said, "That's enough, I have to get you to look forward to something tomorrow."

"OK then let's turn around slowly," she said.

I slowly did a Williamson Turn, and headed back toward the bed. I felt like perhaps I should have gone for the hallway but Instaflate beckoned. I felt triumphant yet lazy at the same time. I settled in with my back to the bed as they unstrapped me and helped me into Instaflate. The horror of the seventh floor was now behind me. Walking and pissing in two days, it didn't get better than that.

The next day Emma returned and said that the leather contraption was a thing of the past. I could graduate to a walker with a couple of straps on it.

"Do you think you can support yourself with your arms?" she asked.

This was a big graduation day, and my anxiety rose thinking it would just be me going out into the cruel hallway. How would my body react to such a new endeavor?

"I really don't know," I told her. I knew I had to try to try.

The strapping took a fraction of the time the leather monster did but I felt a little more on my own. My spindly arms were going to have to work double time on this one. As I was slowly assisted to a seated position I noticed my neck muscles had strengthened, and my grip felt a little firmer. I once again put one foot in front of the other, and then, yes, I was walking out that door. The hallway, it was a strange place. I was finally on my own outside my room unassisted. It took a while to get used to the turns of the wheels on the walker, but I was slowly finding my way.

There was a lot of racket going on as some workmen were occupied with a door frame, and were letting it have it with some pneumatic tool. It felt like they were in another dimension, handling heavy equipment, standing for long periods, and me learning how to walk. I only got three doors down on this day until my arms and shoulders started to give a little. The hallway looked so familiar just like the one with the post-partum rooms when we had all of the Babies. These thoughts confused me a bit. I was beginning to believe that I would walk in through my door, and see Becky in the bed with a bassinet beside her. The memory was so clear. However, when I rounded the corner and entered the room there was no one there.

The next day went along much better. I was walking a little further this time past the workmen. My parents were accompanying me, and I was feeling so much better and confident. I knew I was going to be back at that moment, however since I was still in the hospital I was still considered sick. I was weak but I was getting stronger.

As my bladder began to awaken more and more I needed to use the bathroom more and more. Big Daddy assisted me on one occasion which I found odd that my seventy-five--year-old father would be assisting me to the bathroom. I was hoping only that it would be a long while before I was doing the same for him. I leaned on his shoulder, and I would barely make it to the toilet as he unceremoniously threw my flexi-seal aka tail with the bag of shit attached to me in after me. A few times he would shut the door on it. After a few reprimands from my mom, and the realization of the mess he almost made he would be sure to clear the door but toss it in nonetheless. These few times there was more confidence, fewer tears, and a dry floor.

***

FLEXI-SEAL DON'T TELL NO LIES[149]

The unplugging continued for on this day, the day I had been waiting for, my flexi-seal aka the tail would no longer be an appendage, and yes, Sir Flagyl would no longer be in my life. I would no longer fear it being twisted around me, getting smushed in the door, any infection coming from it, the disturbing yet sometimes invigorating cleaning, the overall weird sound and feel of it, or best of all the feeling that my ass was going to be ripped out as I was lifted up in the bed. However, I would start having to go to the bathroom for real like a sucker. It was finally coming out, and Lord knows I learned the hard way what was used to keep it in must have been some sort of super Gorilla Glue. For on this day a team of four nurses was rounded up and entered my room.

So strange and foreign this novelty must have been for nurses far and wide that a head nurse said, "Come on in, I need to show all of you how to remove one of these." The bottom line was that four young ladies were staring at my ass as a tube was removed. That thing was a part of me so I was a bit nervous over the force that would be needed to separate it from my back way.

"Lie on your side please," a female voice said.

As I did a hundred times but never really got used to, I rolled over, and the weight of my body once again crushed the bone in my non-existent shoulder. I could still see the yellowish streak in the console, someone had not cleaned this bed very well. I still meant to say something about it.

The tugging commenced. It felt like someone was literally pulling duct tape out of my ass, giving me the old reverse Ned Beatty. The feeling was horrific, and the hairs were unwilling to let go. I gritted my teeth, and let the nurse get on with it. I imagined the chief puller with her feet off the floor pressed against the bed railing, pulling with all of her might.

"OK, you have to keep pulling after you have applied this," she said.

Oh, this was unpleasant. Finally the seal was ripped free, and there was an exclamation from the group as if they and Geraldo Rivera had actually found something in Al Capone's vault.

The head nurse said, "So that's what was causing the trouble."

I had not a clue to what she was referring but just lay there letting my new found freedom sink in.

"Would you like to see what the trouble was?" she asked hopefully. I could imagine she was holding what looked like a dead mink on the end of a piece of tape or simply my ass scalp.

I said, "What?" Was she talking to me?

"I have it right here."

Have what, some sort of gerbil or memo sticking pin? Million to one shot nurse, million to one.

I really didn't want to see any more, especially something with my hair all covering it in front of the four ladies so I said, "No thanks." So with that she was gone, and my relationship with the thunder box began anew.

***

YOU GOTTA MOVE[150]

My free ride was over, they were going to start making me bathe myself, the horror of this. A young girl came in with a tray one morning. No one was there but me; she was a gregarious gal, had to be in her first couple of years of college.

"It's bath time," she said cheerfully, as I quickly tried to look busy with my imaginary screwdriver.

"OK," I responded.

She set the familiar looking basin on the tray table, handed me the wash cloth, and then sat down. It was clear that she was not going to do anything else.

Why you lazy so and so, making me clean myself, and not even wrapping the washcloth around a stick. Where are the cameras, where's the press? I thought.

But I suddenly realized that was the way it was going to be. I made up my mind that this was good, no more rough treatment, and I could go at my own pace. I really couldn't reach anywhere so I just made an effort to get where I could, as I threw the wash rag around like a lazy ninja with cotton nunchucks. Then she just began to talk about anything that was on her mind, sports, the weather. I was a little annoyed that she was hanging around. I felt like I was being treated like a shut-in. Well, I guess I did meet all of the basic and preferred requirements of a shut-in.

She mentioned a show on ESPN, *Rome is Burning*, and asked if I had ever seen it. I said no, and that I pretty much don't like those shows, they are all a bunch of people screaming at each other. She looked deflated when I said that so I backtracked, and said, "I really haven't seen it yet so I can't really say that." She then described it for me. All of this talking to strangers was still new to me. I still think Mr. Rome changed his last name for show naming purposes. Too convenient. Too catchy. A conspiracy riddled mind.

When I was done with my high effort/low yield bathing she refastened my gown and told me about this one guy she had to move once. He grabbed her arm, and wouldn't let go. It took a couple of other nurses to get her free.

I said, "That sounds terrible."

She replied, "Yeah," and matter of factly added, "He died."

I was shocked that someone died, and that this young girl saw that probably every day. The enormity of where I was hit me, and I wanted out at once. This ain't a hotel, death happens here, I had to keep reminding myself.

Sensing that she had said something a little too grave she changed the subject, and the conversation turned light hearted once again. My pulmonologist came in while we were laughing. I had not seen him before, he was an older guy. He looked so much like a doctor that if one was to draw a picture of a doctor it would look just like him. He had the bald spot with hair around the edges that was graying, was jowly, and had reading glasses on. He could have been wearing a silk tank top in place of the white lab coat. It didn't matter, that man looked like a doctor.

He looked official, and he announced, "I have taken a look at your X-rays, and your lungs are looking better but there's still scarring."

I nodded, and said, "Thank you," and suddenly he looked uncomfortable, and left the room like he was interrupting, and we were about to say a joke at his expense. We talked some more, and I had a few jokes that popped into my head, none at the doctor's expense. She hung out longer, and said, "Well, I'm off, feel better," and left the room.

The next morning she returned, and I knew the drill this time and began with the lazy ninja routine. She sat down and we began talking. I told her about my wife, kids, and family. I enjoyed her company more this time, and then as if on cue the same doctor walked in from yesterday with some more X-rays, and said, "Mr. Hoover, I have reviewed your X-rays and your lungs are looking better but there's still scarring."

I nodded, and said, "Thank you," and he left.

It was like the scene with Leslie Nielsen in *Airplane*, when he kept wishing the pilot good luck during the emergency landing. The young nurse didn't think it was strange but I did, didn't he just come in? We talked more, and she left. A couple of hours later she returned, and said, "My shift's over, I just wanted to say good bye." I bade her farewell giving her all the credit for my thinking that I had a skill at wonderful joke telling. It was a good morning.

***

THERE IS A MOVEMENT AFOOT

My last nurse on the third floor was Dennis. He always liked to punctuate what he said with some sort of weird punch or kick to the air. I found this amusing while he found it to be something he just did. They knew I was ready for rehab but they were trying to get insurance to clear my move. Dennis would tell me that in the hospital you were treated as sick while in rehab you were treated as well. I didn't know how well "well" was so I was not wanting to make any grand predictions on what my performance would be. I just didn't want them to be mean to me. It's fine to be demanding when one is bedridden but when the time comes for becoming a normal human being it can be an anxious time, perhaps what normal was before this will not be what normal was after this.

As the time drew nearer I didn't know what I was expecting, some sort of a Parris Island to get this lazy ass patient out of me or what. The time was coming for me to put up or shut up. During my time in the hospital I had grown accustomed to my private rooms. However to have a private room in the hospital was a rare commodity especially for a stay that was by now at five weeks. Representatives from rehab as far back as my stay in MICU would describe it to Becky as dormitory-style living with four beds to a room. I did not like the sound of that even though I had done it at the Academy when they threw four of us strangers into a room smaller than my room at home. While that room had been shut for a month with the windows closed without climate control during the summer this would hopefully be different. If I had no freedom then, then I definitely had no freedom now, so private was my hope. Perhaps it was the King or Queen of England in me. That was what I hoped awaited me.

Dennis put a lot of work into getting me cleared for rehab. He would go to find something out, and it felt like he would be gone for hours but he would always have an update. Finally he returned, and said, "You have been cleared to go, I think your departure may be some time this evening." He punctuated this statement with a karate chop to some invisible foe. It was happening; the Parris Island of the hospital awaited me. God I hoped I did well.

Later that morning a man in a wheelchair came into the room, and introduced himself, "I'm Dr. Scott, the doctor in charge of the rehab unit where you'll be staying. I just wanted to come and introduce myself, and see what your particular needs will be during your stay."

He didn't yell at all. Maybe this wouldn't be too bad but then again I had been wary of this in the past. Even with his pleasant demeanor, I was apprehensive about going someplace new, even though it meant my departure from here.

He checked me over, and his gaze went to my infamous Instaflate. He noted the length of it, and said, "We'll be able to get you a bed extender so you won't be cramped up like this anymore."

My jaw dropped, in my head, I didn't want to exude too much happiness. Regardless, Alleluia.

Next, he examined my feet which were still dark purplish in the extremities, especially the toes, and said, "You have some dead tissue here. When you come in we'll get a solution going to soak these in to remove all of the dead tissue."

I was hoping that the removal would not include the toes themselves, floating in some briny solution. As for the toes, no one could really give a definitive answer on whether they would stay or not. They seemed to be functioning properly when I walked, however they felt numb and sensitive at the same time. Plus they looked like hell.

Dr. Scott then departed by saying, "We look forward to having you in rehab; I'll see you soon."

I still was suspicious. Would he be nice up here and mean down there? I was not willing to give in to new people especially during the transition times. I was not sure about the length of my rehab stay, no one was really sure. The initial estimate was one month inpatient and three to four months outpatient. It sounded like a long road, and that I would be calling the place home for quite a while but as long as I was working to get better, and not in the hospital everything was headed in the right direction.

Dennis finally came in that evening, and announced, "It was great having you as a patient; transport is now here to take you to rehab. They're going to work you there," as he did a roundhouse kick to the air.

Big Daddy then chimed in, "He went through Indoc twice, he'll be able to make it." In reference to my going through the indoctrination period at the Academy not once but twice, thankfully not thrice like in the nightmares I still have, due to a whole lack of readiness on my part. I felt like Big Daddy was writing checks that my buttocks might not be able to cash. I had no choice but to make it, I had to, this was more important even than Indoc. Also this was the first time Becky hadn't been around for a room move. Luckily my parents had arrived with my aunt and uncle after a leisurely dinner at I am sure a four-star restaurant in the hospital. They were going to be worked right now getting my load of crap onto carts, and getting me the hell out of here. I was still too weak to sit in a wheelchair for a prolonged period so I was laid on a gurney. I said a long last farewell to my Instaflate. Old

Blue and I had been through hell. During that time we had hated and loved each other. We were there together nonetheless through thick and thin.

Farewell you old bastard, I shan't forget you, I thought as I peered over my shoulder at it, and the still present phlegm stain that I had really meant to tell someone about, *take care of the next one like you did me.*

The caravan headed out of the room, to the elevators, and down through passageway after passageway, until it came to this very long windowless tunnel. It seemed that the rehab unit was in a wholly separate building from the hospital so this tunnel connected the two. The tunnel seemed to go on for a mile as we slowly and silently made our way past the demarcation line. I could feel that now was the time I would prove myself. It was in my hands now.

Part V: Closer to My Home[151]

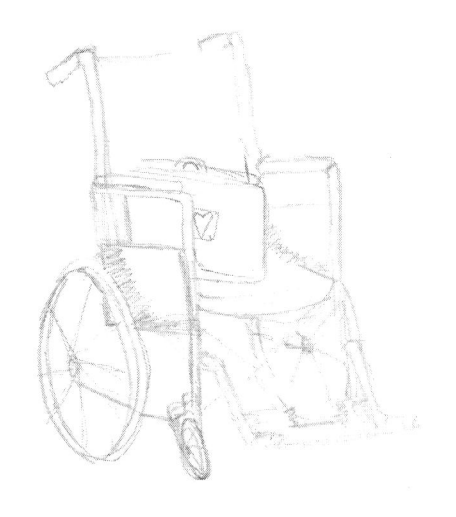

CHAPTER 35

Final Steps

Vasopressors are second line agents in the treatment of severe sepsis and septic shock, intravenous fluids are preferred as long as they increase perfusion without seriously impairing gas exchange.[152]

FEBRUARY 18 - 25, 2009

REHAB, BABY, REHAB[153]

The tunnel ended, and we were led to a bank of elevators as I was taken to my new home. I had already set in my mind that I would be sharing a room now but the reality of the situation didn't hit me until we got to the nurse's station to find out what room I would be in.

The nurse said, "He's in Room 234A." As in, if there is an A there must be a B.

My mom gave an exasperated look mostly for me, and for her since she wasn't ready to visit a multi-person room. I was rolled into the new room, and there it was, two beds. The one bed was not occupied. I figured it would be a matter of time before I was bunking with someone else. Which bed to choose? I knew as soon as I made a choice I would regret it. Luckily the choice was made for me as I was moved to the bed closest to the door which looked a bit like my old Instaflate. True to Dr. Scott's word a bed extension was brought in, and it was the most luxurious I had felt in a long time. No more scrunched up legs. I couldn't believe it, no more hanging off the bed. No more Ned from *One Fish, Two Fish, Red Fish, Blue Fish*. I was giddy with excitement.

Another new-found freedom I was privy to was the hospital gown was no longer the uniform of the day, civilian active wear was, including tennis shoes. Of course I didn't feel too active so it was more of a name than anything. Becky arranged for my parents to bring those items. I didn't really want to see my tennis shoes; before the hospital they were used mostly for everyday use and not so much exercise. I remembered them looking not unlike the shoes that Phil Collins and Phillip Bailey wore in the *Easy Lover* video. I figured they were not very becoming, probably white and scuffed. Nothing too inspiring. When my parents took them out of the bag, I couldn't believe how cool these shoes were. I had completely forgotten that they were black and grey with black laces. I could see myself doing some serious kick-ass rehab in these things, the black laces guaranteed that. I was excited as hell. Also there were my sweatpants, some sweatshirts were in the mix, some I recognized and some were new. I did not see the Chippewas sweatshirt that I spent my last moments in the house wearing, but as I and Homer Simpson's Nuclear 101 professor liked to say, "out with the old, in with the nucleus."

My parents put these away in the wardrobe next to the other bed. I was wondering how I would get back to get them with a new roommate but I was excited nonetheless. I had always figured that the unknown made me more nervous. Now that I was seeing the room and the atmosphere I realized this place wasn't too bad, so far. Maybe they

PART V: CLOSER TO MY HOME[151] - FINAL STEPS

wouldn't be making my life too hard. We would wait until tomorrow to discover if that was true. After my parents, aunt, and uncle had unpacked they said farewell, and I was left on my own in a new place.

The one distinction was that I was now a student and no longer a patient.

***

AS I START OUT THE CLIMB[154]

That morning I was awakened at 5:00 a.m. by the sound of a cart being wheeled into the room, the hall light had the impact of the midday sun. To add insult to injury the fluorescent light over my bed was then turned on. It was my phlebotomist and fortunately not Lady IV to take my blood, and Lord knows what else, oh yes the shot in the stomach, of course. I did not enjoy this. I never did, but it was a no nonsense stop, and he was gone immediately afterward. I hoped to God that there was improvement, and that my blood would be the bringer of good news.

Around 7:00 a.m. breakfast was served, and I found that I was anxious about what was to come, and once again had trouble eating. Later a nurse dropped off my schedule for the day. It had the day blocked off with a few forty-five-minute classes including physical therapy, occupational therapy, something called power builders, and recreational therapy.

Since the original prognosis was one month in rehab with three to four months of outpatient rehab, I was raring to get started. Later that morning someone came into the room while I was still trying to get my bearings. She introduced herself, "Hello my name's Karen; I'm your occupational therapist, and we'll be working together to get you up and running again."

"Hello, nice to meet you," I said relieved that a smiling face was greeting me.

She was blond, young, and she reminded me of one of Becky's sorority sisters.

She said, "So first things first, you'll be getting your shower."

"A shower? Is it really that time?" I couldn't believe that it was happening.

"Yes, a shower, I'm sure you've been looking forward to that," she replied, fully appreciating the shock in my voice.

"I have but I don't know how I'll make that happen," I said uncertainly.

She said, "Easy, we'll get you in the bathroom, I'll get your clothes, and you can get that hospital gown off once we get you in there. Can you walk into the bathroom on your own?"

At this point I was sitting on the bed leaning on the tray table. "I don't know."

"No problem, if you could get into a wheel chair, I'll get you into the bathroom."

I said, "Certainly." I was getting stronger so I was able to sit up in the wheelchair as she pushed me into the bathroom.

"OK, let's get you up and into the shower, there's a seat in there if you need to sit on it."

I did, and I took full advantage of its paddedness not thinking of the many asses that had passed over it before my own. I handed her my gown through the curtain, and she turned on the water. It felt so foreign to me, and it woke me up. I started talking like Steve Martin's description of a Chatty Kathy Doll in *Planes, Trains, and Automobiles*,

PART V: CLOSER TO MY HOME[151] - FINAL STEPS

and like his assertive comparison of the doll to Del Griffith, played gracefully by John Candy, I was the one pulling the string. I told her about my home, my family, where I went to school, you name it I was blabbing. The water was acting like Wonder Woman's lasso of truth.

Finally Karen said, "Look, you don't need to tell me your life story."

This completely rolled off my back as I thought, *I'm sorry. You gave me the gift of shower so you have to abide by all the privileges offered therein.*

I was hesitant to do much in there, I was afraid if I bent a certain way I wouldn't come out of whatever position I was in. After she turned the water off I was shivering and exhausted. I was ready to get back in the bed. "Is that unusual?" I asked.

"Not at all, it's just the change in temperature in your body that's tiring you out."

She helped me get out of the shower while I held a towel around myself. I got back into the wheelchair, and sat there like a lump. "OK," she said, "once you get dressed, someone will be here to transport you to your first class."

Once you get dressed? What the hell? I guess I really wasn't a patient anymore.

I slowly got myself dressed in a seated position, while Karen stepped out and closed the door. It was an adventure putting on underwear for the first time in a long while. I could barely raise my arms to put on my shirt, and the pants were an exercise in tight rope walking. I looked in the mirror at myself for the first time since I discovered my face was intact. I was emaciated, I wasn't myself, I was bearded, my hair was long, and my face looked years older. I still couldn't believe what I had gone through. I just knew I had to be patient until I got discharged.

Once I was able to dress myself in normal clothing for the first time in weeks, I was ready to face the day. Karen came in to make sure my first attempt at dressing myself was a success. I did require assistance pulling a shirt over my head; my shoulders felt like they would snap in two from the effort.

***

I'M FIT WITH THE STUFF TO RIDE IN THE ROUGH [155]

Transport brought me to the gym for my first look at the world of rehab. My wheelchair was parked in a gathering of patients. There were about ten of us waiting in a pack near the door. As I looked around the room I thought I was a spy or some interloper that would soon be discovered. I was still surprised, and still thought that there was no way I should be in here but here I was. Time to take it one step at a time. I had to calm myself down, this wasn't the evil dojo from *The Karate Kid*, and that beach-boy bully wasn't here smirking at me.

In the group were people of mostly advanced age; however it was the younger ones that especially struck a chord with me. There was one young girl who looked like she was in her twenties and had been in an accident. She was paralyzed from her neck down, in a wheelchair. She had the halo to immobilize her neck, a device I first read about in that SI article about Darrel Stingley in 1983. However with the deck stacked against her she still maintained a positive attitude with the staff when they would address her. She just never seemed down, it was obvious that she was thankful to have survived whatever she had been through and always had a smile on her face.

PART V: CLOSER TO MY HOME[151] - FINAL STEPS

Another guy a few years younger than me had no wheelchair and was walking freely, but it was obvious from his partially shaved head that he had had some sort of brain surgery. He was being walked around the room as his therapist had him recite the months.

I saw a lot of hard work going on here. People that were working to get back some semblance of their life, to be independent, but it was obvious for a few that this was as good as they were going to get. I couldn't believe my utter fortune with not having lost fingers, hands, toes, feet, and limbs. Actually the jury was still out on the toes. I just felt so blessed to have come this far, there was no way I was going to give up on this.

One by one a therapist came by to get one of the patients in the group until I was one of the last ones left. It felt like some bizarre junior high dance. Finally a tall woman came over and introduced herself.

"Mr. Hoover, I'm So and So your physical therapist for today," she said. She then looked down at my chart, and said, "Good grief I was looking for someone who was forty-one. You don't look forty-one."

You flatterer you. You do mean that I look younger than forty-one don't you? I thought. I just took the compliment assuming it was a compliment.

She brought over a walker for me. I was able to raise myself off the wheelchair and take it ever so gingerly in my hands. It was a tough walk but I eventually got to a flat therapy table that was padded. She raised it up a little.

"Now we're going to do a little benchmarking, and see how well you do. I want you to sit down on this bench, and raise yourself up into a standing position as many times as you can in two minutes. Again, you cannot push off from the table with your hands."

Ringo was back in me head and responded, *how's about with me feet?* She might as well have asked me to bend the table with my mind.

I saw all the other patients out there in the gym working, and I focused on the task at hand. I sat down, and tried to stand up. My ass was caught in some sort of anti-gravity shield; it wasn't going up but it wasn't going down. My thighs were screaming to lift me up, waiting for something to push me over the edge. I finally was successful, time to call in the parade organizers. *I wonder what float they'll put me on*, I thought.

"One," she said. I then lowered myself back down to the so comfortable seated position. Again I tried, and got another one. Not surprisingly, it was getting very difficult. I was able to do two more for a grand total of four and that was it. Four stand and sits in two minutes. There was room for improvement.

***

IT FEELS LIKE YEARS SINCE IT'S BEEN CLEAR[156]

After my physical therapy session Karen took me for a little while in the wheelchair where we worked on some fine-motor-skill activities. Afterward she wheeled me out of the gym. She said, "We have a little time left, and I have some paperwork to do, and it's really beautiful outside. Would you like to go outside?"

I was speechless, I hadn't been outside in over a month, just unbelievable; and I said, "Am I allowed?"

"Certainly," she laughed. "As a matter of fact when you start getting a little more independent you can start going out on your own."

I was in a state of shock over this. I couldn't believe it. I felt like I was getting away with something. She wheeled me outside, and indeed

PART V: CLOSER TO MY HOME[151] - FINAL STEPS

it was a gorgeous day. We went to a landscaped area with benches behind the building, and I could see to my right the hospital towers that I had called home. I was happy to be away from there, there were people in there now, fighting for their lives. She wheeled me around, and I sat in the wheelchair with my face in the sun in disbelief that I was almost out the front door. I said, "This is unbelievable."

I got chatty again, and she was really unable to do any of the paperwork she had planned. She told me where she was from, somewhere near Detroit. I told her about my family, and I told her even though I am right handed I brush my teeth better with my left hand. She paused with her work, looked up, and said, "I have to hear the reason for this."

I said, "It all started in the fall of 1997; they were heady times. *Austin Powers* fever had swept the nation, radio stations were making us listen to Ben Folds Five, and U2's *Pop* had tanked. One night I was looking through our wedding photos when I noticed my gum line on my left side was higher than my right side. I of course attributed this to overzealous brushing so from that day on I decided to brush with my left hand."

She looked at me, and laughed, "That's a very strange story but a reasonable answer."

After more attempts at trying to be quiet, and watching her write in folders she said, "All right, I'm finished here so unfortunately that means that it's time to go in."

I felt like a five-year-old whose recess was over, "Do I have to?"

"Yes, but we can come back again some other time."

I was just happy with the chance to go outside; I felt like I was human again.

***

I KNEW SOMETHING WASN'T RIGHT, I COULDN'T FIND IT[157]

"Power Builders" was one class that I thought I would enjoy. It certainly showed how weak I had really become. Susan was my therapist in this class. We were in a group, and we would rotate stations. The first station she took me to was the curling station which was a Universal contraption with the pulley and weight. She had me maneuver the wheelchair over to the station, and grab the metal handle.

"OK, I'm going to put this on the lightest weight for you, and see how you do."

I grabbed the handle, and made the movement of a curl. Nothing happened. Really, nothing happened, and it was on the lowest setting. My pencil arms were not up to the task.

"How are you doing?" she said as she came over to check on me.

"I can't move it," I said with a look of surprise.

"Really? That's only five pounds."

I really didn't need to hear that.

Then she said, "Let me give you this,"

She handed me a dumbbell that was the type old people walk with. I guess I shouldn't have been surprised, I was barely able to lift small vials of saline a couple of weeks ago but I was still disappointed.

"How much is this?" Not really wanting to hear the answer. The anticipated answer was, "It's so light that earth's gravity has no effect on it." Fortunately, "Two pounds," was the reply. It was doable but still not easy. When I was in high school we played an away game against a team that listed the bench press and squat weights of each player in the program. This weight would not have been listed.

PART V: CLOSER TO MY HOME[151] - FINAL STEPS

She said, "You can keep those, and work on them in your down time."

I knew I needed the extra work so I squirreled them away in the back of my wheelchair, and worked on them when I had the chance back in my room. Eventually I moved up in weight, and by the following week I had my revenge on that five pound setting, that magnificent bastard.

***

HEY, HEY, HEY. WHAT'S IN YOUR HEAD, IN YOUR HEAD?[158]

On my schedule was a class called "Psychiatric Eval" or something to that effect. I kept re-reading it to make sure it didn't say "Psychotic Eval." I was to report to a particular room number for this session at 11:00 a.m. When the time came I was wheeled to the hallway where the office was. The door was closed, so transport left me to cool my heels until someone showed up.

A nurse came up, and said, "Would you like something to read? She might be a while."

"Yes," how thoughtful. I chose an issue of *Rolling Stone* since I hadn't seen one in ages, and began thumbing through it. It was not lost on me that I was able to hold a magazine in comfort without being fidgety and unable to focus on the articles or cleavage. I saw in this issue there was an article where the "experts" actually ranked the top one hundred singers in rock. I found this utterly ridiculous but of course I had to look. I began to thumb through it to see where the Beatles placed. Paul was in the high twenties, and John was in the top 5. I shouldn't have been surprised, Rolling Stone has always been pro-John. They should be he appeared on the cover of the first issue. George and Ringo were nowhere to be found, and Bono was in the teens. I forgot who was top, perhaps Moon Unit Zappa.

My focus on the article was interrupted momentarily by a noise from behind me that sounded like a person struggling to get an automated wheelchair steered properly. Seeing that this was a rehab center it really couldn't have been anything else. I could hear the person breathing heavily, and a male voice walking alongside talking in an encouraging tone. I didn't want to turn around and stare to call attention to the patient's plight and kept reading. The voice and the breathing were slowly getting closer. My curiosity was getting the better of me but I didn't turn around. Finally when the sounds were right on top of me my chair was heavily bumped from behind.

The voice said, "OK, that's OK you just need to straighten it back up." Then addressing me he said, "Please excuse us."

At first I was going to say something smart ass like, "For a moment I thought I was invisible," but thought better of it. This was a patient that had a long road ahead of him, I didn't want to joke so I said, "That's OK," and returned to my article.

Finally the door opened, and a lady wearing glasses said, "Mr. Hoover?"

"Yes."

"You can come in now. Can you make it on your own?"

"I think so."

I hadn't done it before yet I managed to steer myself through the office door. I was nervous about what they expected from me.

PART V: CLOSER TO MY HOME[151] - FINAL STEPS

She said, "Roll up to this desk please. I'm going to ask you a few questions, and we're going to do some activities to see what your mental state is."

"That'll be fine."

She then said, "OK, I would like for you to write out a check for this amount, and sign your name."

I took a pen, and held it correctly but I was shaking, and I was only able to scribble some chicken scratch that was legible. Not neat by any means. I hoped she wasn't going to make me balance the checkbook next. I could barely get enough force on the pen to make a good mark.

"OK, great." I guess I passed that test, and then she said, "I want you to tell me what numbers you see."

This was more difficult as I had to discern the colored numbers from a similarly colored background. I had done this before but this seemed a little more challenging. Next was shape matching or something like that. After a few more activities each more fiendish than the last, she said, "OK, I'm going to read a passage to you, and I want you to tell it back to me as best you can."

I was worried about this. I have never received the Nobel Prize in listening before I got sick, especially when I am being read to. That is a weakness, so I was determined to pass this one. She said, "Are you ready?" I nodded.

She read a passage about a man named Steven that brings a present to his wife named Mary. The present was a ring, and somehow it had gotten broken and lost, and there was anger, and then a solution was thought of that they both could live with. As she read the story I played it in my head like a movie, and when she was finished, it was my turn to tell her what she read so I played the movie back in my head, and told her basically what I was seeing.

I don't know where this talent came from, was it something that was with me the entire time, and I just uncovered it? I suppose I felt everything was on the line, and I knew I really had to nail this portion of the *Howard Becomes Free Show*.

When I was finished she looked dumbfounded, and said, "I have never had anyone tell me that back in such detail. Excellent job." Another hurdle jumped.

***

BLESS YOU, WHOEVER YOU ARE

That afternoon after lunch my parents had arrived, and I was relaxing in my room, actually in the bed since I was not too comfortable sitting yet. We were talking about rehab, and how different it was from the hospital. First and foremost I felt I had more freedom, and it was the opposite of what I thought it would be. There was no one laughing at me or trying to shame me. I felt I could handle the external stuff, it was just the mental and physical challenge of doing it. I was deep in this thought when all of a sudden who should walk in the door but Becky!

"Hey!" I said excitedly in a high-pitched squeal. She was a sight for sore eyes. She was back with me for the final push out of here. I was very excited about the future. She seemed a little agitated when she came in as everyone was who tried to find the building, but she immediately cheered up when she saw me.

"Hello! I shouldn't get too close to you in case I'm still sick. I do have a surprise for you," she said as she took out a bag. She produced three T-shirts for me, all to inspire my recovery: a Superman T-shirt, a Mr. Incredible T-shirt, and a Guinness T-shirt. "I have also gotten *The*

Incredibles T-shirts for me and the Babies," she said. I was so happy to see her, and to have a re-invented T-shirt collection.

As we were catching up on the last three days there came another knock on the door. I said, "Yes, come in." Nothing could ruin my mood.

An older lady popped her head in, and introduced herself as a volunteer member from Local Episcopal Church. She immediately asked, "So what are you in here for?" with a light hearted tone.

I said "Sepsis," finally remembering the term.

She then said dismissively, "Oh, been there, done that," as she waved her hand in a dismissive tone, and tore on into the room like she owned the place.

I immediately wondered what the fuck she was talking about. *This isn't a fucking headache lady.*

I then could see out of the corner of my eye Becky cross her arms. She turned to Becky, and said, "And you are," as if she demanded an explanation of her presence.

Becky just replied, "Becky."

My parents introduced themselves. She wanted more details about my sickness as if I was willing to tell. She said she had sepsis, and was in the hospital for three days once. I grew tired of this woman as soon as she had walked in. She dismissed what I had been through, and talked about herself only. I didn't hear anything about church or God or anything at all in what she said. I wanted her to leave; actually we all wanted her to leave. She was rude. After not really wanting to tell her anymore, she took her leave. We were none too happy to see her gone. I guessed my mood did take a hit.

CHAPTER 36

Closer

AND I CAN DO ANYTHING[159]

Dr. Scott would make his rounds through the gym in the morning. He had another doctor with him, and the two of them would meet with each student to see how they were doing. He had a very disarming quality, always had a kind word to say, and was very encouraging. I always felt as he came over to me that this was temporary, and I would soon be out of it. Again, this was the place that made me feel fortunate every day. He would see me, come over, and say, "How's it going today?"

"Great, very good."

"Are they treating you right?"

"Yes, absolutely I'm so happy to be here, and to have come this far."

"Good."

The other doctor would check my vitals and then my trach wound. "Progressing nicely," she would say. "How are you feeling otherwise, any lightheadedness?'

"No, not yet but I haven't done much yet either."

"You have done plenty with what you've been through."

Then they would say good bye, and be on their way to the next student. Every morning he would come over, and as I started to wear the super hero T-shirts that Becky bought for me he would say, "That's the right attitude."

I would say, "The attitude's super but the arms are weak." Or some other witticism. I always made him laugh, or maybe he was just being polite.

The next day I had on the Mr. Incredible T-shirt, and he complimented me on that, and I had something else witty to say and told him how the family was decked out in them. Then the next day I had on a plain white T-shirt, and I was going to say something about being the Fonz but he wasn't there that day. Oh well, I hadn't really developed anything good to say. I was hoping the T-shirt would carry the day, and I had nowhere to go after saying, "Ayyyyyyyy!!!!!", and adding "amundo" after every word.

Rehab was not what I had expected. There was no "Drop and give me fifty!" here, only encouragement. The only fifty they would have gotten had I dropped would have been moans.

***

PICK UP THE PIECES, WHOO[160]

Not only did Dr. Scott order me a bed extender, but true to his word he had my feet soaked as well. The nurse came in the first night, and wrapped my feet in some sort of lotion-covered towels then inserted my feet in a bag of water with air forced through it. It made noise yet it was rather soothing. I only wondered what would happen when I would have to go to the bathroom, and how long it would take to get out of this thing. The catheter did have its benefits. Luckily my first night in the bag went uneventfully, and I was able to sleep with a bubbling bag on my two feet. I don't know how, but I did it.

When the bag was removed that first morning I was shocked to see how soft and malleable my feet had become. The dead tissue was starting to fall off like pulled pork from the bone making way for the living tissue to come in. I never knew how close I was to losing my toes, and even my feet until a nurse came in to look at them. I asked her why this happened to my feet, and she replied, "Because in these situations the body dies from the outside in."

"Oh," I said.

Letting that sink in the nurse then said in an excited tone, "Dr. Pick will love to see this; she'll definitely want to come in to see you. She loves to pick at dead tissue and remove it."

I wasn't sure I was excited to see Dr. Pick. If she wanted to do that, and if that was her bag, then so be it.

That afternoon Dr. Pick came in to look at my feet. They were still a gangly purple. Putting on shoes and socks seemed to be an exercise in frustration especially since I didn't know if I would continue to have feet for much longer. Dr. Pick was a tall woman with curly hair and glasses. She appeared to be in her late forties, and had the white coat giving her instant credibility. She came in and said, "My name is Dr. Pick, and I'm here to look at your feet."

I said, "The nurse said you would want to see them."

"I know. I couldn't pass it up. It's just something I'm good at." She uncovered them and began to examine them from all sides. She began to pick at them with an instrument I guess she used for picking called a "Picker." Some of the picking was getting a little painful but she was very focused. I realized if there was pain, there was hope. After about fifteen minutes when I thought I could take no more picking she received an urgent call and had to leave. Dr. Pick was never to return but the bubbling bag would.

For three nights I had the bubbling bag on and sometimes my mind would control my bladder in the middle of the night. I would say over the intercom, "Howard needs to use the restroom, his bladder's full…full of urine!"

The nurse came in, looked shocked, and a little aggravated that she had to disassemble the bubbling bag. I grabbed hold of her as she led me into the bathroom, her evening having gotten a little more interesting.

Afterward, I was off the bubbling bag for a couple of nights, and then one night I was suddenly back on it. When I complained about this, that perhaps the bubbling bag was not for me anymore the nurse said, "It's written down in the chart so I need to give it to you."

Even something as small as getting back on the bubbling bag would make me feel as if I hadn't advanced at all; at least they weren't sticking the bubbling bag up my ass.

***

THE GIFT YOU GAVE IS GONNA LAST FOREVER[161]

One afternoon early during my stay I was lying in the bed watching TV before another one of my classes when a knock came on the door. Two female faces poked their heads in smiling. "Hello," they said. "We're Sally and Doris from the MICU, we wanted to see how you were getting along."

"Hey, nice to see you," I said sitting up a little more not recognizing them at all but having the urge to have a screwdriver on hand to look busy.

I tried to sit on the side of the bed, and they said, "You don't need to do that. You probably don't remember us, we were there early on when you weren't conscious yet, we're so happy to see you doing so well."

"Thank you so much," I felt a little ashamed though. Here they come all this way to see just me, and I am lying in the sack. My fear was that they were expecting a little more activity from me. I should have been sitting in a wheelchair or something. I should have been showing them more than just this, lying in the bed. I swore I had done stuff, let me juggle for you!

We talked a little more about how my stay was, and how I was feeling. I felt very lucky to have had them watching over me. They seemed like they were very bright and energetic. I wanted to do a trick or something for them without letting on that I was showing off. They said, "It was great seeing you, and please say hello to Becky for us; she was by your side every night. You have a wonderful wife."

I replied, "Thank you so much for stopping by, and I do, I really do."

***

EVERYBODY'S WORKING FOR THE WEEKEND[162]

I was disappointed when I was told on Friday that on weekends the rehab center closes down. I was making such progress I really didn't want it to cool down for two days. There was however a couple of classes that I could take on Saturday morning. When this was offered to me I said, "By all means. Whatever you have available."

I arrived at 10:00 a.m. for the class, still needing someone to walk me over to the gym. The class met in a room right off the gym, and when I entered I realized I was the youngest by thirty years. I certainly didn't feel like I belonged here, yet I felt I had the most to gain to get out. I tried to make small talk with some of the elders in there with me but it didn't go too far. I did see those famous socks from the hospital on a couple of the patients that I refused to wear once I got into rehab. Even though my socks from home were a little rough on my purplish feet I didn't want to take a step back with wearing those cursed hospital socks.

The instructor was a young lady with brown hair pulled back into a pony tail. We went over some breathing exercises, and some basic arm movement exercises which when demonstrated I thought would be very easy, however I underestimated the strength of my shoulders, and I soon found myself challenged. My therapist had said that I should feel free to hold dumbbells when I signed up for the class, thinking I was more advanced than I was. She also warned me that there would be people of different ages and abilities in the class so I should just look at it as getting more work in and not as a put down. Putdown? Hell, I would work out in a class with Hitler, Mussolini, Miss Devil, and Rick Astley if it got me home sooner.

After class we were pulled out into the hallway to await our transport except my transport decided I should try to start moving the wheelchair myself, like a sucker. I did this very gingerly at first, and it took a little while. She took over for stretches but I was getting the hang of it more and more. Another step.

***

I'M HEALTHY, I DO DECLARE[163]

There was a definite sense of more freedom in rehab. I guess the freedom was actually being able to get out of the bed when I requested to go to the bathroom. I would call on the intercom, and the nurse would come in, and I would lean on her as we walked into the can. There was no way I could make it on my own yet but she would leave me once I got on the toilet, and leave the door open a smidge.

It had never been a habit of mine to talk to anyone through the bathroom door. Even at home if the kids were to yell through the door that the dog was on fire, walking through the curtains I would keep my mouth shut. Not to say I wouldn't be alarmed, but not conducting a social faux pas seemed to be more important. One had to have focus. I certainly was talking away here those first couple of nights. Plus just sitting at a sink to brush my teeth had its moments too. All of the pieces of a normal life were being given back slowly to me. There was a process though while sitting on the toilet. The flexi-seal had left me a wasteland down there in the nether region so when I went, regular toilet paper was out of the question; special care had to be taken. Then getting off the toilet was an adventure as I pushed up from the sink, and held on to the bars. I was not a leg-only guy yet.

As time went on I felt more and more confident getting up from the bed. The nurses always told me that I had to wait for them to do anything in the middle of the night even to go to the bathroom. Just call them, they would repeat. My freedom, however, got a bit more of a lift from the necessity in fixing an annoying, recurring problem. My new Instaflate seemed to have an attitude, well not the Instaflate itself but the extender. Frequently I would wake up to find the hose had become detached from the main bed and the noise it made was not comforting. The first couple of times I called the nurse on the intercom and the problem was fixed. The next time it was taking the nurse a little longer to come in so I decided to try rectifying the situation on my own. I sat up and reached down to re-attach the hose, hoping I could find the correct hole to insert it while not tumbling out of the bed. After a few nights of this the confidence in my physical abilities began to increase.

One night I woke up with my bladder just aching, and I called on the intercom. There was no time for the "full of urine" gag, which, by the way, never got old. I repeat. Never got old.

"Yes," came the reply from the intercom.

"I need to go to the bathroom," Like a first grader in class.

"Someone will be right in."

I waited forever and a day, and no one seemed to be coming so I decided to go it alone. I got up into a sitting position, somehow found my slippers, and reached with my feet to get them on. Slowly I stood. I was very wobbly at this point. I was thinking I should re-think this yet something kept pushing me to go on, my full bladder mainly. I felt like I did after an hour and a half of heavy sleep at home, and one of the Babies would wake up. In other words I felt like the aforementioned drunk eighty-five-year-old man but there was no brown liquid, Sinatra, or Flamingo and certainly no Lawford.

I was swaying as I saw the dark doorway loom larger and larger. I made a Frankensteinesque stroll toward it, grabbed hold of the door frame and turned on the light switch. I could see that other person in the mirror that was pretending to be me. I sat ever so gingerly down while holding the sink and let go. I was sitting, and I was loving it, and

I was going to the bathroom without anyone looking on. The act that amazed me as a three-year-old was amazing to me again.

My blissfulness and pats on the back were interrupted when the door opened, and the nurse came in, "What are you doing up?" she said incredulously like a first-grade teacher.

"I couldn't wait," I said innocently.

"Someone has got to be in here in case something happens, if you fall we wouldn't know," she said firmly.

"I know, I'll call next time," I said guiltily but underneath I was happy as hell. I looked into the abyss, and I saw yellow.

***

SEE THE CHILDREN RUN AS THE SUN GOES DOWN[164]

The Babies came to visit me over the weekend. I hadn't seen them since the seventh floor, long before Becky went out of town. I was in show-off mode as I displayed my new found ability to get in the wheelchair. However, that was where my ability ended as Becky had to push me through the hallway while they took turns helping her. In normal times the fighting over who got to push my prone figure would have been annoying but it was sweet music to me.

We went outside to the landscaped garden behind the Rehab building where Karen had taken me earlier. It was great to see them outside the hospital room. I watched them running and playing, running up the stairs, and rolling down a grassed embankment into the courtyard. It was a beautiful day. Actually, it would have been a beautiful day had it been raining and nasty.

They kept asking me, "Come on Daddy, come up here with us on the top of the hill."

I saw those stairs, and I knew there was no going up that hill. I replied, "Not right now, in a little while maybe I will."

I knew a little while would not be on this day, but I did manage to get out of the wheelchair. Without any straps or any braces I grabbed the back of the wheelchair, and did a lap around the garden path very shakily and with a strong resemblance to Mr. Potter's henchman. It was great to be outside, and to be with them again. I couldn't believe my fortune that I had made it this far.

***

SUNDAY WILL NEVER BE THE SAME[165]

Sunday was a day where absolutely nothing was happening, so with this free time I did manage to finally start reading again. When Bob visited I requested from him a list of books about football that he could recommend. He sent this list post haste to my parents who then printed the list out for me. I selected *The Blind Side* before Sandra Bullock ever won the Academy Award. I snobbily still have not seen the film, and *A Civil War*, a book about the Army/Navy football rivalry.

It popped in my head when I received these books what I was reading prior to my illness, *A Tale of Two Cities* by Charles Dickens. Talk about having your ascot on too tight, and with a depressing read no less. A story about an old man that's suffering from dementia? The familiar beginning, "It was the best of times, it was the worst of times," as well as the dementia was absolutely creepily applicable to what I had been through over the past few weeks. However, I didn't think I would add on to the "worst" side of that ledger by continuing with Mr. Dickens's take on the French Revolution.

In my quest to prove that I could get my mind back as well as my body, I read both my new books simultaneously. Of course, not by holding both books and reading them at the same time but putting one down then picking the other up.

The Twilight series was big at this time. Becky told me she had read the entire series in the MICU. I remember seeing the faint glimmer of the book light going at night. I picked one up, and tried to read it. I only got to page eight. It was creepy and I didn't like the idea of a young impressionable girl being wooed by a vampire. Too unsettling, too unholy. On second thought, that's the way vampires have operated for centuries. Why was I so sensitive to it? I guess the thought of a vampire trying to date Kate or Phoebe would turn me into a holy water splashing madman. The books sat on the desk in the room as they followed me on my journey and every time a nurse came in she commented upon seeing them, "I love those books, how far are you into them?"

I would reply in a slightly braggart fashion, "Oh, I couldn't read those."

"So what are you reading now?"

"*The Blind Side* and *A Civil War*," tightening my ascot.

After explaining what those were I could tell they lost interest, and wanted to hurry up and leave because I was a talker.

The tables turned on me that afternoon as I was sitting in the wheelchair reading and blissfully alone. A knock came on the door.

"Yes?" I asked and looked up, and in walked this elderly lady with her hair up holding flowers.

"Hello, I'm So and So, a church volunteer from Local Episcopal Church here to visit and give you communion."

I thought, *but I was really enjoying the solitude.* Instead I said, "Yes, come in, thanks for coming."

As she stood there she looked me over, and asked, "So what happened to you?"

Dammitt! I had to go through this story again. I was just not in the mood to go over this again, don't they take notes? Maybe I don't want to say, maybe I should have just said that but I didn't want to hurt her feelings coming all this way, and bringing flowers, and whatever else that was she was holding so I told her the story. She put the flowers down and made herself at home taking a seat on my Instaflate. My hopes were dashed for a short visit. We talked about my sickness for a little while longer, and I knew that she wasn't leaving until I had communion but first she had a surprise for me. As with all of the church volunteers you get a mini service in your room before communion. Not only did I get that, I got a re-telling of the sermon from that day from a guest rector that I have heard before, and I must say I didn't particularly care for his sermons. Believe me, his sermons were usually a rambling mess built more to generate laughs than anything. As she proceeded to go through the sermon her interpretation of it was no better. Besides, time from my book was being eaten up. I wanted this to end. I felt badly about that, but I just didn't need these visits from strangers. I am OK alone, really.

After she had re-told the sermon it was time for communion, and once that was given she proceeded to the bathroom to pour something out. I hoped that wasn't the wine yet I didn't wish to argue. Arguing would just prolong everything.

She came out, packed her stuff up, and I thought, *Wonderful I can get back to what I was doing. What, has it been three hours already?*

She then proceeded to sit back down on Instaflate. I was devastated. I felt terrible for feeling that way, but on the other hand my evil self felt like conjuring Gunnery Sergeant Hartman from *Full Metal Jacket* to hear him scream "Get the fuck off his Instaflate!" Still, here she came taking time out of her Sunday to visit me but I wondered then if the visit was for me or for her.

She began to look through the DVDs that had suddenly found their way from home into my room. "What movies do you like?"

I said, "All kinds."

"Are you excited about the Academy Awards?"

"Do they still hold those?" I was being a wee bit of a smart-ass. It was an after effect of the paralytics, I swear.

She looked at me funny to see if I was joking, and saw that I was. "I have made it a point to see all of the nominees for this year. Have you seen any of them?"

"I don't know. What's been nominated? I still remember *A Trip to Bountiful*," I said with humor but really not wanting to extend the conversation yet how could I not with a witty gem like that? I thought of nominees from when I was in high school that no high-school kid would have been caught dead seeing, especially one starring grand dame Geraldine Page. I guessed my opinion was unchanged in early middle age because I still had not seen Ms. Page tear up the screen getting to wherever Bountiful may have been. Plus, admitting that I knew what *A Trip to Bountiful* was had been a harsh burden to bear all these years. I blame Siskel and Ebert.

"There's *Slumdog Millionaire, Milk, Benjamin Button, The Reader, Frost/Nixon*," she said rattling them off as if she had just seen them consecutively in some viewing session from hell.

I still have never known what benefit there is to be gained from watching one of those awards shows. So what if Tilda Swinton has had her career boosted for her work in *Michael Clayton*? That's great for Ms. Swinton but what have I gained from that other than having to deal with more Tilda Swinton in my life?

"No, none of those yet. Usually I get to the animated stuff first with three kids," I said.

"You have three children, may I see a picture?" She asked.

I was thankfully saved from my Tilda Swinton internal commentary. I was fully on board with her request. My pride and love for my children was something from which I did draw great benefit and they so grounded me during this mess.

"Certainly," I said. I showed her the page of pictures that Becky had left with me, still not fully believing that these lovely little people were mine.

"Oh, they're beautiful," she said as earnestly as I heard anyone say anything.

She was OK, and I wanted our time to end right there while we were on a high note. Although talking about my kids excited me for a while, I still found that I had to bite my lip, and endure more of the small talk trying to stay positive while maintaining focus. I was growing tired, and a long conversation with a stranger was not what I had in mind at the moment. She continued the small talk for what seemed like eons. I was polite and that was a difficult attitude to carry. If I was going to be chatty, I would need to go sit on the toilet and talk to her through the cracked door.

Finally she said, "I hope you feel better, and let us know if there's anything else we can do for you."

I said, "Thank you, it was nice visiting with you and have a nice day."

I thought that this was more motivation to get out of the hospital to make these visits stop. I am a horrible person.

Becky came in later that afternoon, and I complained to her about the church volunteer situation. "Please don't have them come back. I'm really fine right now. I made it, and I'm just trying to get back to normal, and the visits aren't making me feel normal. I'm just tired of having these people older than Methuselah coming here to make me feel better when they're actually depressing me. I don't want to feel like I have to open up to strangers. It makes me feel wrong."

"This is a delicate situation since Cooper runs the program and we think the world of him."

I knew he was there when things were bad and helped us through, and I would certainly welcome visits from him but these Johnny Come Latelys were kind of annoying me.

Becky said "I'll e-mail him about it."

"I feel bad for feeling this way, to reject help might be bad for recovery."

"It's your call. You're the one that went through all of this. It's your recovery and they should honor your wishes."

That made me feel better yet I still I felt like an ingrate. What if in the future I needed help, what then?

***

TELL ME LIES, TELL ME SWEET LITTLE LIES[166]

On Monday morning during occupational therapy with Karen, I was working on my fine-motor skills, trying to sort small items into different piles. My hands were still shaking and it was hard to control

PART V: CLOSER TO MY HOME[151] - CLOSER

them. I sat concentrating when Karen spoke up, "You know we had our meeting this morning, and it was recommended that you could go home on Thursday."

I sat there stunned, and paused from doing the sorting. I was speechless.

She continued, "What do you think about that?"

I had waited for this moment for so long that I didn't know how to react; I just felt that if I showed too much emotion they might make me stay. I thought, *it's a test, it might be within your grasp but this isn't going to happen. They're playing games.*

I was just still paranoid about the entire situation. I thought I would never see home again, and was strangely getting used to life here. So I said the first thing that popped into my mind, "I think you're lying."

As soon as I said it I kicked myself. Real damn smooth Howard. You get the news you have wanted to hear for weeks, and that's what you say. And to Karen no less. Nurse Half Ass or Effeminate Curtis, fine, but not Karen. It's just like what your first words were to Cherry Soda Girl, you blow it. Even as I realized this, I showed no change in my outward demeanor.

She seemed a little shocked, and said, "Oh no I'm quite serious. You have progressed far enough since last week that we think you'll be ready by then. We also think that being at home will do more good for you than anything you can do here."

It suddenly dawned on me that they were going to let me go no matter what, whether I said offensive things or not. The moment I had been waiting for. I was in no condition to resemble the guy that got up out of the wheelchair, and whistled his way out of the hospital, but that was fine, this would do. After I mulled it over I was just able to choke out a "Thank you."

***

YOU KNOW ITS GONNA MAKE IT THAT MUCH BETTER, WHEN WE CAN SAY GOODNIGHT AND STAY TOGETHER[167]

It was Monday, and I had gotten the good news that I would be home on Thursday. After a long day at school Becky brought the Babies again to see me. Once they got there I wanted to show them how I could walk, so I got out of the bed under my own power, stood up with nothing and no one assisting me, and slowly walked to the door and out into the hallway. Kate was on my left, and I was able to look down at her slowly lest I lose my balance. She looked up at me with her big grin while she held my hand. I felt terrific. We were all here. I was whole and I could finally walk with them. I was so proud of them. We got a lot of stares in the hallway, looks of admiration at my beautiful family. It was a wonderful feeling to beat something so terrible and slowly get what you missed back.

After we walked to what I referred to as "Times Square," we came back to my room. The demand for TV or a movie was great except the TV was not as advanced as they remembered at my previous stops. It looked like it had spent a former life in a Western Auto waiting room. To add insult to injury there was no DVD player but I did have my laptop and *The Simpsons* third season DVDs. I popped one of the discs in and they started watching. I guessed letting them watch it dashed any hopes I had of winning father of the year. We watched and watched. It was wonderful even though Tramp wasn't around this time to kill that rat.

PART V: CLOSER TO MY HOME[151] - CLOSER

After a few shows, it was now time for them to go. It had been dark for a while and they had school tomorrow. Kate and Phoebe both gave me a kiss, but Henry was still hanging around the side of my bed. Becky said, "Come on Henry we need to go now, Daddy needs to rest."

Henry was not coming. He finally said to me, "Come on Daddy, you're coming with us." Apparently he had had enough of this and was ready for me to come home. He began pulling on my arm repeating, "Come on Daddy, you're coming home, you're coming with us."

I was near tears as my almost three-year-old had finally given up on being patient with the situation, and was ready for it to be over. I said as bravely as I could, "I can't Henry, they haven't let me go yet, I'll be home soon though."

"No, Daddy you're coming now," he said as he kept tugging on me more forcefully.

The little guy was persuasive. I nearly said, "You're right Henry, enough's enough, let's get the hell out of here."

Luckily before I started to break down, Becky intervened, and said, "Daddy'll be home soon, it'll just be a little longer that's all, he'll be home in a couple of days."

Henry, not seeming convinced yelled, "I'm tired of this! I want him home with us!"

I continued to reassure him, "I'll be home soon, and I'll no longer be here, and you'll no longer have to come visit me. I'll be with you soon and I won't leave."

This seemed to make him feel better but he was still upset about the situation. He was tired of the visits and the well-meaning visitors in the house. He wanted things to be as they were, I could tell. They left the room, and I felt really bad but really loved.

***

BEEN DOWN ONE TIME/BEEN DOWN TWO TIMES/I'M NEVER GOING BACK AGAIN

I was getting more and more paranoid about re-catching something, be it a virus, infection, bacteria, Dog Person mauling, or retelling of the tuna fish story before I got out and had to be rolled back into the MICU. The main focus of my fears was the dressing on my trach wound. I was not going to let that go, and if a day passed without them changing the dressing I was on them. This of course was a mixed wish. On one hand I knew I needed a new dressing to prevent further infection but on the other hand the idea that they were opening the dressing to expose the hole in my throat freaked me out.

Henry was always the first to comment on this dilemma, "Daddy, why do you have a band aid on your neck?"

I would tell him, "Because they had to cut a hole in there for me to breathe."

"You mean you have a hole in your neck?"

"Yes, Henry I have a hole in my neck."

"Daddy has a hole in his neck; you need to cover that up so it feels better," he would say as he grabbed a blanket, and put the edge over my throat.

During those times when the dressing was changed I could feel the air rushing around the hole when it was opened. I did not want to know what it looked like. I would ask hopefully "Getting better?"

"Yes," the nurse that looked like a female version of The Cars front man Ric Ocasek would say after a slight pause, "Getting there."

I was wondering if she felt too grossed out about it to speak but then again she is a nurse, she must see all sorts of crazy stuff. I just knew that I was going to have to deal with it once I got home. I didn't know if I could handle that. It's not like shaving in the mirror. I mean I would have to look at this hole in my fucking throat. I didn't know if I could do that. Heal you bastard, Heal! Nurse Ocasek showed me the different dressings she was using, and one was a compression foam fitting that looked like it sort of fit down in the wound. If I had to do that with my current hand shaking coupled with my innate squeamishness, the trach wound would be the least of my worries.

I decided to confide in Nurse Ocasek about my latest visit from the church volunteer, how I felt about the situation, and also to take my mind off the trach wound. She said something to the effect that people visit when they want to make themselves feel better or they pry when they don't know what else to say. I took her words to heart since she had probably seen a lot of those situations arise with heavy handed visitors and upset visitees. I thought to myself, *of course someone who had written the poignant "Drive" would have such insight.*

***

THE SIMPLEST THINGS SET ME OFF AGAIN[168]

Karen came in on Tuesday morning to get my shower stuff ready. She glanced down at the tray table, and saw the pictures of the Babies. "Oh, are these pictures of your kids?" she exclaimed.

I said, "Yes they are, that's them."

"May I look at them?"

"Sure," came my reply. I was so proud of them.

As she looked at them she saw the picture of me and Phoebe, and remarked, "Wow, is this you in this picture."

I said, "It sure is."

"You look so young. When was this taken?"

I was a little confused myself so I looked at the date on it, November 2008, "Gosh, I guess only three months ago," I remarked.

"No kidding, I can't believe it, you look so young without the beard, if I were you I would lose it."

Here I was, bearded, wearing glasses, with longer hair, and just only having realized a week ago that I had not lost half my face that vanity set in and the challenge was accepted.

Younger? Could this be? So against my Uncle Barry's recommendations to keep the beard, since it must have made me look like a college professor holding court in the local café on the meaning of logic, and things that are logical, I decided to rid my face of it. I didn't want to be that logical guy so I went about taking the time I had free after my last class that day to get rid of the beard. It was only logical.

When I returned to the room that afternoon I was determined to shave, and was determined to look like I did in that picture. I went about gathering the items that my sister had purchased for me so long ago that had gotten little use: shaving gel and a Schick razor. Neither were my brands of choice. I wheeled myself into the bathroom, and began to spread the gel around my face. My hands were still shaking quite a bit so I knew it would be a new adventure. The beard was long but I had time.

As I proceeded with my immediate task I was reminded of a TV movie from the 70s about a guy who comes home from the Vietnam War with a long beard, long hair, disabled, and unrecognizable to his children. Compounding the children's inability to recognize their father was his inexplicable wearing of sunglasses indoors, which I didn't really understand unless he wanted to show the kids that Daddy wasn't a square, man. In the next scene he shaves and triumphantly yells his achievement so the entire house can hear him. That scene stayed with me when I was a fourth grader so when I saw it again a couple of years ago I was surprised to see that the two scenes looked like a high school play but no less was the impact in my head. I thought that if that actor playing that guy could do it then so could I. I could even have taken off the sunglasses on my own, if I had any. I was apprehensive as I took the first swipe, and the tugging commenced. It took four or five swipes with the hand shaking heavily and the uncooperative hairs. Needless to say I gave the trach wound a very wide berth. Re-application of the gel was necessary. It was slow going and I had to rest a few times. I couldn't bring myself to cut too high on the sideburns. I decided that would be the signature look of post hospital Howard, longer sideburns, to always remember. However I would stop short of greasing my hair and pushing around scrawny shopkeepers.

After a while, the razor became too clogged with hair to continue. As a result, after an hour and a half of struggling, instead of seeing the Howard from the picture I was seeing more of a skinny GI Joe doll from the late 70s with mange. As a last resort I attempted to use one of the hospital issue razors but I would have had more luck using the edge of my imaginary screwdriver. So I quickly got on the horn to Becky to bring in my razor with extras to finish the job. I was lucky to have the forethought to not undertake this when I had one more class to go in the day. They may have tacked on another two weeks to my stay had they seen the horrors of horrors that would have wheeled itself into the gym with Kung Fu grip fully engaged.

Becky came in that night with my razors. I was truly thankful. "What are you doing?" she asked.

"Shaving off ten years, that's what I'm doing." I finished the job after fifteen minutes, and I looked at myself. *Getting closer,* I thought.

CHAPTER 37

Vanity

I STILL CAN'T SEE CLEARLY NOW[169]

Speaking of vanity, and wanting to get back to that picture of me two months before I got sick I decided that the shaving would not suffice. I needed to get rid of the glasses too so I had Becky bring in my contacts so I could try getting those back in which must have come as a surprise since I was refusing my glasses for so long in the MICU. Not really treating the contacts as a serious alternative to my glasses at the moment, I decided I would take the hour and a half between lunch and my next class to get them in.

    I mustered up my courage and rolled into the bathroom. I took the contact container; my hands were shaking like it was holding that vibrating dumbbell, and realized that my coordination was going to be a challenge. If the therapists were looking for a true test of fine-motor skills then they need have looked no further with this task that I was imposing upon myself. I somehow managed to get the contact on the tip of my finger after repeated drops on the sink and re-washings. The next step was getting the damn thing in my eye. Usually I have to be two feet away from the mirror to see to get them in properly but with the wheel chair and the sink I was four feet away and blind as a bat. Plus my eyes don't open that wide requiring two hands to be able to keep the eyelid open. Now I may sound like a creature from Middle Earth with this description but I was still human at this point.

As my hand approached my eye, the shaking wouldn't stop, and my abnormally long Gloria Swanson eyelashes prevented any sort of proper seating of the contact. I was beginning to get upset. I had to do it, I had to be the guy in the shorts getting up and walking out of here.

After an hour and half of struggling I heard my parents come into the room. "Howard? Are you in here?"

I said, "Yes," in a distressed manner.

They walked into the bathroom and asked, "What are you doing?"

"I'm trying to get my goddamn contacts in! They won't go in, this sucks!"

Big Daddy said, "You have to take it slow on this, it all doesn't come back overnight. You'll be able to get them in but you have other things you need to be doing to get better."

I felt beaten but knew he was right, I just couldn't do it now. Some other day I would have the dexterity to handle it. I then shut up the case, and forgot about it finally remembering what Ms. So and So P.A. had said in the alcove. The whistling guy would have to wait.

***

MORE FREEDOM

I remembered Karen saying if I wanted to get out of the room or go outside at any time just let the desk know so they knew where I was. My quest for freedom was unlimited, and as I was getting quite adept at the wheelchair I decided to test this offer. I rolled out into the hall, and went up to the front desk and said, "I would like to go outside if I could."

The nurse looked at me strangely, and said, "Really?"

"Yes, I do."

Not because I really wanted to but because I felt I had to.

She said, "Go to your room, and I'll have someone come by."

A few minutes later I was all dressed in my sweatsuit expecting the nice day I had experienced outside with Karen. It was a little later, about 4:30 p.m., and it was getting dark out. The nurse came in, and I had *A Civil War* and *The Blind Side* at the ready.

I said, "Can I go out to the landscaped area?"

"No, we would rather you didn't without a staff member or visitor with you, but you can go to the interior courtyard."

I said, "OK, that'll be fine."

She rolled me into the cafeteria and through an exterior door. It was a bit nippy out there.

She said, "OK, it's cold out so I'll check on you in thirty minutes."

I had no watch so I was going to have to trust her on that. The shadows had grown long, and the sun was going down as I began to read. I suddenly felt like I was back in college in New York, and it was 1985. It had a 1985 feeling to it, this area. I can't really explain it. Other than it felt like 1985! I had nothing else to offer as proof than this scene. It felt so much like 1985 that I had this feeling that soon a Delorean would pull up, spit out a Goonie who would offer me a New Coke while boasting about the Chicago Bears' 46 defense, and in the next breath proclaim that Tears for Fears was a thinking man's band and insist that I see *Vision Quest*. Damn know-it-all Goonie. 1985! I was now beginning to think that Rehab was giving the MICU a run for its money in making me crazy.

I read and read, switching between books thinking that certainly thirty minutes had passed. The wind was whipping, and I was not feeling very comfortable. How was I going to get through thirty minutes? I was determined; my thirst for freedom must be quenched. Was it really freedom if I was forcing myself to do it? After mulling this over in my head I decided that while I enjoyed 1985, the courtyard and I had had enough of each other, so I decided to roll up my tent and call it a day.

I rolled myself over to the cafeteria door, grabbed the handle, and son of a bitch the door would move only an inch. Even at my fittest I didn't think I could have opened this thing from a seated position. I kept trying but the door kept hitting the wheelchair. I was going to perish out here all because I wanted to go outside. Where was that nurse? It had to be an hour by now. I saw people inside talking on the other side of the cafeteria. At first I knocked quietly trying to draw attention yet not trying to draw excessive attention that would just be socially awkward. Then my knocking turned to banging.

One of the workers saw me and hurried over to the door, "My, you're going to catch your death out there, this door's heavy no way you could get through that. I can't believe they have no handicapped access to the courtyard of a rehab center."

I said, "There was no way I was getting through that door. Thank you so much."

"Not a problem, they did look into getting an automatic opener for that door but a quote came back that was so high they shelved it."

"Is it OK if I read in here?"

"Of course, make yourself at home."

I pulled myself up to a table, and began to read knowing I could get back to my room at any time. I really felt normal at that point.

The nurse came back eventually, and said, "Were you done already?" I guess that was thirty minutes, my internal clock was still broken.

***

GETTING STRONG NOW, WON'T BE LONG NOW[170]

I had a class called "Gait," and I suppose it was the pre-requisite for "Strut." It usually occurred after lunch and this time I was in with a group of other students. There were about five of us, and we took turns walking around the gym. While I was getting stronger, the walks around the gym could be tiring so I was happy to get to my wheelchair. I had water with me at all times, and when I would fill up at the water fountain my hands would shake uncontrollably. Once Susan, my Power Builder instructor, had noticed this and said, "You're shaking like a leaf! What's wrong?" in a less than serious manner.

My smart-ass self wanted to say, "Because you're near," but decided that was wrong on so many levels, plus I must not let them think they have that much power.

As I would continue with the class I was just a little put out when I saw that the guy that had brain surgery didn't require a wheelchair. He was walking quickly and getting up from his chair quickly as well. I really admired the way he was so energetic and his attitude to get to work. I knew that I would have to lose the wheelchair in time but I just wasn't ready to do that yet and besides who knew how long it took him to get to this point. I had to just worry about myself, and remind myself that this was not some competition. *Now, somebody get me out of this chair so I can show Braino who's boss!*

Another student in the class was an older lady; she had the oxygen tank and the tracheotomy tube in her throat. It was not lost on me that I had those accessories just a week ago, and the freedom and fortune that I felt no longer needing them was overwhelming. We had been in a couple of classes together already when she asked me, "What happened to you? Were you in a car accident?"

"No, I got really sick, and went into toxic shock, and nearly died here."

"So you were in the ICU awhile, I was there too for five weeks."

I instantly felt a bond with her, and wanted to talk to her more about the ICU, and how it drove me crazy being in there but it was my turn. I didn't get to talk to her again. Strangely, I was beginning to feel a part of this group though I knew my time was growing short.

***

CAN YOU TAKE ME HIGH ENOUGH?[171]

One thing that I found strange was getting used to my height, after all that time looking up at people I was finally looking down. I felt at all times like I was walking on a ledge. I threaded the needle on one walk around the gym by squeezing through the therapist that had taught the weekend class and a table very shakily. She looked up at me with fear in her eyes like I was going to topple over her at any moment. It also didn't help that my therapists were often times very short. I felt like I was on stilts and that disaster awaited me. Having been bed bound for so long, and effectively three feet tall for weeks, my normal height was taking some getting used to. I had a very far way to fall, and I was scared. In other words I was afraid of my own height.

The therapists other times would take me over to a king-size bed they had in the gym. I would ask, "Are you going to have me change the sheets, and make it up?" I asked.

They laughed, and said, "No, we just want to see you lie down, and if you can get up from a regular bed." Yes, I repeated the same joke to multiple therapists.

I would lie down, and strain to get into a seated position. I finally used my momentum by rocking and rolling a bit to a seated position. My core strength was a thing of the past and I was lucky to be able to do what I did.

Other times during the class I would be asked questions about my house, and what kind of layout it was. I had one word, "Steps. I have steps everywhere."

"Is your bedroom on the first or second floor?"

"Second floor and there are two right angle turns on it. I also have steps into the kids' playroom and into the sitting room, there's a step from the kitchen to the breakfast room."

"How about the front yard?"

"There are steps all over the damn place, why did I buy a house with so many damn steps in it?"

The therapist laughed, and said, "OK, we'll work on steps then."

They had a staircase with about four steps in the gym that reached a small landing, and a ramp that went down to the floor. I tried going up the steps and I was holding tightly on to the handrail. I would then with great relief walk down the ramp. I did laps in this way until I had satisfied the therapist that I was OK going up.

The next day she added the descent of the steps. This was a real challenge since I still was not used to my height, and the act of standing on one foot while the other descended challenged my balance to no end. I felt dizzy a few times like I was going to fall but I recovered. I did a few laps of that.

The next day she wanted me to let go of the handrails

"That I can't do," came my reply.

"Sure you can. I'll walk with you, and catch you if you start to falter."

It was painful, and it was harsh, the steps and the balance came with greater difficulty. I couldn't believe that I had done this with such ease before. It really seemed impossible at this point. I did it and it was difficult. She then had me descend the steps with no handrails. I felt like I was going to fall through the earth with no hope of landing safely. My balance was not up to this, and we had to wait until another day to try it. My advancement though to this stage surprised even me, so I wasn't as down about the descent as I thought I would be, it was coming back.

The next day I arrived in the wheelchair again. I was getting the hang of turning it, and it was also boosting my arm strength. I couldn't believe I was mobile without assistance in such a short time. I was not ready to go on any wheelchair basketball teams by any means but I did like to show off my newfound skills to all visitors.

Susan, my Power Builder instructor, saw me roll into the gym, and stay seated as I waited for my therapist. She asked me to get up and walk to her. I did that and stopped in front of her.

She said, "You don't need to be in the wheelchair anymore. I'm going to update your chart that you don't need that."

Not have my wheelchair? I couldn't possibly be without my security.

My therapist arrived and said we would walk through the halls today, and go to the real stairs. I was nervous about the real stairs. Talk about unforgiving. She had me turn my head from side to side, and then hold it to one side which made me think of the old "Eyes Right" at the Academy. That was so long ago. I was surprised how difficult it was to do and how way back then I didn't walk into the visiting dignitary during the "Pass in Review" portion of the program. It was usually some old guy wearing a ribbon. I think they kept them in storage and brought them out for special occasions. Then she had me look up and down while walking in a straight line. Too bad the dignitary didn't see that skill.

We got to the stairs out in the hallway, and the steps seemed to go on forever. This was the real deal, and a fall here would be the end. I grabbed the hand rail for dear life and the therapist said, "Take one step at a time, and don't think about the next one until you get down the one you're dealing with."

I walked down like a two-year-old, making sure both feet were secure on a step before I tried to descend again. I was scared, I was scared of this height, and it was not a good feeling. It went a little more smoothly the more times I ascended and descended the steps, but I was spent by the time we got back to the gym and just lucky to be out of there before the tumble came. I felt like I had conquered Everest although I still respected it.

What I didn't get to do or even see and what I had wanted to do for so long was get in the rehab pool. There was the door. I would pass it all the time on the way to the gym. Just a quick dip to get that MICU desire out of me, yet it was never offered and I never asked.

Other exercises we did were walking around cones while being timed, and then we would pass a ball back and forth while side stepping. The most challenging one however was the walk to the cone, bend down, pick it up, and return it to the starting line. I didn't think I was going to come back up, my hips felt like they were locked in concrete. My back felt like a column. I swayed back and forth on the bend down like a crane that had lost his way, and was flapping his wings to get back to an upright position. There always seemed to be a new wrinkle of movement that I had not tried yet. Simply bending down to pick up my kids, I had done that before but this cone challenge was a new adventure.

Through all of this I would look up from time to time, and see Karen monitoring my progress. I was trying, I was getting there.

***

ONE NIGHT AT THE FAIR BUT STILL YOU WANT IT ALL[172]

My appetite was back in full force. I was eating again like a sixteen-year-old. I just couldn't get enough. Every morning, a nice staff member named Ellen would come in, and tell me that day's menu. I had about three choices for every meal and she delivered it with a smile. I remembered her name because she would always tell me it whenever she came in. It was plainly obvious by this point that I was bad with names however even I had to bring attention to how she had finally gotten her name through my thick skull.

She came in one day, and before she could say anything I said, "Hello Ellen."

She was taken by surprise but looked delighted that I remembered her name. So I was comforted by the fact that I hadn't sounded like

Hannibal Lecter when I said it. I then had to compliment her on last night's pulled pork BBQ and turnip greens and added, "Whoever added the packet of vinegar was a genius. I could have eaten another plate of it." I really shouldn't have been throwing around the word "genius" like that.

She replied, "If you wanted more you could always get more."

"I didn't know this, I'll have to take you up on that."

But dinner was at 5:00 and by 8:00 I would be starving again. At one point I asked the nurse's station if I could get something to eat. I was sure they were delighted when a patient had a healthy appetite. They were very accommodating. A nurse went all the way back to the main cafeteria because the one in the rehab center was closed and bought me a roast beef sandwich. I must admit my sixteen-year-old appetite was almost defeated by this dense sandwich. It was so dense light could not escape it. It might have been the same one that was capable of eating that old lady in the dialysis center.

A couple of nights later an offer was made by Becky's and my friend, the real Dannette, that her husband, Brian, could bring me something and what would I like. I said immediately, "A newsmagazine, and Wendy's, two singles with mustard, ketchup, lettuce and cheese, and French fries."

I went ahead and ate dinner that night anyway, and awaited Brian's arrival. It was a Tuesday night so he had to stop by here after work. I was beginning to realize that there was a world going on outside the hospital and my little world yet that did nothing to diminish my hunger, and that trumped all. Brian finally showed up and told me the trouble he had getting in the place. I had no idea where I was much less how to get in. He couldn't find a newsmagazine, so instead he gave me a commemorative Lincoln magazine. Before I looked at it I told him the hell of the last dialysis when I was tortured by the CNN report from the Lincoln Museum. He was getting nervous that I would be disgusted by the magazine he brought but I was not. I pored over it in the days to come. At the end of the visit I was actually full, and could not finish. My sixteen-year-old appetite had finally been vanquished.

***

I HEAR SOMETHING IN THE SHADOW/DOWN THE HALL[173]

It began as an inconvenience but now I was getting more and more tired of it. As usual the door would open around 5:00 a.m. letting in the harsh hallway light, and then the bed light's fluorescence would light up Instalate waking me up. It was time to have my blood test. This really wasn't the way I liked to start my day with the vampires coming in and the blood builder shots in the stomach. With each day I got more used to the actual blood drawing and the dart throwing into my gut. And with each passing day it seemed to get less and less painful. I always sent my compliments to the vampire that that was the least painful one yet.

Even though the moments were less painful they were still not pleasant and I would await the arrival with fear. I had this habit of waking up at 3:00 a.m., going to the bathroom with no assistance, returning to bed, and listening to music on my Ipod. I suppose it harkened back to my first memory in the MICU wanting to hear music and not being able to communicate. Well, now I could and so I did. Then I would try to force myself to go back to sleep but to no avail. My head was full of thoughts of excitement and going home. It felt like I was eight years old and it was the week of Christmas. Then eventually the door would open and the light would stream in.

***

IT'S ALL I CAN DO, TO KEEP WAITING FOR YOU[174]

Recreational therapy was the best time of the day. There was Bocce, video games, and other tons of fun like that thing and the other thing I did but I can't really remember. Unfortunately, there were no bouncy castles or networking with strange clowns and the subsequent being chased by strange clowns. I felt like a kid when I would walk in there. It was a large room with storefront facades on two of the walls and the other two exterior walls were all glass. The natural night lent a cheerfulness to the room. While I was still in the hospital a recreational therapist came to my room to ask what my interests were. I felt really good about this place.

One day I had just recreational therapy left to wrap up the afternoon. I was feeling good when Nurse Ocasek came in and said, "And it's so hard to take, there's no escape without a scrape.[175] Your blood work came back, you're low on magnesium so I'll need to give you an IV when you get back from your class."

I don't know why I felt crushed, I just did. I thought I was done with all that, I didn't want to go back to IVs, and needles, and such. The whole thing was really depressing me. Here I was leaving in a couple of days yet it felt like I was being forced to stay another two weeks. I went to recreational therapy not feeling too cheerful. Today, I was playing Bocce against the young therapist. I lost in all games to her but I didn't care even though I had her on the ropes a couple of times, dammitt. Not even the Wii balance game could have cheered me up. I needed to snap out of it, and just do it. I was weary of infection and having anything else in me. It was an unreasonable fear yet a reasonable fear in my book.

I walked back to the room with the wheelchair in front of me since I still needed that crutch, full of dread. Then Nurse Ocasek came in.

I said, "If you have trouble finding a vein please don't let me know if there's a problem."

She said, "That'll be fine, I can do that."

I also wanted to tell her that after several listens *Heartbeat City* isn't all that objectionable and certainly not that I found Benjamin Orr to be the more capable singer in the group.

As I had predicted Nurse Ocasek did have trouble finding a good vein in my thread-like arm. It took a couple of times but at least she was true to her word and wasn't doing a play by play like Lady IV up in Progressive. After a couple of minutes there was success and I would just have to endure hopefully this last "setback."

CHAPTER 38

Farewell

FEBRUARY 26, 2009

RESTART AND RE-BOOT YOURSELF/YOU'RE FREE TO GO[176]

I have had four commencement days in my life, and this was the fifth and by far the most important to me. I was so excited the night before I could barely sleep. This was it, my dream of leaving the hospital was about to come true. The nurse said I would be discharged around 10:00 a.m. so I should be ready to go when breakfast came.

Becky came in that morning saying, "Hello! Hello! Today's the day!"

"I know, I know, this is unbelievable, it's here," I said not sounding like John Travolta.

She busied herself with packing up my belongings. A nurse came in, one that I hadn't seen before, to give me my discharge papers and instructions for when I got home. There were a lot of instructions and a lot of appointments to be kept with my primary doctor, Dr. Phillips,

OutPatient Rehab, and more blood builder medicine at the injection clinic, at least that's what I called it.

Where was the cap and gown? Where was that weird ginger ale fruit punch? Where was the gauntlet of slow clappers? Where was the sheepskin diploma rolled with a sheepskin ribbon encased in a sheepskin case? It seemed anticlimactic as I got into the sheepskin wheelchair, and said farewell to my last room at General Hospital. The end of the line. The Babies were in school so they would have a coming home gift….that would be me.

My parents had arrived for the commencement, and helped with the packing. Big Daddy was trying to pack the box that my beloved flexi-seal came in and for some strange reason kept following me around. I jokingly got on him, "What have you got there? Throw that thing out or I'll have them put it in you."

"I just thought you would want to remember it," he replied.

I should have saved it, and wrapped it up for him for next Christmas along with a complimentary installation and a year's supply of Sir Flagyl.

I think I was at a point where home care was not needed. I was fortunate for that so there would be no Effeminate Curtis prancing me up and down the street mockingly sprinkling flower petals in my path. As I went out into the hallway the only gauntlet of humanity I could see was the one in my head full of the doctors, nurses, and therapists that got me out of here. I also provided the slow clapping for the full effect. I did get some strange looks.

We went downstairs. Becky got my beloved blue minivan, yes beloved, and I was helped in. While I wasn't the guy in the tan shorts and T-shirt at this moment, and I couldn't, and still can't whistle anyway, that didn't matter. I was going home.

PART V: CLOSER TO MY HOME[151] - FAREWELL

I can't believe it, my eyes deceive me
That I'm back in your arms, away from all harm
It's like a dream, to be with you again
Can't believe that I'm with you again[177]

EPILOGUE
A Suitable Ending, I Think[178]

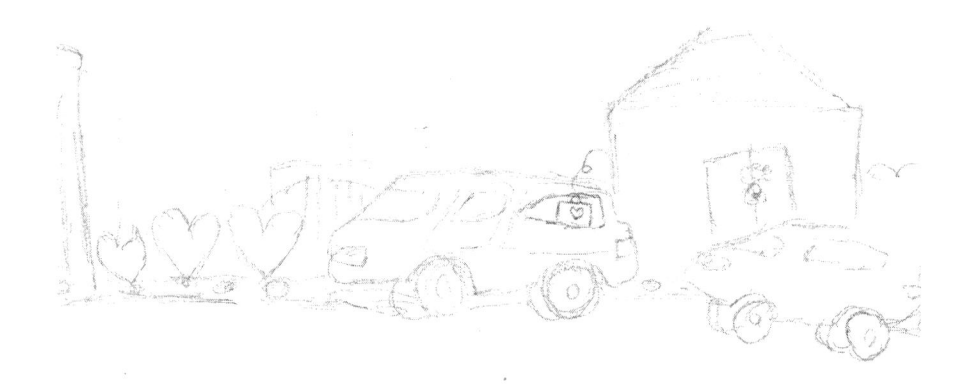

TOP OF MOUNT HALEAKALA, MAUI

JANUARY 15, 2010, 5:00 A.M. HST

It was dark, cold, and windy. The van that had picked us up at the hotel at 2:30 a.m. dropped us off in the parking lot of the visitors' center at the top of Mount Haleakala, and was not letting us back on. As I packed for Maui I didn't take seriously the warnings of windy conditions with temperatures in the low thirties, but I did pack adequately.

For the one-year anniversary of the beginning of my travels through a toxic shock nightmare Becky wanted to know what I would like to do to mark the milestone. I said I didn't know yet I was certain that I wanted to be surprised and I wanted to get as far away from the MICU of General Hospital as possible. So with this being no small request short of going to a MICU in Beijing, she passed with flying colors. Even though a return address on an envelope that arrived a week before our departure had spoiled the surprise of the destination, I was still excited to do something we had never done before: celebrate life by riding a bicycle down a volcano to the north coast of Maui.

But first Becky had figured out that the exact time of sunrise at the top of the volcano was when I went into the emergency room EST.

We waited in the darkness for what seemed forever for the sunrise but even in the miserable cold we were not to be denied. Seeing the sun rise over the earth marked for us a time when just a year before such a trip was unlikely to happen. We wanted to recognize health, love, happiness, freedom, togetherness, and escape from such a horrible time. As we stood there with our arms around each other, I could see the upper edge of the sun coming over the horizon, and I knew that I was home.

EPILOGUE - A SUITABLE ENDING, I THINK[178]

***

AMELIA ISLAND, FLORIDA

FEBRUARY 3, 2010

"You guys clean up nicely," the lady said to us as we made our way through the reception area outside the hotel ballroom.

"It takes a while but we get there," I replied, trying to hide my nervousness.

"We'll wait out here a few more minutes until they're ready for you inside. Are you ready?" the lady asked as I sat there with Becky, Kate, Phoebe, and Henry

"I think so, I'm all rehearsed up," I replied. Just then some other representatives came over to greet me and my family. As the greetings were being exchanged a technician came over.

"All right we'll need to wire you for the microphone."

Good idea. This was one class operation. I didn't want to be yelling my message.

We had just finished our first full day of our visit to the Ritz Carlton on Amelia Island as invited guests of a California based company. The company, I learned five months before, had developed and manufactured the Presep catheter that identified my condition as sepsis in the emergency room at General Hospital that drove the treatment that ultimately saved my life. I had been in contact with them since September 2009 as possibly having my story told and how my case could be used as a primary example of the importance of early detection of sepsis. The plan was that our story would be told via a professionally made video that would be shown at the company's national sales conference [and is now available on YouTube], and afterward I would come to the stage and say a few words. Just two weeks before a crew had come to our house to film interviews of me, Becky, and the kids, and show us in our daily routine. During my interview I found it difficult to compress and express all I wanted to say in a few meaningful words, so I struggled while Becky did a sterling job.

To eliminate my mumbled thoughts from two weeks before, I really wanted to say in as few words as possible the most powerful message I could get across that conveyed my appreciation. I wanted to recognize the importance of the Critical Care Division of the company, and how they truly are making a difference in developing partnerships with hospitals to establish sepsis awareness programs. While the other factor that saved me was living less than two miles from a hospital, luckily it was one that had such a program in place that saved my sorry ass. In other words I owed these people my life, and I was going to do anything they asked me to do. If that meant having a four-day all-expenses paid weekend at the Ritz Carlton on Amelia Island then so be it.

When word came we were led into the ballroom which was filled to capacity with what must have been over 500 people and were seated near the front. Perhaps I was sensitive to it but I could feel a quiet come across the room as we walked in. I knew what I was going to say I just hoped I would remember it all.

The company representative sat down next to me, and asked, "Are you nervous?"

I shook my head in a half convincing fashion. I could say anything up there but I knew I would have to say something significant. This was a big deal since they helped save my life.

EPILOGUE - A SUITABLE ENDING, I THINK[178]

Carl, the director of Critical Care for the company, talked for a little while about the advances Critical Care had been making and said, "Now we have a video to show you of one of those cases that really illustrates what our company's all about, and what we're ultimately trying to do."

The lights went down and I heard a familiar voice say, "My name is Howard Hoover, I am from Charlotte, North Carolina and I survived sepsis."

Top Eleven Things I Learned During My Time with Toxic Shock Syndrome

---

11. I now look at Medical ID Badges with the same affection as Regan did when she saw the priest collar at the end of *The Exorcist*.

10. Do not drink Nehi grape soda with a Flexi-Seal attached.

9. General Hospital's official policy is to not allow Dog People in as visitors. As employees, maybe. Definitely not as visitors.

8. The swirling red liquid of the dialysis machine does not mean it also serves Icees.

7. The symbol for medical waste is not an evil devilish alien creature mocking me.

6. The foot of the bed does not show the date of birth and death of my relatives or give flight information. It only says "Instaflate Activated."

5. *Roman Holiday* starring Gregory Peck and Audrey Hepburn is not ideal MICU viewing because it keeps patients awake with its pedestrian and predictable plot. And that ending!

4. Everybody that has visited me has not decided to go to medical school.

3. You cannot have anyone fired by pushing a button on the footboard of the bed.

2. Delicious Sir Flagyl, even with the adjective "Delicious," will never be offered as a topping at Ben and Jerry's.

1. Hospital gowns are not sold in the hospital gift shop.

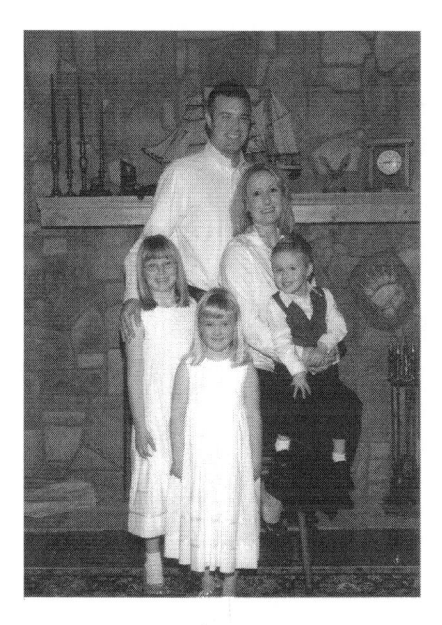

March 29, 2009

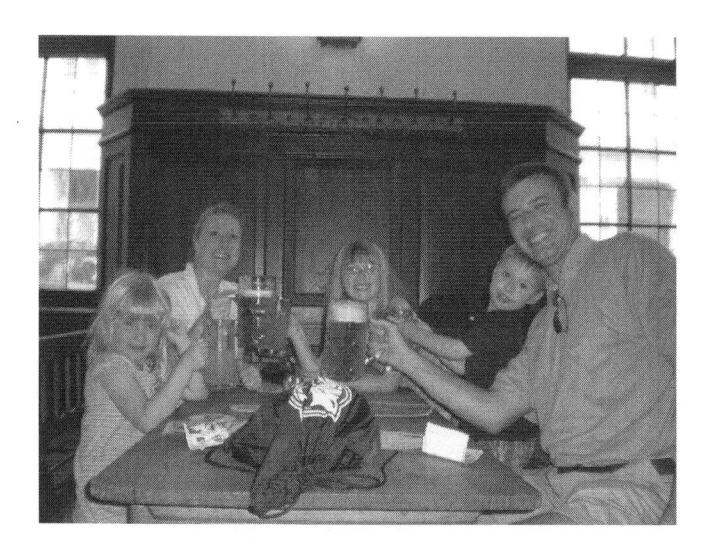

June 29, 2009

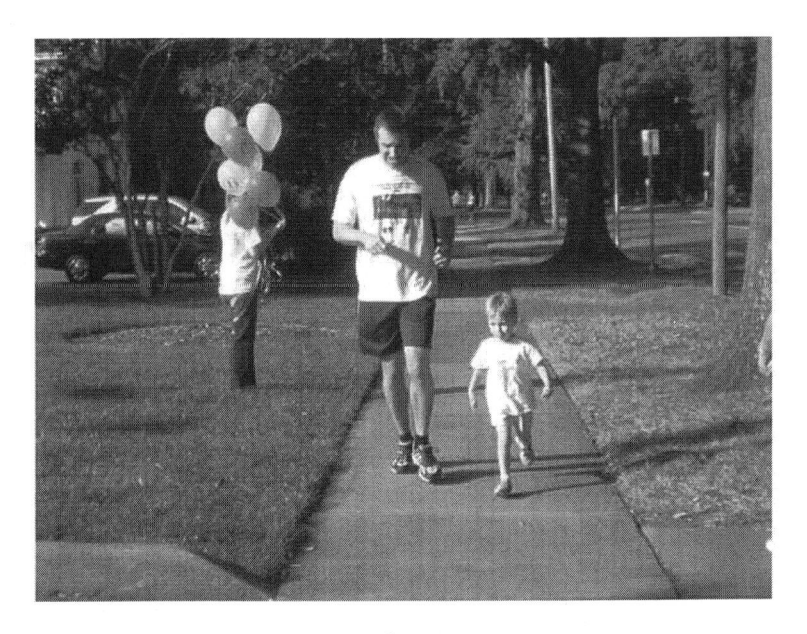

September 9, 2009

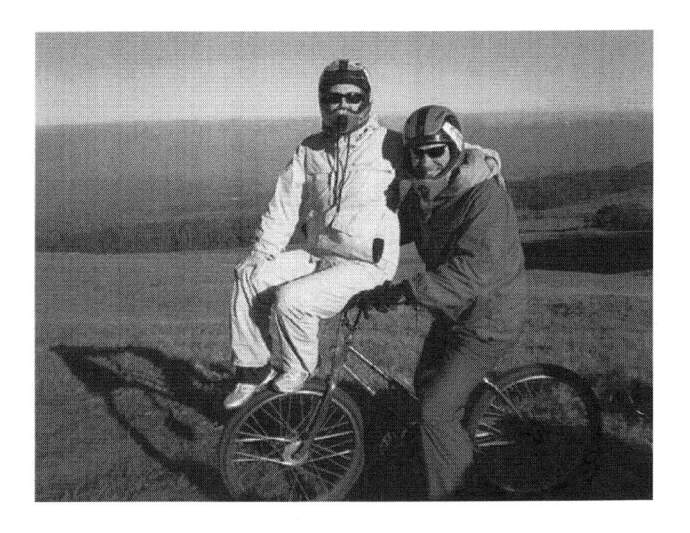

January 15, 2010

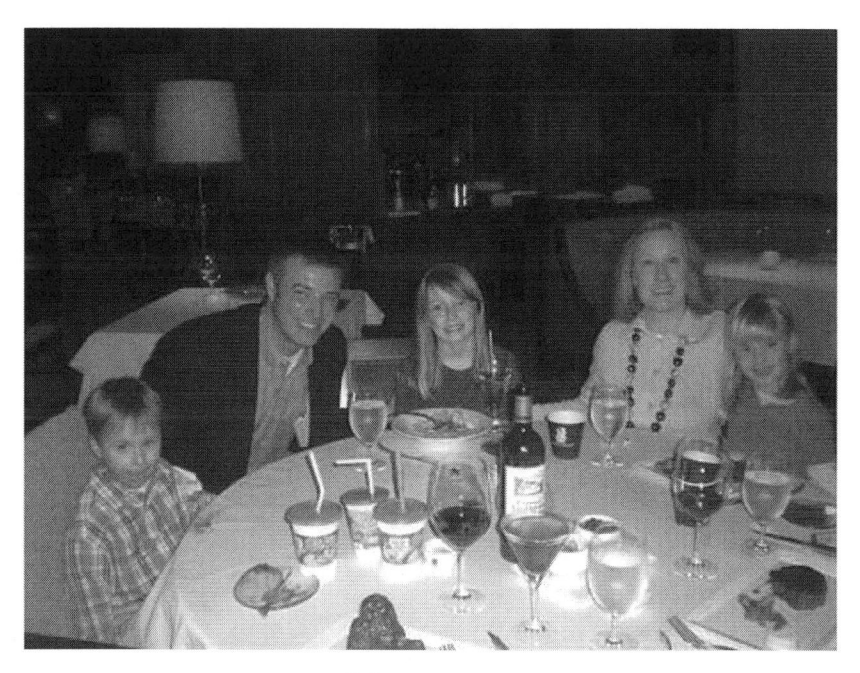

February 3, 2010

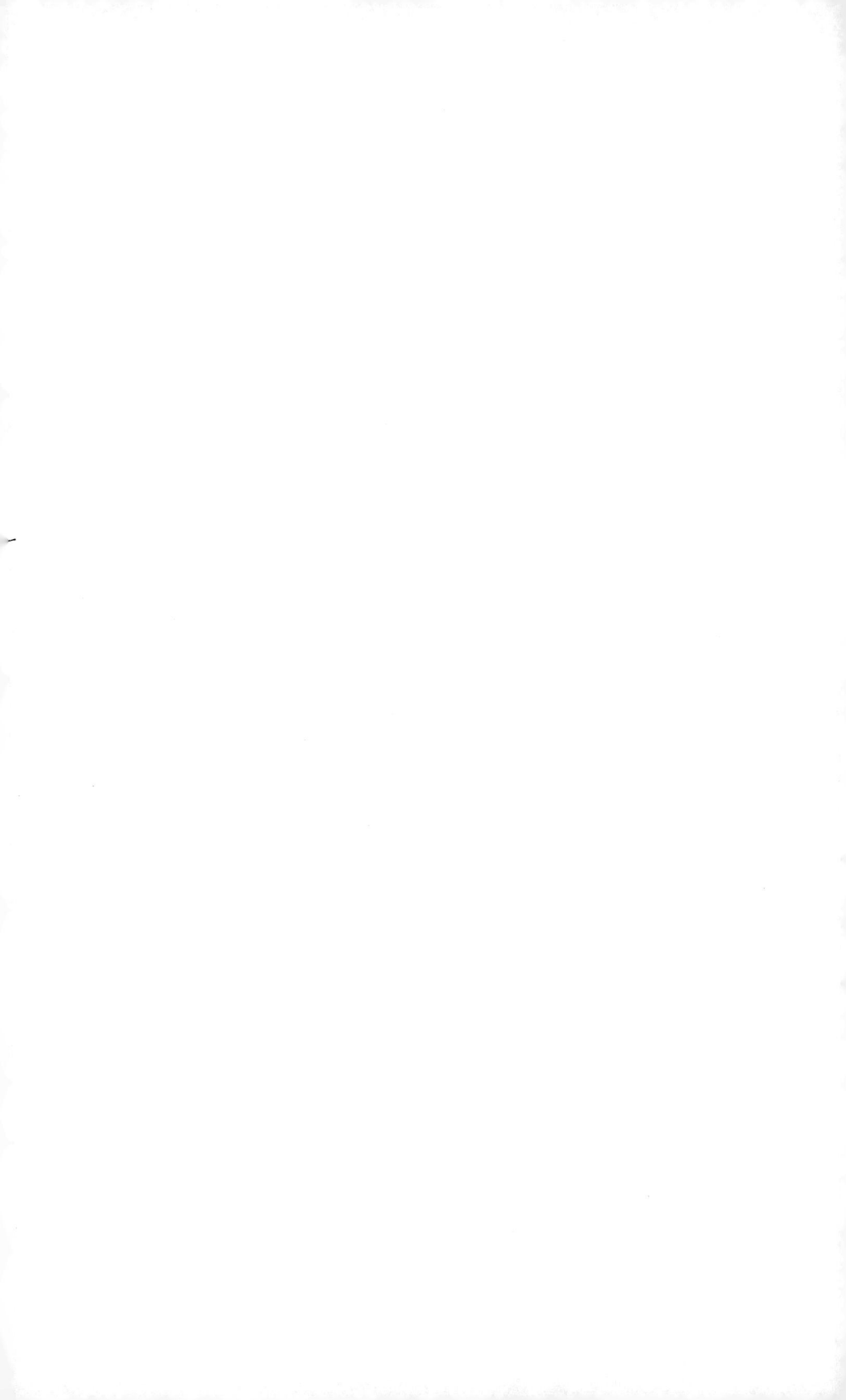

Afterword

On January 15, 2009 US Airways Flight 1549 bound for Charlotte, NC crash landed on the Hudson River with incredibly no loss of life, and was known thereafter as "The Miracle on the Hudson." Unbeknownst to the passengers and crew, I was beginning my own miracle at the same time in the emergency room of General Hospital in Charlotte, NC. As they were unaware of what I was experiencing, in my unconscious state I had not a clue of what they were experiencing either. I am not a medical person; I have attained some CPR training through school, and learned secondhand medical advice from pediatric nurses at ungodly hours of the night that might make me dangerous at a cocktail party. Nothing on earth could prepare me for what I was going to go through that day, and the days to follow.

During my time at General Hospital I decided to write down what I remembered from my journey through sepsis, and its awful descendants septic shock, and toxic shock syndrome when I was in a semi state of consciousness/unconsciousness for my own gallows humor amusement. Subsequently this turned into writing a full-fledged book after one of my neighbors who brought over a meal for the family shortly after my return home said to me, "You should write a book." I didn't take her seriously at the time but as the days, and months followed I began to think more and more about it, and began to add details to my journey. To my surprise the words kept coming in describing my experience since it was still so vivid. I tell those that ask about the book that it is a cross between Pink Floyd's *The Wall*, and the early 80's *St. Elsewhere* or *Trapper John MD*." *Trapper John MD*? That would be too far out there.

Of course, I have taken liberties with the dialogue; nevertheless it is as close as I can remember. It is an accidental-tourist version of a healthy person waking up to find that he has been the sickest person ever seen by his doctors and nurses, and to make it home in one piece. As a forty-one-year-old healthy male at the time getting ill so quickly still makes me think about it every day, and how it lends proof to the general suddenness of life.

Flight 1549 finally made its way to its final destination in Charlotte on a flat-bed truck after two and a half years in storage. Thank God we both had our miracles.

Acknowledgements

I am so grateful to have been able to finish this book and finally get it out after five years. Writing it has been both blessing and burden. My thanks and love to those that helped make it possible.

To Becky, I would not be here to tell this story were it not for your sense, love, and devotion. Thank you.

To Kate, Phoebe, and Henry, I'm so glad you had each other and I know I had you with me. I am very proud of you and love you very much.

To the first responders of the Charlotte Fire Department, your ability to think on your feet saved me.

To the EMTs, and in particular, the ambulance driver, thanks for making the call on my destination.

To the doctors, nurses, therapists, technicians, and staff of that wonderful hospital I was taken to in Charlotte, thank you for your attention, consideration, and knowing how to do your jobs. I won't forget you.

To my parents, Betty-Bruce and Herbert Hoover, thanks for getting to Charlotte at a moment's notice; you set a new record for packing for six weeks. Your love and support made all the difference.

To my mother-in-law, India Van Brunt, thanks for keeping watch over the Babies, and keeping everything running smoothly at home.

To my brother, David, and my sister, Lorraine, thanks for dropping everything to get to Charlotte.

To all my family, friends, and neighbors who visited me, prayed for me, thought of me, helped my family, or asked about me. Thank you.

I spent a lot of time on this book but it never would have seen the light of day until I showed it to a select few. Thanks to John Lawson, India Van Brunt, Becky Hoover, Kaye Cloniger, Scott Lindblom, Sherry Russell, Danielle Hutcheson, Lorraine Hoover Lucey, Herbert Hoover, Betty-Bruce Hoover, Susan Morrow, and that wonderful anonymous book reviewer at Create a Space for your invaluable comments, encouragement, and support. Your input and opinion that I had written something touching and entertaining kept me going even when I had my doubts. Thank you.

Thanks to Scott Lindblom for that wonderful foreword. Your words helped to illustrate a very serious matter.

Thanks also go out to Martha, Catherine, Kathy, Karen, Dora, Dana, Jill, Kelly, Aimee, Holly, Lynne, Jenny, Melissa, Tessa, Hannah, Peggy, Sandy, Lindsey, Patrick, David, Katie, Tiffany, Melissa, Eileen, Christy, Gina, Hang, Justin, Scott, Chester, Jaspal, Lewis, Philip, Nancy, Todd, Scott, Chester, John, Philip, Chris, Gena, William, Danielle, John, Tim, Martha, Chris, Charlotte, Richard, Phillip, Leslie, Nga, Becky, Patricia, Valerie, Mike, Leslie, Natasha, Sarah, Kara, Emily, John, Robin, Brittany, Kiddy, Churly, Chinwe, Melissa, Mary, Jennifer, Jackie, Jewell, Sheila, Dave, Justina, Jessica, Alyssa, Leah, Kara, and Aletta for your care and getting me through to the other side. I am able to type this because of all of you.

Thanks Scott, Lori, Rex, Lisa, India, Julie, Kay, Tim, Kristal, Kim, Laura, Jennifer, Kelly, Shannon, Kaye, Jerry, and John for your visits and others that I have forgotten but whose visits helped to make the difference. I know I gave those that stared and those that shopped a hard time. I would have done the same thing had I been you, probably more. It does not lessen my thanks to you.

Thanks to those from my church that came to visit me: Sally, David, and especially Carter. You provided me with the faith I needed to get through to the other side.

Also thanks to Michael, Carlyn, Amanda, Beryt, Carlos, Josue, Rosa, Gloria, Luis, Monica, Linnette, Carmen, and Jacqueline for the opportunity to tell my story.

Thanks to Cindy, I am happy good timing allowed the opportunity for us to help one another.

Thanks to John, Paul, George, and Ringo and yes, even, no, especially Morris Albert for providing the soundtrack to my travels.

HOWARD HOOVER

Charlotte, North Carolina
February 26, 2014

About the Author

Howard Hoover lives in Charlotte, NC with his family and is a first time author. As a sepsis survivor he has been invited to speak at conferences, hospitals, and manufacturing facilities domestically and internationally. He holds bachelor degrees from the United States Merchant Marine Academy, and the University of South Florida, and a graduate degree from Mercer University. He is a registered professional engineer in Georgia and North Carolina.

The house where the illness almost got him still weighs heavily on his mind for so many reasons. Not a day goes by that he doesn't think about those days but slowly they are retreating behind the good and bad memories of all that has occurred since then. The physical reminders from his travels include the tracheotomy scar that looks and feels mighty weird when he swallows and sings poorly but with great aplomb, scarring of the lungs, pain in his sides from the drainage tubes, and mild tingling/numbness in his fingers and toes.

He still has never been to South Dakota.

Bibliography

Austin Powers: International Man of Mystery. Writ. Mike Myers and Michael McCullers. Dir. Jay Roach. Perf. Mike Myers, Elizabeth Hurley, Michael York, and Mimi Rogers. New Line Cinema. 1997.

Mandel, Jess, MD, and Gregory A. Schmidt, MD. ed. Polly E Parsons, MD, Daniel J Sexton, MD, and Kevin C. Wilson, MD, "Management of severe sepsis and septic shock in adults." *UptoDate http://www.uptodate.com/contents/management-of-severe-sepsis-and-septic-shock-in-adults.* N.p. 25 Oct. 2011, 06 Jun. 2012. Web.

Planes. Trains, and Automobiles. Writ. John Hughes. Dir. John Hughes. Perf. John Candy and Steve Martin. Paramount Pictures, 1987. DVD.

"Sepsis." *Stedman's Medical Dictionary.* 28th ed. Lippincott Williams & Wilkins, 2006.

"Septic Shock." *Stedman's Medical Dictionary.* 28th ed. Lippincott Williams & Wilkins, 2006.

Stevens, Dennis L., MD, PhD. ed. Daniel J. Sexton, MD and Elinor L Baron, MD, DTMH."Epidemiology, clinical manifestations, and diagnosis of streptococcal toxic shock syndrome." *UptoDate, http://www.uptodate.com/online/content/topic.do?topicKey=gram_pos/5335&view=.* N.p. 13 Jan. 2009, 11 Jan. 2010. Web.

"Toxic Shock Syndrome." *Stedman's Medical Dictionary.* 28th ed. Lippincott Williams & Wilkins, 2006.

Discography

Aerosmith. "No More, No More." By Steven Tyler and Joe Perry. *Toys in the Attic*. Columbia Records, 1975. CD.

Average White Band. "Pick up the Pieces." By Average White Band. *AWB*. Atlantic Records, 1974. MP3.

The B-52s. "Love Shack." By Kate Pierson, Fred Schneider, Keith Strickland, and Cindy Wilson. *Cosmic Thing*. Warner Brothers, 1989. CD.

The B Sharps "Baby On Board," Words and Music By Jeff Martin, Shelby Grimm, Harry Campbell, George Economou, and Danny Jordan. *Songs in the Key of Springfield*. Rhino Records. 1994.

Baker, Chet. "My Funny Valentine." By Richard Rodgers and Lorenz Hart. *Babes in Arms*. Fantasy, 1952.

The Beach Boys. "Heroes and Villians." By Brian Wilson and Van Dyke Parks. *Smiley Smile*. Capitol Records, 1967. MP3.

The Beach Boys. "Wouldn't It Be Nice." By Brian Wilson, Tony Asher, and Mike Love. *Pet Sounds*. Capitol Records, 1966. CD.

The Beatles. "A Taste of Honey." By John Lennon and Paul McCartney. *Please Please Me*. EMI/Northern Songs Ltd., 1962. CD.

The Beatles. "Anytime at All." By John Lennon and Paul McCartney. *With The Beatles*. EMI/Northern Songs Ltd., 1963. CD.

The Beatles. "Christmas Time Is Here Again." By John Lennon, Paul McCartney, George Harrison, and Richard Starkey. *Christmas Record for Beatles Fan Club*. EMI/Northern Songs Ltd., 1967.

The Beatles. "Here Comes the Sun." By George Harrison. *Abbey Road*. EMI/Northern Songs Ltd., 1969. CD.

The Beatles. "Dr. Robert." By John Lennon and Paul McCartney. *Revolver*. EMI/Northern Songs Ltd., 1966. CD.

The Beatles. "I'm Only Sleeping." By John Lennon and PaulMcCartney. *Revolver*. EMI. Northern Songs Ltd, 1966. CD.

The Beatles. "P.S. I Love You." By John Lennon and Paul McCartney. *Please Please Me*. EMI/Northern Songs Ltd., 1962. CD.

The Beatles. "Penny Lane." By John Lennon and Paul McCartney. *Anthology 3*. Apple Records, 1967. CD.

The Beatles. "Real Love." By John Lennon. *Beatles Anthology 2*. Apple Records, 1995. CD.

The Beatles "Tell Me What You See." Written by John Lennon and Paul McCartney. *Rubber Soul*. EMI. Northern Songs Ltd., 1965. CD.

The Beatles. "There's A Place." By John Lennon and Paul McCartney. *Please Please Me*. EMI/Northern Songs Ltd., 1962. CD.

Bowie, David. "Modern Love." By David Bowie. *Let's Dance*. EMI America Records, 1983. MP3.

Calloway, Cab. "Papa's in Bed with His Britches On." By Jesse Stone. *Are You Hep To The Jive?* Columbia Records, 1940. CD.

The Cars. "It's All I Can Do." By Ric Ocasek. *Candy-O*. Elektra Records, 1979. CD.

The Cars. "You Might Think." By Ric Ocasek. *Heartbeat City*. Elektra Records, 1984. CD.

The Cast of *Oliver!* "Food, Glorious Food." By Lionel Bart. Tams-Witmark Music Library, Inc., 1960.

Chicago. "Stay the Night." By Peter Cetera and David Foster. *Chicago 17*. Full Moon/Warner Bros., 1984. MP3.

The Church. "Metropolis." By Marty Willson-Piper, Peter Koppes, Richard Ploog, and Steve Kilbey. *Gold Afternoon Fix*. Arista Records, 1990. MP3.

Clapton, Eric. "Heaven is One Step Away." By Eric Clapton. *Crossroads Disc 4*. Warner Bros. Records, 1985. CD.

Concrete Blonde. "Bloodletting (The Vampire Song)." By Johnette Napolitano. *Bloodletting*. I.R.S., 1990. CD.

The Cranberries. "Just My Imagination." By Dolores O'Riordan and Noel Hogan. *Bury the Hatchet*. Island Records, 1999. CD.

The Cranberries. "Ode to My Family." Words by Dolores O'Riordan, Music by Dolores O'Riordan and Noel Hogan . *No Need to Argue*. Island Records, 1994. CD.

The Cranberries. "Zombie." By Dolores O'Riordan. *No Need to Argue*. Island Records, 1994. MP3.

The Cult. "Love Removal Machine." By Ian Astbury and Billy Duffy. *Electric*. Beggars Banquet, 1987. CD.

The Cure. "Boys Don't Cry." By Michael Dempsey, Robert Smith, and Lol Tolhurst. Fiction Records, 1979. MP3.

Damn Yankees. "High Enough." By Tommy Shaw, Jack Blades, Ted Nugent. *Damn Yankees*. Warner Bros., 1990. MP3.

The Del-Vetts. "The Last Time Around." By Jimmie Nelson. Universal Music Publishing Group, Sony/ATV Music Publishing LLC, 1966. MP3.

Dio. "Hungry for Heaven." By Ronnie James Dio and Jimmy Bain. *Vision Quest Soundtrack*. Geffen Records,1985. CD.

Duran Duran. "Save a Prayer." By Duran Duran. *Rio*. Capitol Records, 1982. MP3.

Dylan, Bob. "Lay Lady Lay." By Bob Dylan. *Nashville Skyline.* Columbia Records, 1969. CD.

Electric Light Orchestra. "Mr. Blue Sky." By Jeff Lynne. *Out of the Blue.* United Artists, 1978. MP3.

Fleetwood Mac "Little Lies." By Christine McVie and Eddy Quintela. *Tango in the Night.* Warner Bros. Records, 1987. CD.

The Fortunes. "Here Comes That Rainy Day Feeling Again." By Roger Frederick Cook, Roger John Reginald Greenaway, and Tony Macaulay. *Here Comes That Rainy Day Feeling Again.* Decca Records,1970. MP3.

Garbage. "The Trick is to Keep Breathing," Words and Music by Garbage. *Version 2.0.* Almo Sounds, Inc., 1999. CD.

Grand Funk Railroad. "I'm Your Captain (Closer to Home)." By Mark Farner. *Closer to Home.* Capitol Records, 1970. MP3.

Guns n' Roses "Welcome to the Jungle." By Axl Rose, Slash, Izzy Stradlin, Duff McKagan, and Steven Adler. *Appetite for Destruction.* Geffen Records, 1987. CD.

Harrison, George. "Be Here Now." By George Harrison. *Living in the Material World.* Apple Records, 1973. MP3.

Harrison, George. "Don't Let Me Wait Too Long." By George Harrison. *Living in the Material World.* Apple Records, 1973. MP3.

Hebb, Bobby. "Sunny." By Bobby Hebb. *Sunny.* Philips, 1966. MP3.

Henley, Don. "Sunset Grill." By Don Henley, Danny Kortchmar, and Ben Tench. *Building the Perfect Beast.* Geffen Records, 1984. CD.

Henley, Don. "You're Not Drinking Enough." By Danny Kortchmar. *Building the Perfect Beast.* Geffen Records, 1984. CD.

Herman's Hermits. "There's A Kind of Hush All over the World." By Les Reed and Geoff Stephens. Columbia Records, 1967. CD.

DISCOGRAPHY

Idol, Billy. "Eyes Without A Face." By Billy Idol and Steve Stevens. *Rebel Yell.* Chrysalis Records, 1984. MP3.

INXS. "New Sensation." Words by Michael Hutchence, Music by Andrew Farriss. *Kick.* Atlantic Records, 1987. MP3.

INXS "The Gift," By Jon Farriss and Michael Hutchence. *Full Moon, Dirty Hearts.* Atlantic Records, 1993. MP3.

John, Elton. "Sad Songs (Say So Much)." By Bernie Taupin and Elton John. *Breaking Hearts.* Geffen Records, 1984. MP3.

Lawrence, Gertrude. "Someone to Watch over Me." Music by George Gershwin, Words by Ira Gershwin. *Oh! Kay.* Released as Victor 20331, matrix 36654-3. 1926.

Lennon, John. "#9 Dream," By John Lennon. *Walls and Bridges.* Capitol Records, 1974. CD.

Lennon, John. "Cold Turkey." By John Lennon. *Shaved Fish.* Apple Records, 1969. CD.

Lennon, John. "Crippled Inside." By John Lennon. *Imagine.* Apple Records, 1971. CD.

Lennon, John. "How Do You Sleep?" By John Lennon. *Imagine.* Apple Records, 1971. CD.

Lennon, John. "Watching the Wheels," By John Lennon. *Double Fantasy.* Geffen Records, 1980.

Little, DeEtta. "Gonna Fly Now (Theme from Rocky)." Music by Bill Conti, Words by Carol Connors and Ayn Robbins. *Rocky – Original Motion Picture Score.* United Artists, 1977. MP3.

Loverboy. "Working for the Weekend." By Paul Dean, Mike Reno, and Matt Frenette. *Get Lucky.* Columbia Records, 1981. MP3.

Madness. "Our House." By Chris Foreman and Cathal Smyth. *The Rise & Fall.* Geffen Records, 1982. MP3.

Madonna. "Ray of Light." By Madonna, William Orbit, Clive Muldoon, Dave Curtiss and Christine Leach. *Ray of Light*. Maverick Records, 1998. MP3.

Mazzy Star "Fade into You." By Hope Sandoval and David Roback. *So Tonight That I Might See*. Capitol Records, 1994. CD.

McCartney, Paul. "My Brave Face." By Paul McCartney and Elvis Costello. *Flowers in the Dirt*. Capitol Records, 1989. CD.

Men at Work. "Overkill." By Colin Hay. *Cargo*. Columbia Records, 1983. CD.

The Monkees. "What Am I Doing Hangin' Round?" By Michael Martin Murphey and Owen Castleman. *Pisces, Aquarius, Capricorn & Jones Ltd*. Arista Records, 1967. MP3.

Morrison, Van. "Call Me Up In Dreamland." By Van Morrison. *His Band and the Street Choir*. Warner Bros. Records, 1970. CD.

The Motels. "Only the Lonely." By Martha Davis. *All Four One*. Capitol, 1982. MP3.

Nash, Johnny. "I Can See Clearly Now." By Johnny Nash. *I Can See Clearly Now*. Epic Records, 1972. MP3.

Nicholas, Paul. "Heaven on the 7th Floor." By C. Neil and Paul Nicholas. RSO Records, 1977. MP3.

Nugent, Ted. "Free-for-All." By Ted Nugent. *Free-for-All*. Epic Records, 1976. CD.

O'Riordan, Dolores. "When We Were Young." By Dolores O'Riordan. *Are You Listening?* Sequel Records, 2007. CD.

Palmer, Robert. "Bad Case of Loving You (Doctor, Doctor)." By Moon Martin. *Secrets*. Island Records, 1978. CD.

Planet P Project. "Why Me?" By Tony Carey. *Planet P*. Geffen Records, 1983. MP3.

Plant, Robert. "Little by Little." By Robert Plant and Jezz Woodroffe. *Shaken N' Stirred*. Es Paranza, 1985. MP3.

The Police. "Don't Stand So Close to Me." By Sting. *Zenyatta Mondatta*. A&M Records, 1980. CD.

Quiet Riot. "Cum on Feel the Noiz." By Jim Lea and Noddy Holder. *Metal Health*. CBS Records, 1982.

R.E.M. "Gardening at Night." Words and Music by Bill Berry, Peter Buck, Mike Mills, and Michael Stipe. *Eponymous*. I.R.S. Records, 1982. CD.

R.E.M. "Superman." By Gary Zekley and Mitchell Bottler. *Life's Rich Pageant*. I.R.S. Records, 1986. CD.

The Rolling Stones. "Dandelion." By Mick Jagger and Keith Richards. *Through the Past, Darkly (Big Hits Vol. 2)*. Decca Records, 1967. MP3.

The Rolling Stones. "Happy." By Mick Jagger and Keith Richards. *Exile on Main Street*. Rolling Stones Records, 1972. MP3.

The Rolling Stones. "Sympathy for the Devil." By Mick Jagger and Keith Richards. *Beggars Banquet*. Decca Records, 1968. MP3.

The Rolling Stones. "Waiting on a Friend." By Mick Jagger and Keith Richards. *Tattoo You*. Rolling Stones Records, 1981. CD.

The Rolling Stones. "You Can't Always Get What You Want." By Mick Jagger and Keith Richards. *Let It Bleed*. Decca Records, 1969. MP3.

The Rolling Stones. "You Gotta Move." By Fred McDowell and Gary Davis. *Sticky Fingers*. Rolling Stones Records, 1971. CD.

Rush. "Fly by Night." Words by Neil Peart, Music by Geddy Lee. *Fly By Night*. Mercury Records, 1975. CD.

Scaggs, Boz. "Lido Shuffle." By David Paich and Boz Scaggs. *Silk Degrees*. CBS Records, 1976. MP3.

The Scorpions. "Arizona." By Rudolf Schenker. *Blackout*. Mercury Records, 1982. CD.

Sebastian, John. "Welcome Back." By John Sebastian. Reprise Records, 1976. MP3.

Seger, Bob. "Night Moves." By Bob Seger. *Night Moves*. Capitol Records, 1976. MP3.

Simon, Carly. "Nobody Does It Better." Music by Marvin Hamlisch, Words by Carole Bayer Sager. Elektra Records, 1977. MP3.

Simple Minds. "See the Lights." By Kerr/Burchill. *Glittering Prize*. Virgin Records,1991. CD.

Sinatra, Frank. "Fly Me to the Moon." By Bart Howard. *It Might As Well Be Swing*. Reprise Records, 1964. MP3.

Smokey Robinson and the Miracles. "Tears of a Clown." By Smokey Robinson. *Make It Happen*. Motown Records. 1967. MP3.

Spanky and Our Gang. "Sunday Will Never Be the Same." By Terry Cashman and Gene Pistilli. *Spanky and Our Gang*. Mercury Records, 1967. MP3.

The Spinners. "The Rubberband Man." By Thom Bell and Linda Creed. Atlantic Records,1976. MP3.

Sting. "Fields of Gold." By Sting. *Ten Summoner's Tales*. A&M, 1993. CD.

Stone Temple Pilots. "Trippin' On A Hole in A Paper Heart." Words by Scott Weiland. Music by Eric Kretz. *Tiny Music..Songs from the Vatican Gift Shop*. Atlantic Records, 1996. MP3.

Tears for Fears. "Head Over Heels." By Roland Orzabal and Curt Smith. *Songs from the Big Chair*. Phonogram Records/Mercury Records, 1985. CD.

The Tokens. "The Lion Sleeps Tonight." By Solomon Linda. RCA Victor Records, 1961.

U2. "Get On Your Boots." Music by U2, Words by Bono. *No Line on the Horizon*. Horoscope Records, 2009. CD.

U2. "God Part II." Music by U2, Words by Bono. *Rattle and Hum*. Island Records, 1988. CD.

U2. "I'll Go Crazy If I Don't Go Crazy Tonight." Music by U2, Words by Bono. *No Line on the Horizon*. Horoscope Records, 2009. CD.

U2. "Kite." Music by U2, Words by Bono. *All That You Can't Leave Behind*. Universal International Music BV, 2000. CD.

U2. "Lemon." Music by U2, Words by Bono. *Zooropa*. Polygram International Music Publishing/Island Records, 1993. CD.

U2. "No Line on the Horizon." Music by U2, Words by Bono. *No Line on the Horizon*. Horoscope Records, 2009. CD.

U2. "One." Music by U2, Words by Bono. *Achtung Baby*. Island Records, Inc., 1991. CD.

U2. "One Step Closer." Music by U2, Words by Bono. *How to Dismantle an Atomic Bomb*. Universal International Music BV, 2004. CD.

U2 "Sometimes You Can't Make It on Your Own." Music by U2, Words by Bono. *How to Dismantle an Atomic Bomb*. Universal International Music BV, 2004. CD.

U2 "Ultraviolet (Light My Way)." Music by U2, Words by Bono. *Achtung Baby*. Island Records, Inc, 1991. CD.

U2. "Unknown Caller." Music by U2, Words by Bono. *No Line on the Horizon*. Horoscope Records, 2009. CD.

U2. "When I Look at the World." Music by U2, Words by Bono. *All That You Can't Leave Behind*. Universal International Music BV, 2000. CD.

U2 "Zoo Station." Music by U2, Words by Bono. *Achtung Baby*. Island Records, Inc., 1991. CD.

U2. "Zooropa." Music by U2, Words By Bono. *Zooropa*. Polygram International Music Publishing/Island Records, 1993. CD.

Valli, Frankie. "Can't Take My Eyes off You," Words and Music by Bob Crewe and Bob Gaudio. Philips Records. 1967.

Waite, John. "Missing You." By John Waite, Mark Leonard, Chas Sandford. *No Brakes*. EMI, 1984. MP3.

Walt Disney World's Carousel of Progress. "The Best Time of Your Life." By the Sherman Brothers. The Walt Disney Company, 1964.

Warwick, Dionne. "I Say A Little Prayer," written by Burt Bacharach and Hal David. *The Windows of the World*. Scepter Records. 1967. MP3.

The Who. "A Quick One While He's Away." By Pete Townshend. *A Quick One*. Decca Records, 1966. MP3.

The Yardbirds. "Heart Full of Soul." By Graham Gouldman. *Having a Rave Up*. Columbia Records, 1965. MP3.

Yes. "Long Distance Runaround." By Jon Anderson. *Fragile*. Atlantic Records, 1972. CD.

NOTES
(Endnotes)

[1] The Del-Vetts. "The Last Time Around." By Jimmie Nelson. Universal Music Publishing Group, Sony/ATV Music Publishing LLC, 1966. MP3.

[2] "Sepsis." *Stedman's Medical Dictionary*. 28th ed. Lippincott Williams & Wilkins, 2006.

[3] "Septic Shock." *Stedman's Medical Dictionary*. 28th ed. Lippincott Williams & Wilkins, 2006.

[4] "Toxic Shock Syndrome." *Stedman's Medical Dictionary*. 28th ed. Lippincott Williams & Wilkins, 2006.

[5] Mandel, Jess, MD, and Gregory A. Schmidt, MD. ed. Polly E Parsons, MD, Daniel J Sexton, MD, and Kevin C. Wilson, MD, "Management of severe sepsis and septic shock in adults." *UptoDate http://www.uptodate.com/contents/management-of-severe-sepsis-and-septic-shock-in-adults*. N.p. 25 Oct. 2011, 06 Jun. 2012. Web.

[6] The Motels. "Only the Lonely." By Martha Davis. *All Four One*. Capitol, 1982. MP3.

[7] Stevens, Dennis L., MD, PhD. ed. Daniel J. Sexton, MD and Elinor L Baron, MD, DTMH."Epidemiology, clinical manifestations, and diagnosis of streptococcal toxic shock syndrome." *UptoDate, http://www.uptodate.com/online/content/topic.do?topicKey=gram_pos/5335&view=*. N.p. 13 Jan. 2009, 11 Jan. 2010. Web.

[8] Morrison, Van. "Call Me Up In Dreamland." By Van Morrison. *His Band and the Street Choir.* Warner Bros. Records, 1970. CD.

[9] Stevens, Dennis L., MD, PhD. ed. Daniel J. Sexton, MD and Elinor L Baron, MD, DTMH."Epidemiology, clinical manifestations, and diagnosis of streptococcal toxic shock syndrome." *UptoDate, http://www.uptodate.com/online/content/topic.do?topicKey=gram_pos/5335&view=.* N.p. 13 Jan. 2009, 11 Jan. 2010. Web.

[10] U2. "When I Look at the World." Music by U2, Words by Bono. *All That You Can't Leave Behind.* Universal International Music BV, 2000. CD.

[11] Stevens.

[12] Henley, Don. "You're Not Drinking Enough." By Danny Kortchmar. *Building the Perfect Beast.* Geffen Records, 1984. CD.

[13] Stevens.

[14] Electric Light Orchestra. "Mr. Blue Sky." By Jeff Lynne. *Out of the Blue.* United Artists, 1978. MP3.

[15] The Beatles. "I'm Only Sleeping." By John Lennon and PaulMcCartney. *Revolver.* EMI. Northern Songs Ltd, 1966. CD.

[16] Mandel, Jess, MD, and Gregory A. Schmidt, MD. ed. Polly E Parsons, MD, Daniel J Sexton, MD, and Kevin C. Wilson, MD, "Management of severe sepsis and septic shock in adults." *UptoDate http://www.uptodate.com/contents/management-of-severe-sepsis-and-septic-shock-in-adults.* N.p. 25 Oct. 2011, 06 Jun. 2012. Web.

[17] U2. "Kite." Music by U2, Words by Bono. *All That You Can't Leave Behind.* Universal International Music BV, 2000. CD.

[18] U2. "No Line on the Horizon." Music by U2, Words by Bono. *No Line on the Horizon.* Horoscope Records, 2009. CD.

[19] Madonna. "Ray of Light." By Madonna, William Orbit, Clive Muldoon, Dave Curtiss and Christine Leach. *Ray of Light.* Maverick Records, 1998. MP3.

[20] Smokey Robinson and the Miracles. "Tears of a Clown." By Smokey Robinson. *Make It Happen.* Motown Records. 1967. MP3.

ENDNOTES

[21] Mandel and Schmidt.

[22] Planet P Project. "Why Me?" By Tony Carey. *Planet P*. Geffen Records, 1983. MP3.

[23] Simple Minds. "See the Lights." By Kerr/Burchill. *Glittering Prize*. Virgin Records,1991. CD.

[24] The Rolling Stones. "Happy." By Mick Jagger and Keith Richards. *Exile on Main Street*. Rolling Stones Records, 1972. MP3.

[25] Mandel and Schmidt.

[26] Harrison, George. "Be Here Now." By George Harrison. *Living in the Material World*. Apple Records, 1973. MP3.

[27] Sebastian, John. "Welcome Back." By John Sebastian. Reprise Records, 1976. MP3.

[28] The Cranberries. "Ode to My Family." Words by Dolores O'Riordan, Music by Dolores O'Riordan and Noel Hogan. *No Need to Argue*. Island Records, 1994. CD.

[29] U2 "Sometimes You Can't Make It on Your Own." Music by U2, Words by Bono. *How to Dismantle an Atomic Bomb*. Universal International Music BV, 2004. CD.

[30] Herman's Hermits. "There's A Kind of Hush All over the World." By Les Reed and Geoff Stephens. Columbia Records, 1967. CD.

[31] The Who. "A Quick One While He's Away." By Pete Townshend. *A Quick One*. Decca Records, 1966. MP3.

[32] Men at Work. "Overkill." By Colin Hay. *Cargo*. Columbia Records, 1983. CD.

[33] U2. "Lemon." Music by U2, Words by Bono. *Zooropa*. Polygram International Music Publishing/Island Records, 1993. CD.

[34] Simon, Carly. "Nobody Does It Better." Music by Marvin Hamlisch, Words by Carole Bayer Sager. Elektra Records, 1977. MP3.

[35] Bowie, David. "Modern Love." By David Bowie. *Let's Dance*. EMI America Records, 1983. MP3.

36 The Monkees. "What Am I Doing Hangin' Round?" By Michael Martin Murphey and Owen Castleman. *Pisces, Aquarius, Capricorn & Jones Ltd.* Arista Records, 1967. MP3.

37 Henley, Don. "Sunset Grill." By Don Henley, Danny Kortchmar, and Ben Tench. *Building the Perfect Beast*. Geffen Records, 1984. CD.

38 Stevens.

39 Harrison, George. "Don't Let Me Wait Too Long." By George Harrison. *Living in the Material World*. Apple Records, 1973. MP3.

40 The Church. "Metropolis." By Marty Willson-Piper, Peter Koppes, Richard Ploog, and Steve Kilbey. *Gold Afternoon Fix*. Arista Records, 1990. MP3.

41 U2. "One Step Closer." Music by U2, Words by Bono. *How to Dismantle an Atomic Bomb*. Universal International Music BV, 2004. CD.

42 Stevens.

43 The Who. "A Quick One While He's Away." By Pete Townshend. *A Quick One*. Decca Records, 1966. MP3.

44 The Police. "Don't Stand So Close to Me." By Sting. *Zenyatta Mondatta*. A&M Records, 1980. CD.

45 The Cure. "Boys Don't Cry." By Michael Dempsey, Robert Smith, and Lol Tolhurst. Fiction Records, 1979. MP3.

46 The Beatles. "Real Love." By John Lennon. *Beatles Anthology 2*. Apple Records, 1995. CD.

47 The Beatles. "Real Love." By John Lennon. *Beatles Anthology 2*. Apple Records, 1995. CD.

48 U2. "Zooropa." Music by U2, Words By Bono. *Zooropa*. Polygram International Music Publishing/Island Records, 1993. CD.

49 Chicago. "Stay the Night." By Peter Cetera and David Foster. *Chicago 17*. Full Moon/Warner Bros., 1984. MP3.

50 The Beatles. "There's A Place." By John Lennon and Paul McCartney. *Please Please Me*. EMI/Northern Songs Ltd., 1962. CD.

51 U2. "Zooropa." Music by U2, Words By Bono. *Zooropa*. Polygram International Music Publishing/Island Records, 1993. CD.

52 The Beatles. "P.S. I Love You." By John Lennon and Paul McCartney. *Please Please Me*. EMI/Northern Songs Ltd., 1962. CD.

53 Stevens.

54 U2 "Ultraviolet (Light My Way)." Music by U2, Words by Bono. *Achtung Baby*. Island Records, Inc, 1991. CD.

55 Mazzy Star "Fade into You." By Hope Sandoval and David Roback. *So Tonight That I Might See*. Capitol Records, 1994. CD.

56 U2. "No Line on the Horizon." Music by U2, Words by Bono. *No Line on the Horizon*. Horoscope Records, 2009. CD.

57 Stevens.

58 U2. "God Part II." Music by U2, Words by Bono. *Rattle and Hum*. Island Records, 1988. CD.

59 U2. "Unknown Caller." Music by U2, Words by Bono. *No Line on the Horizon*. Horoscope Records, 2009. CD.

60 U2. "Kite." Music by U2, Words by Bono. *All That You Can't Leave Behind*. Universal International Music BV, 2000. CD.

61 Stevens.

62 Calloway, Cab. "Papa's in Bed with His Britches On." By Jesse Stone. *Are You Hep To The Jive?* Columbia Records, 1940. CD.

63 Stevens.

64 Lennon, John. "Crippled Inside." By John Lennon. *Imagine*. Apple Records, 1971. CD.

65 Waite, John. "Missing You." By John Waite, Mark Leonard, Chas Sandford. *No Brakes*. EMI, 1984. MP3.

66 Mandel and Schmidt.

67 The Scorpions. "Arizona." By Rudolf Schenker. *Blackout*. Mercury Records, 1982. CD.

⁶⁸ The B Sharps "Baby On Board," Words and Music By Jeff Martin, Shelby Grimm, Harry Campbell, George Economou, and Danny Jordan. *Songs in the Key of Springfield*. Rhino Records. 1994.

⁶⁹ Warwick, Dionne. "I Say A Little Prayer," written by Burt Bacharach and Hal David. *The Windows of the World*. Scepter Records. 1967. MP3.

⁷⁰ Stevens.

⁷¹ Valli, Frankie. "Can't Take My Eyes off You," Words and Music by Bob Crewe and Bob Gaudio. Philips Records. 1967.

⁷² Lennon, John. "Watching the Wheels," By John Lennon. *Double Fantasy*. Geffen Records, 1980.

⁷³ Stevens.

⁷⁴ INXS. "New Sensation." Words by Michael Hutchence, Music by Andrew Farriss. *Kick*. Atlantic Records, 1987. MP3.

⁷⁵ U2. "Unknown Caller." Music by U2, Words by Bono. *No Line on the Horizon*. Horoscope Records, 2009. CD.

⁷⁶ Lawrence, Gertrude. "Someone to Watch over Me." Music by George Gershwin, Words by Ira Gershwin. *Oh! Kay*. Released as Victor 20331, matrix 36654-3. 1926.

⁷⁷ U2. "I'll Go Crazy If I Don't Go Crazy Tonight." Music by U2, Words by Bono. *No Line on the Horizon*. Horoscope Records, 2009. CD.

⁷⁸ Stevens.

⁷⁹ U2 "Ultraviolet (Light My Way)." Music by U2, Words by Bono. *Achtung Baby*. Island Records, Inc, 1991. CD.

⁸⁰ Lennon, John. "#9 Dream," By John Lennon. *Walls and Bridges*. Capitol Records, 1974. CD.

⁸¹ Mandel and Schmidt.

⁸² U2 "Zoo Station." Music by U2, Words by Bono. *Achtung Baby*. Island Records, Inc., 1991. CD.

[83] Garbage. "The Trick is to Keep Breathing," Words and Music by Garbage. *Version 2.0.* Almo Sounds, Inc., 1999. CD.

[84] R.E.M. "Gardening at Night." Words and Music by Bill Berry, Peter Buck, Mike Mills, and Michael Stipe. *Eponymous.* I.R.S. Records, 1982. CD.

[85] The Who. "A Quick One While He's Away." By Pete Townshend. *A Quick One.* Decca Records, 1966. MP3.

[86] *Austin Powers: International Man of Mystery.* Writ. Mike Myers and Michael McCullers. Dir. Jay Roach. Perf. Mike Myers, Elizabeth Hurley, Michael York, and Mimi Rogers. New Line Cinema. 1997.

[87] Stevens.

[88] Walt Disney World's Carousel of Progress. "The Best Time of Your Life." By the Sherman Brothers. The Walt Disney Company, 1964.

[89] Sebastian, John. "Welcome Back." By John Sebastian. Reprise Records, 1976. MP3.

[90] Stevens.

[91] The Tokens. "The Lion Sleeps Tonight." By Solomon Linda. RCA Victor Records, 1961.

[92] The Beatles "Tell Me What You See." Written by John Lennon and Paul McCartney. *Rubber Soul.* EMI. Northern Songs Ltd., 1965. CD.

[93] Baker, Chet. "My Funny Valentine." By Richard Rodgers and Lorenz Hart. *Babes in Arms.* Fantasy, 1952.

[94] Mandel and Schmidt.

[95] Hebb, Bobby. "Sunny." By Bobby Hebb. *Sunny.* Philips, 1966. MP3.

[96] Lennon, John. "How Do You Sleep?" By John Lennon. *Imagine.* Apple Records, 1971. CD.

[97] Lennon, John. "Cold Turkey." By John Lennon. *Shaved Fish.* Apple Records, 1969. CD.

[98] Palmer, Robert. "Bad Case of Loving You (Doctor, Doctor)." By Moon Martin. *Secrets.* Island Records, 1978. CD.

[99] Stevens.

[100] The Rolling Stones. "You Can't Always Get What You Want." By Mick Jagger and Keith Richards. *Let It Bleed*. Decca Records, 1969. MP3.

[101] Stevens.

[102] Plant, Robert. "Little by Little." By Robert Plant and Jezz Woodroffe. *Shaken N' Stirred*. Es Paranza, 1985. MP3.

[103] The Yardbirds. "Heart Full of Soul." By Graham Gouldman. *Having a Rave Up*. Columbia Records, 1965. MP3.

[104] Tears for Fears. "Head Over Heels." By Roland Orzabal and Curt Smith. *Songs from the Big Chair*. Phonogram Records/Mercury Records, 1985. CD.

[105] John, Elton. "Sad Songs (Say So Much)." By Bernie Taupin and Elton John. *Breaking Hearts*. Geffen Records, 1984. MP3.

[106] Stevens.

[107] Madness. "Our House." By Chris Foreman and Cathal Smyth. *The Rise & Fall*. Geffen Records, 1982. MP3.

[108] The Beatles. "A Taste of Honey." By John Lennon and Paul McCartney. *Please Please Me*. EMI/Northern Songs Ltd., 1962. CD.

[109] The Who. "A Quick One While He's Away." By Pete Townshend. *A Quick One*. Decca Records, 1966. MP3.

[110] The Rolling Stones. "Sympathy for the Devil." By Mick Jagger and Keith Richards. *Beggars Banquet*. Decca Records, 1968. MP3.

[111] Scaggs, Boz. "Lido Shuffle." By David Paich and Boz Scaggs. *Silk Degrees*. CBS Records, 1976. MP3.

[112] Mandel and Schmidt.

[113] Guns n' Roses "Welcome to the Jungle." By Axl Rose, Slash, Izzy Stradlin, Duff McKagan, and Steven Adler. *Appetite for Destruction*. Geffen Records, 1987. CD.

[114] Quiet Riot. "Cum on Feel the Noiz." By Jim Lea and Noddy Holder. *Metal Health*. CBS Records, 1982.

[115] The Beatles. "Dr. Robert." By John Lennon and Paul McCartney. *Revolver*. EMI/Northern Songs Ltd., 1966. CD.

[116] *Planes. Trains, and Automobiles*. Writ. John Hughes. Dir. John Hughes. Perf. John Candy and Steve Martin. Paramount Pictures, 1987. DVD.

[117] U2. "One." Music by U2, Words by Bono. *Achtung Baby*. Island Records, Inc., 1991. CD.

[118] U2. "Get On Your Boots." Music by U2, Words by Bono. *No Line on the Horizon*. Horoscope Records, 2009. CD.

[119] Mandel and Schmidt.

[120] The Cranberries. "Just My Imagination." By Dolores O'Riordan and Noel Hogan. *Bury the Hatchet*. Island Records, 1999. CD.

[121] The Beatles. "Anytime at All." By John Lennon and Paul McCartney. *With The Beatles*. EMI/Northern Songs Ltd., 1963. CD.

[122] The Cult. "Love Removal Machine." By Ian Astbury and Billy Duffy. *Electric*. Beggars Banquet, 1987. CD.

[123] The Who. "A Quick One While He's Away." By Pete Townshend. *A Quick One*. Decca Records, 1966. MP3.

[124] Dylan, Bob. "Lay Lady Lay." By Bob Dylan. *Nashville Skyline*. Columbia Records, 1969. CD.

[125] The Spinners. "The Rubberband Man." By Thom Bell and Linda Creed. Atlantic Records,1976. MP3.

[126] Mandel and Schmidt.

[127] O'Riordan, Dolores. "When We Were Young." By Dolores O'Riordan. *Are You Listening?* Sequel Records, 2007. CD.

[128] The Cast of *Oliver!* "Food, Glorious Food." By Lionel Bart. Tams-Witmark Music Library, Inc., 1960.

[129] Rush. "Fly by Night." Words by Neil Peart, Music by Geddy Lee. *Fly By Night*. Mercury Records, 1975. CD.

130 Mandel and Schmidt.

131 Nicholas, Paul. "Heaven on the 7th Floor." By C. Neil and Paul Nicholas. RSO Records, 1977. MP3.

132 Aerosmith. "No More, No More." By Steven Tyler and Joe Perry. *Toys in the Attic*. Columbia Records, 1975. CD.

133 Mandel and Schmidt.

134 Duran Duran. "Save a Prayer." By Duran Duran. *Rio*. Capitol Records, 1982. MP3.

135 Mandel and Schmidt.

136 The Beatles. "Christmas Time Is Here Again." By John Lennon, Paul McCartney, George Harrison, and Richard Starkey. *Christmas Record for Beatles Fan Club*. EMI/Northern Songs Ltd., 1967.

137 Idol, Billy. "Eyes Without A Face." By Billy Idol and Steve Stevens. *Rebel Yell*. Chrysalis Records, 1984. MP3.

138 The Rolling Stones. "Waiting on a Friend." By Mick Jagger and Keith Richards. *Tattoo You*. Rolling Stones Records, 1981. CD.

139 The Rolling Stones. "Sympathy for the Devil." By Mick Jagger and Keith Richards. *Beggars Banquet*. Decca Records, 1968. MP3.

140 The Fortunes. "Here Comes That Rainy Day Feeling Again." By Roger Frederick Cook, Roger John Reginald Greenaway, and Tony Macaulay. *Here Comes That Rainy Day Feeling Again*. Decca Records,1970. MP3.

141 Mandel and Schmidt.

142 Seger, Bob. "Night Moves." By Bob Seger. *Night Moves*. Capitol Records, 1976. MP3.

143 Yes. "Long Distance Runaround." By Jon Anderson. *Fragile*. Atlantic Records, 1972. CD.

144 Mandel and Schmidt.

145 Stone Temple Pilots. "Trippin' On A Hole in A Paper Heart." Words by Scott Weiland. Music by Eric Kretz. *Tiny Music..Songs from the Vatican Gift Shop*. Atlantic Records, 1996. MP3.

ENDNOTES 565

[146] *Planes. Trains, and Automobiles.* Writ. John Hughes. Dir. John Hughes. Perf. John Candy and Steve Martin. Paramount Pictures, 1987. DVD.

[147] Harrison, George. "Be Here Now." By George Harrison. *Living in the Material World.* Apple Records, 1973. MP3.

[148] Sinatra, Frank. "Fly Me to the Moon." By Bart Howard. *It Might As Well Be Swing.* Reprise Records, 1964. MP3.

[149] The Rolling Stones. "Dandelion." By Mick Jagger and Keith Richards. *Through the Past, Darkly (Big Hits Vol. 2).* Decca Records, 1967. MP3.

[150] The Rolling Stones. "You Gotta Move." By Fred McDowell and Gary Davis. *Sticky Fingers.* Rolling Stones Records, 1971. CD.

[151] Grand Funk Railroad. "I'm Your Captain (Closer to Home)." By Mark Farner. *Closer to Home.* Capitol Records, 1970. MP3.

[152] Mandel and Schmidt.

[153] The B-52s. "Love Shack." By Kate Pierson, Fred Schneider, Keith Strickland, and Cindy Wilson. *Cosmic Thing.* Warner Brothers, 1989. CD.

[154] U2. "I'll Go Crazy If I Don't Go Crazy Tonight." Music by U2, Words by Bono. *No Line on the Horizon.* Horoscope Records, 2009. CD.

[155] The Beach Boys. "Heroes and Villians." By Brian Wilson and Van Dyke Parks. *Smiley Smile.* Capitol Records, 1967. MP3.

[156] The Beatles. "Here Comes the Sun." By George Harrison. *Abbey Road.* EMI/Northern Songs Ltd., 1969. CD.

[157] Clapton, Eric. "Heaven is One Step Away." By Eric Clapton. *Crossroads Disc 4.* Warner Bros. Records, 1985. CD.

[158] The Cranberries. "Zombie." By Dolores O'Riordan. *No Need to Argue.* Island Records, 1994. MP3.

[159] R.E.M. "Superman." By Gary Zekley and Mitchell Bottler. *Life's Rich Pageant.* I.R.S. Records, 1986. CD.

[160] Average White Band. "Pick up the Pieces." By Average White Band. *AWB.* Atlantic Records, 1974. MP3.

161 INXS "The Gift," By Jon Farriss and Michael Hutchence. *Full Moon, Dirty Hearts.* Atlantic Records, 1993. MP3.

162 Loverboy. "Working for the Weekend." By Paul Dean, Mike Reno, and Matt Frenette. *Get Lucky.* Columbia Records, 1981. MP3.

163 Nugent, Ted. "Free-for-All." By Ted Nugent. *Free-for-All.* Epic Records, 1976. CD.

164 Sting. "Fields of Gold." By Sting. *Ten Summoner's Tales.* A&M, 1993. CD.

165 Spanky and Our Gang. "Sunday Will Never Be the Same." By Terry Cashman and Gene Pistilli. *Spanky and Our Gang.* Mercury Records, 1967. MP3.

166 Fleetwood Mac "Little Lies." By Christine McVie and Eddy Quintela. *Tango in the Night.* Warner Bros. Records, 1987. CD.

167 The Beach Boys. "Wouldn't It Be Nice." By Brian Wilson, Tony Asher, and Mike Love. *Pet Sounds.* Capitol Records, 1966. CD.

168 McCartney, Paul. "My Brave Face." By Paul McCartney and Elvis Costello. *Flowers in the Dirt.* Capitol Records, 1989. CD.

169 Nash, Johnny. "I Can See Clearly Now." By Johnny Nash. *I Can See Clearly Now.* Epic Records, 1972. MP3.

170 Little, DeEtta. "Gonna Fly Now (Theme from Rocky)." Music by Bill Conti, Words by Carol Connors and Ayn Robbins. *Rocky – Original Motion Picture Score.* United Artists, 1977. MP3.

171 Damn Yankees. "High Enough." By Tommy Shaw, Jack Blades, Ted Nugent. *Damn Yankees.* Warner Bros., 1990. MP3.

172 Dio. "Hungry for Heaven." By Ronnie James Dio and Jimmy Bain. *Vision Quest Soundtrack.* Geffen Records,1985. CD.

173 Concrete Blonde. "Bloodletting (The Vampire Song)." By Johnette Napolitano. *Bloodletting.* I.R.S., 1990. CD.

174 The Cars. "It's All I Can Do." By Ric Ocasek. *Candy-O.* Elektra Records, 1979. CD.

[175] The Cars. "You Might Think." By Ric Ocasek. *Heartbeat City.* Elektra Records, 1984. CD.

[176] U2. "Unknown Caller." Music by U2, Words by Bono. *No Line on the Horizon.* Horoscope Records, 2009. CD.

[177] The Who. "A Quick One While He's Away." By Pete Townshend. *A Quick One.* Decca Records, 1966. MP3.

[178] The Beatles. "Penny Lane." By John Lennon and Paul McCartney. *Anthology 3.* Apple Records, 1967. CD.

Made in the USA
San Bernardino, CA
03 September 2014